Foam Sclerotherapy
A Textbook

Foam Sclerotherapy
A Textbook

Edited by

John Bergan and Van Le Cheng

The ROYAL
SOCIETY of
MEDICINE
PRESS Limited

Published by the Royal Society of Medicine Press Ltd
1 Wimpole Street, London W1G 0AE, UK
Tel: +44 (0)20 7290 2921
Fax: +44 (0)20 7290 2929
Email: publishing@rsm.ac.uk
Website: www.rsmpress.co.uk

British Library Cataloguing in Publication Data
A catalogue record for this book is available from the British Library

ISBN 978-1-85315-771-4

Distribution in Europe and Rest of World:

Marston Book Services Ltd
PO Box 269
Abingdon
Oxon OX14 4YN, UK
Tel: +44 (0)1235 465500
Fax: +44 (0)1235 465555
Email: direct.order@marston.co.uk

Distribution in the USA and Canada:

Royal Society of Medicine Press Ltd
c/o BookMasters Inc
30 Amberwood Parkway
Ashland, OH 44805, USA
Tel: +1 800 247 6553/+1 800 266 5564
Fax: +1 419 281 6883
Email: order@bookmasters.com

Distribution in Australia and New Zealand:

Elsevier Australia
30-52 Smidmore Street
Marrickville NSW 2204, Australia
Tel: +61 2 9517 8999
Fax: +61 2 9517 2249
Email: service@elsevier.com.au

Typeset by Phoenix Photosetting, Chatham, Kent
Printed and bound by Krips b.v., Meppel, The Netherlands

Contents

Contributing authors vii

Foreword 1 ix

Foreword 2 x

Preface xi

THEORY

1. **The history of sclerosant foams: persons, techniques, patents and medical improvements** 3
   Jan-Christoph GR Wollmann

2. **Dermatological manifestations of venous insufficiency** 13
   Kurosh Parsi

3. **Sclerotherapy of varicose veins – Guidelines of the German Society of Phlebology** 31
   Eberhard Rabe, Felizitas Pannier, Horst Gerlach, Franz Xaver Breu, Stefan Guggenbichler and Jan-Christoph GR Wollmann

4. **Legal guidelines for use of polidocanol and sodium tetradecyl sulfate for sclerotherapy** 43
   Lowell S Kabnick

PRACTICE

5. **The science of producing extemporary foam and its clinical results** 55
   Alesssandro Frullini

6. **Ultrasound guidance for therapeutic interventions** 61
   John Bergan and Van Le Cheng

7. **A personal method for foam sclerotherapy: technique and results** 69
   Philip D Coleridge Smith

8. **Foam sclerotherapy with and without duplex ultrasound guidance** 79
   Jean-Jérôme Guex and Jean-Luc Gillet

9. **Foam sclerotherapy for varicose veins: medium-term results as assessed by ultrasound** 87
   Kenneth Myers and Damien Jolley

SPECIAL CONSIDERATIONS

10. Varisolve® polidocanol microfoam compared with surgery or sclerotherapy in the management of varicose veins in the presence of trunk vein incompetence: European randomized controlled trial 105
David DI Wright, Jean Pierre Gobin, Andrew W Bradbury, Philip D Coleridge Smith, Harry Spoelstra, David Berridge, Cees HA Wittens, Anja Sommer, Olle Nelzen, Dennis Chanter, on behalf of the Varisolve® European Phase III Investigators Group

11. Ultrasound-guided foam sclerotherapy of large varicose veins 117
JM Barrett

12. Transition from alcohol to foam sclerotherapy for localized venous malformations with high risk 129
BB Lee and John Bergan

13. Treatment of telangiectasias by sclerosing foam 141
Philippe Kern

14. Comparison of polidocanol and sodium tetradecyl sulfate in the treatment of varicose and telangiectatic leg veins 155
Mitchel P Goldman

15. Lesser importance of the saphenous vein in varicose vein treatment 163
Paul Pittaluga and Sylvain Chastanet

16. Efficacy of polidocanol foam compared with polidocanol liquid in sclerotherapy of venous insufficiency 177
Takashi Yamaki

17. Studies on safety of foam sclerotherapy 183
Nick Morrison

18. Treatment of recurrent varicose veins by sclerosant foam 193
John Bergan and Van Le Cheng

19. Vascular malformations 199
Juan Cabrera, Antonio Martinez de la Cuesta and Alejandro Sierra

20. Treatment of venous malformations, Klippel–Trenaunay syndrome and other low-flow lesions with foamed sclerosants 219
John Bergan and Van Le Cheng

Epilogue 225
Index 227

Contributing authors

John M Barrett MBChB FACP
Palm Clinic, Auckland, New Zealand

John J Bergan MD FACS FRCS (Hon)
Vein Institute of La Jolla, CA and Department of Surgery, UCSD School of Medicine, La Jolla, CA, USA

David Berridge DM FRCS
Leeds Vascular Institute, The General Infirmary at Leeds, Leeds, UK

Andrew W Bradbury BSc MB MD FRCSEd
University of Birmingham, and Heart of England NHS Foundation Trust, Birmingham, UK

Franz Xaver Breu MD
Praxis für Gefäßmedizin am Tegernsee, Tegernsee, Germany

Juan Cabrera MD PhD
International Institute of Phlebology, Granada, Spain

Dennis Chanter PhD
Statisfaction Statistical Consultancy Ltd, Bexhill on Sea, UK

Sylvain Chastanet MD
Riviera Veine Institut, Nice, France

Van Le Cheng MD
UCSD Instructor of Surgery, SD Vein Institute, Encinitas, CA, USA

Philip D Coleridge Smith DM FRCS
University College London Medical School, London, UK

Alessandro Frullini MD
Studio Medico Flebologico, Figline Valdarno, Florence, Italy

Horst Gerlach MD
Praxis für Gefässmedizin, Mannheim, Germany

Jean-Luc Gillet MD
Vascular Medicine-Phlebology, Bourgoin-Jallieu, France

Jean Pierre Gobin MD
Cabinet de Medecine Vasculaire, Lyon, France

Mitchel P Goldman MD
Clinical Professor of Dermatology/Medicine, University of California, San Diego; and Medical Director, La Jolla Spa MD, La Jolla, CA, USA

Jean-Jérôme Guex MD FACPh
University of Nice, Nice, France

Stefan Guggenbichler MD
Praxis am Viktualienmarket, Munich, Germany

Damien Jolley MSc AStat
Monash Institute of Health Services Research, Monash University, Melbourne, Australia

Lowell S Kabnick MD FACS FACPh
New York University Vein Center, Division of Vascular Surgery, New York, USA

Philippe Kern MD
Vevey, Switzerland

BB Lee MD FACS
Georgetown University, Washington DC, USA

Antonio Martinez de la Cuesta MD MSc FRCR
Vascular Malformations Area, Clinica Universitaria, Pamplona, Spain

Nick Morrison MD FACS FACPh
Morrison Vein Institute, Scottsdale, AZ, USA

Kenneth Myers MS FACS FRACS
Australasian College of Phlebology, Melbourne, Australia

Olle Nelzen MD PhD
Vascular Surgery Unit, Department of Surgery, Skaraborg Hospital, Skovde, Sweden

Kurosh Parsi MBBS MScMed FACD FACP
Department of Dermatology and Vascular Birthmarks Clinic, Sydney Children's Hospital; and St Vincent's Hospital, Sydney, Australia

Felizitas Pannier MD
Dermatologie Kastanienhof, Köln, Germany

Paul Pittaluga MD
Surgical Chair, Riviera Veine Institut, Nice, France

Eberhard Rabe MD, PhD
Department of Dermatology, University of Bonn, Germany

Alejandro Sierra MD PhD
Phlebology Unit Clinica Universitaria, Pamplona, Spain

Anja Sommer PhD
Department of Dermatology, University Hospital Maastricht, The Netherlands

Harry Spoelstra MD PhD
Therapeutisch Vascular Centrum, Gavere, Belgium

Cees HA Wittens MD PhD
Department of Vascular Surgery, St Franciscus Gasthuis Kleiwed, Rotterdam, The Netherlands

Jan-Christoph GR Wollmann MD
Kreussler-Pharma, Wiesbaden, Germany

David DI Wright MD FRCS
Provensis Limited, London, UK

Takashi Yamaki MD
Department of Plastic and Reconstructive Surgery, Tokyo Women's Medical University, Shinjuku-ku, Tokyo, Japan

Foreword 1

The treatment of varicose veins has a long and rich history. In the 19th century, Friedrich Trendelenburg ligated the saphenous vein to treat varicose veins. Subsequently, saphenous ligation and stripping became dominant. But, like general surgery, the most rapid and exciting developments in treating venous insufficiency have occurred in last quarter of the 20th century.

In general surgery, minimally invasive surgery, including laparoscopic and robotic surgery, transformed the specialty. Now, natural orifice transluminal endoscopic surgery (NOTES) may be about to further that transformation.

In treatment of venous insufficiency, the first change was the application of radiofrequency energy to ablate the saphenous vein. This was followed by the redirection of dermatologic laser techniques to the treatment of varicose veins. Therefore, as the 20th century ended, laser closure of the saphenous vein became dominant just as interest in direct surgery for venous insufficiency waned. Foam sclerotherapy, the subject of this book, developed during the same era but was less supported and promoted commercially. Therefore, it has been adopted more slowly.

This work documents the key role of foam sclerotherapy in treatment of venous insufficiency. A glance at the Table of Contents will demonstrate the broad applicability and easy availability of foam. The chapters show that foam sclerotherapy is greatly aided by duplex technology and ultrasound imaging.

The future of minimally invasive general surgery cannot be precisely predicted. Similarly, no one knows the exact future role of foam sclerotherapy. However, the quiet introduction of foam sclerotherapy is refreshing. Foam therapy is quick, efficient, durable, easy to use and cheap. It may be the first new treatment introduced in recent years in medical care that does not increase, but instead decreases, the cost of medical care. It is easy to predict, based upon these pages, that foam will soon become the dominant mode of therapy for varicose veins.

Mark Talamini MD
Department of Surgery
UCSD School of Medicine
San Diego, CA, USA

Foreword 2

The battle for supremacy between sclerotherapy and surgery, laser, radiofrequency and phlebectomy in treating varicose veins could be compared to the power struggle between the English and French in the Hundred Years' War (AD 1337–1453).

An impartial observer will find both differences and similarities. The obvious difference is that the Hundred Years' War is over, whereas the conflict between sclerotherapy and surgical interventions is not. As for similarities, the supremacy of one method over the other has varied with time. So did supremacy in new weaponry. For example, liquid sclerotherapy handed the advantage to surgery, whilst advances in the use of foam have now tilted the balance back in favor of sclerotherapy. Ultrasound investigation is neutral: it assists advocates of both methods, as long as they are able to master it.

The most notable change is that, until recently, surgeons have almost always used surgical procedures, whilst medical phlebologists have mainly favored sclerotherapy. But now this difference is progressively vanishing as both sides have included at least laser or radiofrequency Closure©, phlebectomy and sclerotherapy in their daily practice. At the 2005 meeting of the Venous Forum of the Royal Society of Medicine in Edinburgh, attendees agreed that to treat varicose veins, the physician had to master all techniques in order to give the patient the best possible treatment.

Amongst the arguments advanced by supporters of classical surgery is that in order to stop reflux from the deep veins to the saphenous trunk, it is mandatory in most situations to perform high ligation, or more precisely high ligation of the saphenous termination flush with the femoral vein, and resect the upper several centimeters of the saphenous trunk. But ultrasound investigation has proved that the terminal saphenous valve is competent in more than 50% of patients with saphenous trunk insufficiency. Furthermore, endovascular procedures without high ligation have given results as good as those with classical surgical high interruption. This has retrospectively explained the satisfactory results obtained with liquid sclerotherapy in the past.

> The myth of compulsory high ligation has fallen.

Now, returning to foam sclerotherapy, the question is this: Will it become the first choice for treating primary superficial venous insufficiency and perforator reflux?

Until that question is answered, what is clear is that the replacement of liquid sclerosants by foam is a real advance; and that is the subject of this book.

Throughout this book, the advantages and drawbacks of this very promising method are described in detail. Clearly, the odds are in favor of foam because of cost, which is crucial in evaluating healthcare methods, the rarity of postprocedure complications, the easy repetitiveness, and the minimally invasive nature of the technique.

Yet natural circumspection compels me to reserve judgment on foam sclerotherapy until we have data from long-term, multicenter trials. At the same time, I recognize that high-quality, prospective, randomized control trials comparing foam with other procedures will be very difficult to carry out.

Michel Perrin
Lyon, France

Preface

Recently, much has changed in the world of phlebology. Amongst the most important, and most powerful, of the changes has been the advent of foam sclerotherapy. This is destined to be the most important tool available to phlebology in the 21st century. Just as surgery has evolved to become more minimally invasive, so has the treatment of varicose veins. While telangiectasias have always been the target of treatment by needle, it is now true that even the refluxing great saphenous vein and clusters of large varicose veins are yielding to the pressures of needle management. It is the properties of foam that make this possible, and the foam, acting neither quite like a solid nor quite like a liquid, pushes blood in the veins aside and acts directly on the endothelium. When this happens, the vein is sealed, and can be sealed permanently if all of the endothelium is denuded. This book, chapter by chapter, explains this phenomenon.

First, the Forewords by Mark Talamini and Michel Perrin set the stage for what follows. Then Jan-Christoph Wollman of the Kruessler Company in Germany recites the history of sclerosant foam. From Sydney, Kurosh Parsi has supplied an overview of the dermatologic manifestations of venous disease. The German Society of Phlebology, always well organized, has laid down guidelines for the use of sclerosant foam, and the latest of these guidelines are discussed by Eberhard Rabe.

In the United States, the use of polidocanol has always been controversial, as the Food and Drug Administration has not approved this agent. Yet it remains the best sclerosant in the world and the most used. Lowell Kabnick explains the legal connotations of its use.

Always at the forefront of foam therapy is Alessandro Frullini, who explains the science of producing extemporary foam and its early results. He was amongst the first to preach the use of foam in sclerotherapy.

Ultrasonography has been an important part of the treatment with foam sclerotherapy, and we explain here how ultrasound can be used optimally during, after, and before foam sclerotherapy. Foam sclerotherapy is so new that there are only very individual ways of applying it. Fortunately, chapters have been written by Jean-Jérôme Guex, Ken Myers, and Philip Coleridge Smith, each of whom presents his own viewpoint from a depth of knowledge and a wealth of personal experience. In the background, commercial foam is being developed by the Provensis Company, and its medical director, David Wright, describes its first European trial of foam sclerotherapy.

Amongst the earliest physicians to describe personal experience with foam was John Barrett of New Zealand. He has analyzed treatment of varicose veins of various sizes and even large varices in order to provide a chapter describing this experience. BB Lee, now at Georgetown, adds his own experience in transitioning from alcohol, with its manifold complications, to foam.

Philippe Kern, from Switzerland, has conducted a thorough scientific investigation of the treatment of the most common of venous abnormalities, telangiectasias. His work is quite convincing in proving the need for compression after treatment. Mitchel Goldman provides a comparison of polidocanol and sodium tetradecyl sulfate foam in the treatment of varicose veins.

It appears that, in the future, the saphenous vein will not be the target of therapy that it is today. In this respect, Paul Pittaluga, amongst the most forward-thinking of vascular surgeons investigating this issue, presents the lesser importance of the saphenous vein in treatment of varicose veins.

This is a truly international volume. From Japan, Takashi Yamaki describes the experience of use of polidocanol foam compared with liquid sclerotherapy. On the other side of the world, it was learned that adverse events characterized the early experience with foam sclerotherapy. Nick Morrison has studied this phenomenon in depth, coming to some conclusions about how these events can be aborted.

Our own experience in San Diego has been extraordinarily good with foam, and our chapters describe the treatment of recurrent varicose veins and vascular malformations. But the real pioneer in this area was Juan Cabrera, who has prepared an excellent chapter on the Granada experience with vascular malformations.

All in all, this is a book for the future that describes experiences of the past. We, who have assembled this knowledge, sincerely hope that those who use this book for patient care will do their jobs well and that the patients will be the better for it.

John Bergan MD, La Jolla, CA
and Van Le Cheng MD, Encinitas, CA

THEORY

1 The history of sclerosant foams: persons, techniques, patents and medical improvements

Jan-Christoph GR Wollmann

Today's method of sclerotherapy of varicose veins and other conditions using sclerosant foams has evolved from a long series of individual independent steps, or "building blocks." The development of a particular building block may well have been motivated by dissatisfaction with existing varicose vein treatments. But some other improvements to available options were, in fact, the result of pure coincidence. What is clear though is that sclerotherapy, an inexpensive and increasingly popular treatment, would probably not be available today were it not for the inventive thinking and personal commitment of a number of pioneers in specific areas such as development of sclerosing agents, injection devices, ultrasonography and foam manufacturing technology. Still, modern "endovenous chemical ablation" or – to use another term – "endovenous nonthermal elimination of varicose veins" has only become feasible by combining the individual building blocks and identifying existing interrelationships.

Over the past 15 years, preclinical and clinical research findings, improvements in sclerotherapy techniques, and harmonized treatment recommendations have all contributed to greater safety overall and efficacy of sclerotherapy. Modern electronic communication, which was not available until quite recently, has greatly facilitated rapid dissemination of new insights. In fact, findings predating the Internet are less widely known because they are not easy to track down. But they are still there. In addition to medical publications, development of foam sclerotherapy has also relied on input from other fields of science and technology. This chapter presents the individual "building blocks."

Injectable sclerosing agents

The first injection of a fluid into a human body probably dates back to Elsholz (1623–1688), and the first injection of a medicinal product for sclerosing evidently dates back to Zollikofer in 1682. The French surgeon Charles Gabriel Pravaz (1791–1853) invented a small syringe, the piston of which could be driven by a screw, thereby allowing exact dosage. A sharp needle could be introduced into the vessel, making a dissection unnecessary. He initiated the development of various new types of syringes made of either glass or metal combined with glass, thus allowing the widespread use of injections for sclerotherapeutic purposes. Pravaz himself used his syringe for the obliteration of arterial aneurysms and injected ferric sesquichlorate. In the years that followed, numerous sclerosing agents were tried, including substances that were later classified as detergent-type sclerosing agents.

Sodium morrhuate, the oldest representative of the detergent group, was used for the first time in 1930 by Higgins and Kittel. A few years later, Biegeleisen in New York described the use of ethanolamine oleate (1937). Reiner introduced sodium tetradecyl sulfate in 1946 and, 20 years later, Henschel (1913–1999) described the first results of sclerotherapy with polidocanol. Like many inventions, polidocanol owes its discovery not directly to specific research, but to the deliberate and consistent integration of casual observations from other research results. At the end of the 1940s and into the early 1950s, the search was underway for better injectable local anesthetics, including various representatives of "alkyl polyglycol ethers." During tests of systemic tolerability, it was noted that intravascular injections of higher concentrations of polidocanol caused irritation of the vein wall. Credit goes to Henschel, who suspected in 1963 that this side-effect might have a sclerosing utility. He then specifically developed the observation further, and Lunkenheimer, a friend of his, had a chance to test it between 1963 and 1966, after which sales of polidocanol solution began. To the best of our knowledge, no other sclerosing solutions were developed after 1966.

Only the detergent-type sclerosing agents offer the possibility of being foamed. Consequently, before 1930, when the first detergent agent was introduced, no one really thought about changing the injection of an ordinary liquid sclerosant to foam. Almost a decade after the beginning of use of sodium morrhuate, McAusland described in 1939 the novel use of foam in the injection treatment of telangiectasia.[1] He used sodium morrhuate in the form of a "froth," obtained by "shaking up the rubber-capped bottle" and aspirating the foam into his syringe. He explained the benefits of using foam instead of liquid for the treatment. These were: better treatment surveillance "... froth can be seen travelling along the small venules" and could be felt as crepitus; better manual treatment enhancement "... and the froth ... can be made completely to traverse an area of about two square inches"; and a better visual quality control of the treatment "... the veins suddenly go pink, sometimes ... retract and almost disappeared at once ...." Ethanolamine oleate has been used in the form of foam since 1944,[2] and Polidocanol was used as a foam even before it entered the market.[3]

Methods of foam production

Improvement in sclerotherapy

The development of foam production technologies began long before the development of foam sclerotherapy back in 1939. Foams were needed for a wide variety of different purposes, for example, in fire-fighting. Therefore, a number of inventions and discoveries were made in this as well as in other fields of engineering and technology. The utility of a fine-bubble fire-extinguishing foam that could be made from soap solution and air or another gas was described as early as 1929.[4] The use of small sieves or filters for foam production was described in 1936. Gas and a soap solution will form a foam if their passage through porous bodies is sufficiently rapid.[5] In 1964, Wilmsmann introduced a production method that involved a plastic brush rotating at a constant speed in a detergent solution to form foam.[6] In 1979, Cunningham addressed the problem of the variability of different foams, particularly the impact of different air-to-liquid ratios on foam density, average bubble sizes, and foam half-life.[7] In 1989, Poizot filed a patent application for another device suitable for the formation of foam of consistent quality that produced foam using a fine filter assembly (pore sizes of 10–250 μm), through which the gas and liquid were passed simultaneously.[8] In general terms, Poizot reconfirmed that the distribution and spread of a product were easier to control if present in the form of a foam.

As already mentioned, McAusland[1] started the development of methods specifically designed for the production of sclerosing foams in 1939. At the same time, sclerotherapy was continually improved through patented inventions and by the application of simple medical procedures that may well have been accomplished without any awareness of the long history of the development of foam sclerotherapy. Besides the use of foam, McAusland recommended injecting into an "empty vein" as obtained by elevation of the leg prior to injection. He preferred to combine lithium salycylate and a chinine–urethane mixture because, after mixing both agents in vitro, he noted that these substances were "incompatible," forming a "sticky, semi-solid substance" that was "always certain of producing sclerosis." This is, without having been noticed, the first mention of increased efficacy of treatment if viscous agents (not necessarily foams) are used instead of liquids.

Although frequently cited, Orbach's 1944 publication did not deal with foam.[9] Instead, he used two "conventional liquid" techniques for his patients: smaller veins were punctured and treated whilst the patient was standing ("full vein technique"), whilst, on the other hand, he used the "empty vein technique," in which varicose vein segments with a large diameter were first isolated between two tourniquets. Then, after venipuncture, the leg was elevated by 45–90°. By releasing the proximal tourniquet, blood could flow into the central or more proximal direction, whilst the distal tourniquet reduced or eliminated the supply of new blood from the distal direction. This technique caused less dilution of the liquid sclerosing agent.

However, Orbach sometimes noticed therapeutic failures. Then he had the following "great idea." In order to intensify contact between the sclerosant and the endothelium, not only should the diameter of the vein be reduced as far as possible prior to injection, but the vein should also be free of any blood. Therefore, he injected a small amount of air into the venous segment to be treated in order to displace completely the remaining blood. Clinically, he used this "air-block technique" only for small and medium-sized varicose veins. The maximum amount of air injected was 3 mL, a limit that became an orientation for most physicians using the air-block technique.[10,11]

In the same year as Orbach's publication, a book by Robert Rowden Foote[2] was published in London. He wrote about the treatment of spider veins: "The best injection fluid is the soapy froth obtained by shaking up 1 cc of Ethamoline (ethanolamine oleate) in a 2-cc syringe." The sclerosant-to-air ratio of 1 plus 1 described by Foote suggests that the dispersion was very fluid, so that it could not be used for displacing the blood in veins of a larger diameter.

In 1949, Karl Sigg took up the air-block technique described 5 years earlier.[12] He used the new technique for larger veins and reported more than 4000 treatments performed "without problems." Sigg described the rationale for the use of the air-block technique in a similar manner as Orbach and Foote: "The purpose is to prevent the dilution of the solutions for injection in the vein by the blood and to ensure that the sclerosant gets in contact with the intima of the vein in a rather concentrated form. (...) Even with this small-scale use, the air bubble chased the blood before the injection fluid arrived and thus cleared the way for a closer contact of the sclerosant with the venous intima." Later, Sigg combined Orbach's air-block technique and Foote's foam application and thus introduced a new idea into the therapeutic options known to that date: "Orbach's method becomes even more beneficial if foam is injected instead of air. (...) This foam is less rapidly washed away in the varicose vein than it happens with the pure injection of air."

In 1950, publications by Orbach revealed the first attempt to compare the efficacy of foam with the efficacy of fluid sclerosants.[10,11] The efficacy of the foam generated by agitation of the syringe or drug vial was increased approximately 3.5-fold to 4-fold compared with the same amount of "conventional" fluid. He also observed a "marked vasospasm" after injection of foam.

After 1953, Ree[13] departed again from the air-block or foam-block technique and injected 2–7 mL of "pure" foam, corresponding to an amount of air of up to 6.6 mL. With his technique (agitation of a detergent solution in the vial and subsequent aspiration of the bubbles into the syringe) he treated a series of 50 patients very successfully.

In 1956, Flückiger[14] recommended the technique known as "retrograde sclerotherapy", a technique characterized by leg elevation and sclerosant injection into saphenous veins from a proximal injection site in a distal direction. Thus, the sclerosant could reach all incompetent collaterals and the saphenous vein with one injection. He obtained better results by using sclerosing foam than by using fluid sclerosants: "Basically, the procedure consists of injecting ... Varsyl (ethanolamine oleate) foam into an appropriate vein. Due to the buoyancy, the foam has only a low tendency to move in central direction with the blood flow. (...) After removal of the needle, the location of the 'foam seal' can be determined by palpation. (...) The foam usually spreads in the surrounding of the injection site in distal and proximal direction. After injection, the intravascular foam depot ... is displaced by manual massage against the periphery."

Flückiger additionally postulated and discussed further treatment-relevant foam properties for the first time: "It is obvious that a given amount of sclerosant in the form of foam has a much larger surface than it has in an unchanged, fluid state: the smaller the bubbles of the foam are, the greater the surface. Since damage to the intima ... is based on the contact of the intima with the sclerosant, the use of foam allows an extended sclerosation with a small amount of sclerosant. The preparation of a homogenous, fine-bubbled foam is an important condition for the success of the procedure." Flückiger considered the various known (sclerosant) foam manufacturing procedures, and suggested his own new technique: "In order to obtain a homogenous fine-bubbled foam, the procedure consisting in the agitation of a syringe filled with air and sclerosant [Orbach's technique of 1950] is completely inappropriate. The drawing of air through a sclerosant in the syringe [Sigg's technique 1949] does not yield a small fine-bubbled foam either. (...) A perfect, fine-bubbled foam is obtained by the simultaneous aspiration of sclerosant ... and air through a thin injection needle. (...) The thin injection needle (the narrower the lumen, the finer the foam) ... is introduced into the ampoule in such a way that approximately two thirds of the opening of the bevel are imbibed in the fluid. When drawing back the plunger, the syringe fills with Varsyl foam under a sizzling noise, the foam remaining stable for several minutes."

A milestone regarding the improvement and standardization of sclerosing foam was the 1957 publication by Mayer and Brücke.[15] They described the first device that had been developed specifically for the preparation of sclerosant foam, a special syringe with a double plunger. "Before the main plunger, there is a second, thin plunger with numerous holes, whose piston leads to a central bore of the main plunger and protrudes it. When the main plunger is fixed, the plunger provided with holes can rapidly be moved forward and backward and Phlebocid (ethanolamine oleate) can be mixed with the air contained in the syringe. A fine-bubbled, viscous foam develops. (…) We have tested most sclerosants of similar composition and selected Phlebocid, which provides the stiffest foam upon agitation with a homogenous distribution of air bubbles. (…) We consider the greatest advantage of the use of foam … to be the homogenous distribution of the sclerosant …." Clinically, they stated after administration of foam: "We never observed complications after foam filling such as air embolisms or skin necroses."

In 1962, Flückiger[16] described another technique for the preparation of foam: pumping of air and sclerosant back and forth between a drug vial and the attached syringe. The foam was very fine-bubbled and of a creamy consistence. Furthermore, Flückiger[14] changed some points since his first publication in 1956. He proposed leg elevation not only during sclerotherapy, but also for some minutes thereafter in order to allow the foam to degrade. He warned therapists to be cautious while "stroking" the foam seal in a peripheral direction in order to prevent any unintended movement of foam into the deep venous system. Today, it is recommended to wait some minutes after the foam sclerotherapy of large veins before applying compression or muscle activation.[17–19]

Gillesberger's technique, published in 1969, was based on the generation of a negative pressure in a syringe so that air could enter through the capillary gap between the syringe piston and the plunger and thus generate bubbles.[20] In 1984, Hauer[21] patented a twin-syringe set for foam preparation: two parallel syringes, one filled with air, the other filled with sclerosing solution, are simultaneously emptied into a "mixing chamber," where foam develops during injection.

All technical developments until between 1939 and 1984 or 1986* were performed without the possibility of using modern ultrasound imaging techniques.

Use of air and other gases

McAusland[1] injected air (in the form of foam) for the first time for therapeutic reasons in patients with varicose veins. The amount of injected air is not known. Orbach later injected pure air as a bolus and limited the amount to a few milliliters.[9–11] Larger amounts of air up to about 40 mL were injected by Meyer and Brücke in 1957 – without problems of embolism or stroke.[15] At about the same time, gases other than air were used in a different area: radiology. Durant, Oppenheimer and colleagues and many others published papers about the safety of intravascular carbon dioxide and the use of X-ray visualization of intra-cardiac structures and blood vessels.[22,23] This opened the door to carbon dioxide angiography, which was used primarily in patients likely to encounter problems with ordinary contrast agents. In 1990, Hess published an article about the possibility of using other gases, and stated that nitrogen was not as good, whereas oxygen and carbon dioxide were better because of their better solubility in the blood.[24] Cabrera then decided to use oxygen and/or carbon dioxide in addition to or instead of air.[25,26] In 1999, Garcia Mingo described the use of helium and other gases in his "Foam Medical System."[27,28]

Ultrasound and duplex

B-mode ultrasound and Doppler ultrasound had been used for diagnostic purposes for quite a while when in 1974 the combination of both techniques was described for the first time by Barber and colleagues.[29] This so-called duplex ultrasound was ideal, particularly for diagnostic purposes in vascular medicine, but was then also used for therapeutic purposes in phlebology, for the first time in 1989 by Knight, Vin and Zygmunt.[30] Basically, their idea was to increase safety during injection sclerotherapy, that is, to avoid "literally blind injections" in which intra-arterial injections sometimes happened, to visually locate the best position for needle placement, and to detect inadvertent extra vascular injection of the

* A 2002 publication by Belcaro comprises information about an event which is reported to have happened as early as 1986.[55] This paper says that in 1986 Grigg demonstrated a new foam production procedure: the principle was the generation of a turbulent flow between two syringes, connected via a plastic infusion tube, so that fluid and air could be pumped forward and backward, thereby mixing.

sclerosant. Even today, most of these ideas are still valid and have been adopted in guidelines for sclerotherapy.[17–19]

In 1993, an additional important step was described by Schadeck.[31,32] He mixed his detergent sclerosing agent with air and recognized that the small foam bubbles would serve as an ideal contrast agent within the vein, allowing the passage of sclerosant agent to be followed visually from the point of injection on its way via the junctions to the deep venous system. In a similar way to Knight et al, Schadeck did not primarily intend increasing the efficacy of the treatment: he wanted to improve the possibilities of monitoring the injection himself – and was successful. In June 1994, Juan Cabrera[25] submitted his patent application concerning an "injectable foam." One year later, he published his first personal series of ultrasound-guided treatments of saphenous veins with his sclerosant foam.[26] From a historical point of view, he combined the beneficial aspects of foam sclerotherapy with the possibilities of real-time ultrasound guidance and surveillance.

Cabrera's patent application was not published until 1999. Only after 1999 was it known that he obtained his foam by stirring with a high-speed rotating brush (a modified dental bur) – like cream with a food mixer – and the facultative addition of carbon dioxide and/or oxygen as carrier gases. The patent application, submitted by the British company BTG/Provensis, included his method of foam preparation with any sclerosing agent, but also the use of "microfoam" in phlebology in general.[25] Because of literature published before the submission of his patent application, the patent was finally declared void. But following Cabrera's publication of 1995, several circumstances coincided, which promoted the speedy propagation of foam sclerotherapy supported by the current technical options:

- A considerable number of phlebologists had the technical prerequisites (e.g., a duplex scanner) to perform ultrasound-guided sclerotherapy.
- Modern means of communication and research possibilities contributed to rapidly propagating the new ideas.
- Some had a basic interest in Cabrera's treatment approach, possibly without having had any knowledge of the long history of foam sclerotherapy development up to that point.
- Because of the delayed publication of the method of foam production of the "microfoam" that Cabrera had submitted, details of his personal technique remained unknown to any other phlebologists for many years. This led to the search for, and development of, "new" personal techniques of foam production.

Recent contributions to foam sclerotherapy

In 1997, Monfreux presented his method of foam production, and the needs of a number of the phlebologists were met, at least temporarily.[33] The "*Méthode MUS*" was taken up, especially by French phlebologists. The principle was similar to Gillesberger's technique: generation of a negative pressure in the glass syringe filled with sclerosing solution, and thus inlet of air through the fine gap between syringe barrel and plunger with corresponding pearling of the solution and transformation into foam. Besides French phlebologists, some Italian colleagues tried this technique, but were not entirely satisfied.[34] One and two years later, respectively, Sadoun and Benigni[35] and Santos Gaston[36] published their variations of the Monfreux method.

In 1999, Garcia Mingo[27,28] described another specific device for foam preparation. The "Foam Medical System" is a sterilizable and reusable device that generates foam by the introduction of helium, carbon dioxide or other gases from a pressurized gas cylinder into a second chamber containing the sclerosant solution, and the subsequent passage of the mixture through a fine foaming element.

In December of the same year, Tessari presented a video documentation of his famous "Tourbillon technique," which for the first time allowed the preparation of a very dense and creamy foam without special equipment, but solely with the use of standard medicinal products (ordinary syringes and a three-way tap) and some pumping movements.[37] Italian colleagues rapidly adopted this technique, since the foam was much better than what could be obtained with the low pressure techniques.[38,39] A more detailed description of the pumping procedure (at least 10 times) to improve the standardization of the foam was given in 2001.[39]

In 2000, Frullini improved the technique developed by Flückinger in 1962 and made it usable for disposable syringes by adding a special adapter.[40,41] In the same year, a patent was submitted by Osman, Flynn and Wright (BTG/Provensis), an improvement of the first patent application by Cabrera.[25,42] The application was about a pressurized foam can, a variety of "physiological gases," polidocanol and, amongst others, the double-piston syringe from 1957.[15]

When searching for a suitable technique for the preparation of a more standardized, but still cheap, foam it was noticed that the methods available up to 2000 all had the disadvantage that reproducibility was poor.[43] The foams all had a different consistency and an inhomogeneous flow behavior if minor changes were made during preparation. Therefore, a preparation variant was searched for that was as simple and fast as the original Tessari method, but especially even more reproducible. In a laboratory experimental series, the variables that possibly affect the stability of the foam were changed systematically, and efforts were made to find the best possible combination of connector type, syringe size and type, liquid-to-gas ratio, sclerosant concentration, and manufacturing instructions.* The result is known as "DSS" (double syringe system) or "Tessari-DSS."[3,43,44] In 2002 and later, experimental data were presented about the different variables and their consequences on foam stability and blood-displacing effects (Figures 1.1 and 1.2).

The same year (2001), Gachet published his aspiration technique, which is, as regards foam preparation, very similar to the description of Flückiger's method of 1956.[14,45] Also in 2001, a third European patent was submitted by Harmann, Pollock and others (BTG/Provensis), this time mainly describing a system with two cans (one for the sclerosant and one for the gas) and

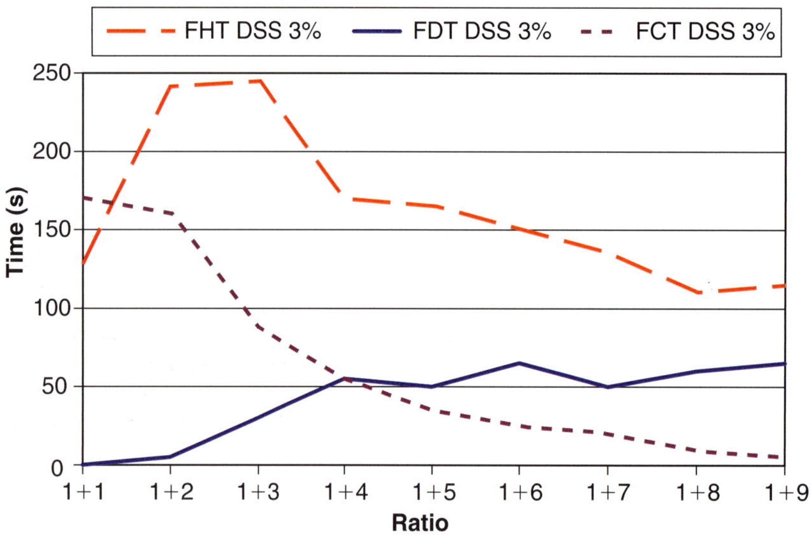

Figure 1.1 Different measures for determining foam stability. All values are in seconds for 3% polidocanol foams prepared by the DSS method with various liquid-to-air ratios. FHT, foam half-time: the time until half of the liquid used to produce foam has drained back to the liquid state. Liquid foams (ratios of 1 + 2 or 1 + 3) have a long FHT. FDT, foam drainage time: the time until visible drainage within the foams begins. The more liquid the foam is (especially ratios of 1 + 1, 1 + 2), the shorter the drainage time and the less stable the foam. In dry foams (ratios of 1 + 4, 1 + 5, etc.), visible drainage starts much later, and the foam is more stable. FCT, foam coalescence time: the time until visible bubbles appear within the foam. The more liquid the foam is (ratios of 1 + 1, 1 + 2, or 1 + 3), the longer the FCT and the more stable the foam. Dry foams rapidly develop large visible bubbles. The "best ratio" as a result of FCT, FDT and FHT is a compromise between all values. A ratio of 1 + 4 has quite a high FHT and a still fairly good FCT and FDT

* The most stable, homogenous and fine-bubbled foam was obtained according to the instructions. Required material: 10 mL syringe (Omnifix), 10 mL syringe (Inject) (each with a Luer-Lock connection), one female–female adapter (Combidyn) and a 0.2 μm filter (for sterilization of air). Exactly 8 mL of air are drawn into the Inject syringe via the sterile filter; afterwards – after removal of the filter – exactly 2 mL of sclerosant. The two syringes are connected to the adapter. First, five pumping movements are performed against resistance (by firm thumb pressure onto the other syringe piston) until the two components are well mixed. Afterwards, the foam is pumped again quickly forth and back seven times between the two syringes without resistance like in the original Tessari technique, until a homogenous foam has formed.

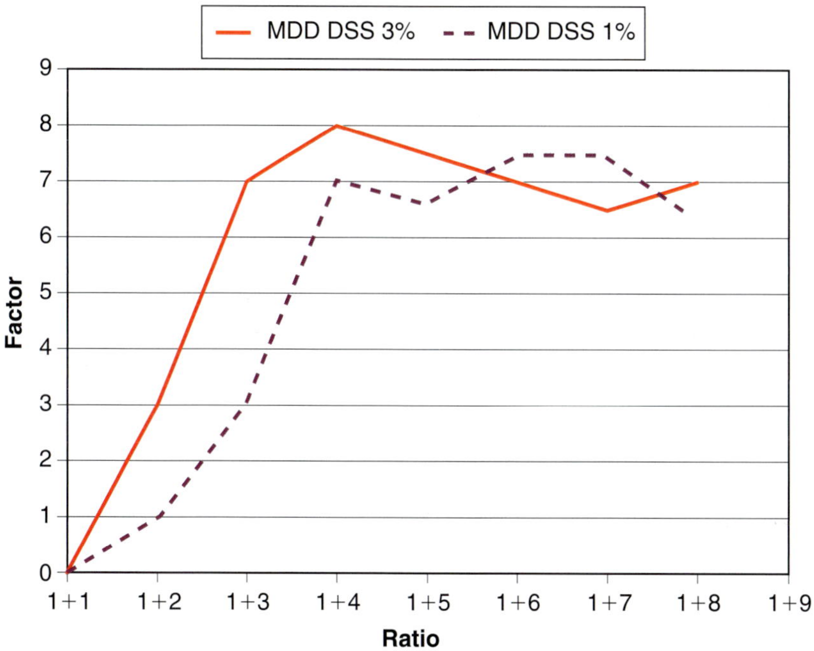

Figure 1.2 Displacing capacity of double syringe system (DSS) foams. MDD, maximum displacement distance of DSS foams with polidocanol, that is, the ability to displace liquids out of tubes. "Factor" is the multiple n in the formula of a virtual cylinder with diameter D and length $n \times D$ (i.e., n is a multiple of the diameter) in a water-filled tubing system from which the water can be completely displaced by an adequately large foam volume. A factor of 0, for instance, means that no displacement takes place; a factor of 5, for example, means that, upon injection, water is displaced from the tube segment (a cylinder) 5 times the length of the tube diameter. Wet foams (1 + 1, 1 + 2) have a substantially smaller displacing effect, and foam floats along the upper side of the tube. Especially in 1 + 2 and 1 + 3 foams, the foam concentration matters a lot: 1% foams have a poor displacing effect, 3% foams have a good displacing effect. Dry foams of ratio 1 + 4 or greater are equally excellent displacers regardless of concentration (1% or 3%). As a summary of Figures 1.1 and 1.2, 1 + 4 foams have the best properties (stability and displacing effect)[43]

a connector to transfer the gas into the sclerosant can.[46] This and/or a later type of "Varisolve" foam has been or is being tested clinically.[47] This is detailed elsewhere in this book. Also in 2001, Onorati presented a variation of the double-piston syringe. A computerized mechanical system to agitate the DSS system with defined power and duration (TurboFoamer) was presented by Hamel and Desnos in 2001. Soon thereafter, Hamel-Desnos and co-workers started the first prospective, randomized multicenter study, comparing a low-volume, single-shot foam sclerotherapy session for great saphenous vein insufficiency with conventional liquid sclerotherapy.[44] This is also described elsewhere in this book.

Early in 2002, Wollmann and Schliephake (Kreussler Pharma, Wiesbaden, Germany) proposed a foaming device to obtain sterile foam using filtered room air and a sclerosant cartridge.[48] In the following year, both proposed another device to obtain foam using sterile room air and a special sclerosant cartridge.[49]

An improved foam can with a "bag in valve" construction was presented in 2003 by Wright and Harman (BTG/Provensis, London, UK).[50] The problem both intended to solve was mainly degradation of polidocanol, which can occur if exposed to oxygen for a longer period of time. Commercially available GMP-conform polidocanol ampoules or vials therefore contain no oxygen, but have a nitrogen atmosphere instead.

In 2005, a modified and advanced version of the Tessari/DSS system was presented by Wollmann (Kreussler).[51] The "EasyFoam" kit contains the gas component in the necessary amount in one syringe. The ratio of liquid to gas was changed slightly from the DSS ratio to allow better blood-displacing effects in veins of a larger caliber. Also, special syringes with a very small amount of silicone and a special two-way restrictor valve-adapter are part of the EasyFoam system. The kit has successfully been tested in a multicenter randomized and controlled clinical trial.[52]

For more or less the same reasons as in 2003, helium was included in a fifth patent application in 2004 by Wright and Harper (BTG/Provensis).[53] As helium can be detected easily, a loss of gas from the pressurised gas containers is discovered more quickly during storage.

To the author's knowledge, the most recent publication of a foaming device dates from 2006 by Gobin and Benigni, who published their "Sterivein" technique.[54] The technique uses one syringe and an air filter, and foam generation is performed through pumping movements, in a similar way to Frullini or Flückinger.

Summary

Foam sclerotherapy has changed methods of treating veins dramatically. Development and improvement in understanding are still underway, but knowledge and standardization of the treatment have made enormous progress in the last few years. Foam sclerotherapy has a good chance of remaining the cheapest treatment by far, and the potential of even becoming one of the best treatments for varicose veins. At any rate, "Foam is the future of varicose vein treatment" (John J Bergan, Bologna 2003).

References

1. McAusland S. The modern treatment of varicose veins. Med Press Circular 1939; 201: 404–10.
2. Foote RR. The Injection treatment. In: Foote RR, ed. Varicose Veins, Haemorrhoids and Other Conditions. London: HK Lewis & Co., 1944: 13–44.
3. Wollmann JC. Schaum – zwischen Vergangenheit und Zukunft. Vasomed 2002; 16: 34–5.
4. Minimax Act.-Ges. Verfahren und Vorrichtung zum innigen Mischen von Flüssigkeiten, Gasen oder Dämpfen oder von Flüssigkeiten mit Gasen oder Dämpfen, insbesondere zur Erzeugung von Schaum für Feuerlöschzwecke. Deutsches Reichspatentamt, DE 477204A; 25.10.1929.
5. Waldschmidt E. Device for producing foam. United States Patent Office, US 2043599A, 09.06.1936.
6. Wilmsmann H. Schaumbestimmung von Tensiden mit einer Reibschaummethode. Fette, Seifen, Anstrichmittel 1964; 66: 955–61.
7. Cunningham CJ. Method and apparatus for producing foam. European Patent Office, EP 11381A1, 16.10.1979.
8. Poizot F. Device for producing foam. European Patent Office, EP 379818A1, 20.12.1989.
9. Orbach EJ. Sclerotherapy of Varicose Veins – Utilization of an intravenous air block. Am J Surg 1944; 66: 362–6.
10. Orbach EJ, Petretti AK. The thrombogenic property of foam of a synthetic anionic detergent. Angiol 1950; 1: 237–43.
11. Orbach EJ. Contributions to the therapy of the varicose complex. J Int Coll Surg 1950; 6: 765–71.
12. Sigg K. Neuere Gesichtspunkte zur Technik der Varizenbehandlung. Ther Umsch 1949; 6: 127–34.
13. Ree A. Etamolin foam in the treatment of varicose veins. A new method. Acta Dermatovenerol 1953; 33: 435–36.
14. Flückiger P. Nicht-operative retrograde Varicenverödung mit Varsylschaum. Schweiz Med Wochenschr 1956; 48: 1368–70.
15. Mayer H, Brücke H. Angiologie – Zur Ätiologie und Behandlung der Varizen der unteren Extremitäten. Chir Prax 1957; 4: 521–8.
16. Flückiger P. Beitrag zur Technik der ambulanten Varizenbehandlung. Die med Welt 1963; 12: 617–21.
17. Breu FX, Guggenbichler S, Wollmann JC. 2nd European Consensus Meeting on Foam Sclerotherapy, April 28–30, 2006, Tegernsee, Germany. VASA 2008; 37 (Suppl 71): 3–32.
18. Breu FX, Guggenbichler S. European Consensus Meeting on Foam Sclerotherapy, April 4–6, 2003, Tegernsee, Germany. Dermatol Surg 2004; 30: 709–17.
19. Rabe E, Pannier-Fischer F, Gerlach H, et al. Guidelines for sclerotherapy of varicose veins (ICD 10: I83.0, I83.1, I83.2, and I83.9). Dermatol Surg 2004; 30: 687–93.
20. Gillesberger W. Die Ausrüstung des phlebologisch tätigen Dermatologen. Z Hautkrankheiten 1969; 44: 669–74.
21. Hauer G. German Patent DE 34 17 182 C2. Zwillings-Spritzen-Set. 1984.
22. Durant TM, Stauffer HM, Oppenheimer MJ, Paul RE. Safety of intravascular carbon dioxide and the use for roentgenologic visualization of intracardiac structures. Ann Intern Med 1957; 47: 191–201.
23. Grosse-Brockerhoff F, Koch D, Loogen F, et al. Kohlendioxid als Kontrastmittel für die Röntgendarstellung des Herzens und der Gefäße. Fortschr Röntgenstr 1957; 86: 285–91.

24. Hess H. Digitale Subtraktionsangiographie mit Kohlendioxid: eine Alternative zur Extremitätenangiographie mit jodhaltigen Kontrastmitteln. Fortschr Röntgenstr. 1990; 153: 233–8.
25. Cabrera J, Cabrera Garcia-Olmedo JR. Injectable microfoam containing a sclerosant agent. European Patent Office, EP 656203A1; 21.06.1994.
26. Cabrera J, Cabrera Garcia-Olmedo JR. Nuevo método de esclerosis en las varices tronculares. Patologia Vascular 1995; 4: 55–73.
27. Garcia Mingo J. Esclerosis venosa con espuma: "Foam medical system". Rev Espan Med Cirugia Cosmet 1999; 7: 29–31.
28. Garcia-Mingo J. "Foam medical system": a new technique to treat varicose veins with foam. In: Henriet JP, ed. Foam Sclerotherapy: State of the Art. Editions Phlebologiques Francaises, 2001: 45–50.
29. Barber F, Baker D, Nation A, et al. Ultrasonic duplex echo-Doppler scanner. IEEE Trans Biomed Eng 1974; 21: 109.
30. Knight RM, Vin F, Zygmunt JA. Ultrasonic guidance of injection into the superficial venous system. In: Davy A, Stemmer R, eds. Phlébologie. Paris: John Libbey Eurotext, 1989: 339–41.
31. Schadeck M, Allaert FA. Duplex scanning in the mechanism of the sclerotherapy: importance of the spasm. Phlebology 1995; Suppl 1: 574–76.
32. Schadeck M. Echo-sclerose de la grande Saphene. Phlebologie 1993; 46: 673–82.
33. Monfreux A. Traitement sclérosant des troncs saphéniens et leurs collatérales de gros calibre par la méthode mus. Phlebologie 1997; 50: 351–3.
34. Cavezzi A, Frullini A, Ricci S, Tessari, L. Treatment of varicose veins by foam sclerotherapy: two clinical series. Phlebology 2002; 17: 13–18.
35. Sadoun S, Benigni JP. The treatment of varicosities and telangiectases with TDS or lauromacrogol foam: video tape. UIP World Congress of Phlebology, Sydney, 1998.
36. Santos Gaston M. In: Santos Gaston M, Santos-Gaston Orus M, eds. Esclerotherapia de varices. Madrid: Vegalon, 1999: 73–7.
37. Tessari L. Nouvelle technique d'obtention de la scléromousse. Phlebologie 2000; 53: 129.
38. Frullini A, Cavezzi A. Echosclérose par mousse de tétradécyl-sulfate de sodium et de polidocanol: deux années d'expérience. Phlebologie 2000; 53: 431–5.
39. Tessari L, Cavezzi A, Frullini A. Preliminary experience with a new sclerosing foam in the treatment of varicose veins. Dermatol Surg 2001; 27: 58–60.
40. Frullini A. New technique in producing sclerosing foam in a disposable syringe. Dermatol Surg 2000; 26: 705–6.
41. Frullini A. Sclerosing foam in the treatment of recurrent varicose veins. In: Henriet JP, ed. Foam Sclerotherapy: State of the Art. Editions Phlebologiques Françaises, 2001: 73–8.
42. Osman T, Flynn BS, Wright DD, et al. Generation of therapeutic microfoam. European Patent Office, EP 1637127A2; 26.05.2000.
43. Wollmann JC. Herstellung und Eigenschaften von Sklerosierungsschaum. Vasomed 2004; 16: 24.
44. Hamel-Desnos C, Desnos P, Wollmann JC, et al. Evaluation of the efficacy of polidocanol in the form of foam compared with liquid form in sclerotherapy of the long saphenous vein: initial results. Dermatol Surg 2003; 29(12): 1170–5.
45. Gachet G. Une nouvelle mèthode simple et économique pour confectionner de la mousse pour sclérose échoguidée. Phlebologie 2001; 54: 63–5.
46. Harman AD, Harper PV, Pollock N, Sinclair GS. Generation of therapeutic microfoam. European Patent Office, EP 1337238B1; 23.11.2001.
47. Wright DD, Gobin JP, Bradbury AW, et al. Varisolve polidocanol microfoam compared with surgery or sclerotherapy in the management of varicose veins in the presence of trunk vein incompetence: European randomized controlled trial. Phlebology 2006; 21: 181–90.
48. Wollmann JC. The history of sclerosing foams. Dermatol Surg 2004; 30: 694–703.
49. Wollmann JC, Schliephake D. Device for producing a medical foam. European Patent Office, EP 1572336B1; 13.11.2003.
50. Wright DD, Harman AD. Container for the production of microfoam. European Patent Office, EP 1507718A1; 23.05.2003.
51. Wollmann JC, Schliephake D. Gerät zur Herstellung eines insbesondere sterilen Schaums. Deutsches Patentamt, DE 20201168U1; 26.01.2002.
52. Rabe E, Otto J, Schliephake D, Pannier F. Efficacy and safety of great saphenous vein sclerotherapy using standardized polidocanol foam (ESAF): a randomised controlled multicentre clinical trial. Eur J Vasc Endovasc Surg 2008; 35: 238–45.
53. Harman AD, Wright, DD. Therapeutic Microfoam. European Patent Office, EP 1597171A2; 07.01.2004.
54. Gobin JP, Benigni JP. Stérivein: Un nouveau procédé de fabrication de mousse sclérosante. Phlebologie 2006; 59: 73–6.
55. Belcaro G, Geroulakos C, Cesarone MR, Nicolaides AN. Comparison among treatment schemes for varicose veins: surgery, sclerotherapy, foam-sclerotherapy and combined options. A 10-year, prospective, randomised, follow-up study. In: Belcaro G, Geroulakos G, Cesarone MR, Nicolaides AN, eds. Sclerotherapy in Venous Disease. Torino: Edizioni Minerva Medica, 2002: 96–104.

2 Dermatological manifestations of venous insufficiency

Kurosh Parsi

Introduction

Foam sclerotherapy can treat a range of venous conditions that may present with a variety of clinical manifestations. Skin changes are one of most important reasons why patients present to practitioners requesting treatment. Correct identification of these skin changes can aid in making the right diagnosis and an appropriate plan of management. Given the significant overlap between phlebology and dermatology, it is essential for phlebologists to be familiar with skin manifestations of venous disease. This chapter discusses the dermatological manifestations of venous insufficiency as well as other forms of vascular ectasias that may present in a similar fashion to venous incompetence.

Patients with venous disease often exhibit dermatological changes. Sometimes these skin changes are the only clue to an appropriate list of differential diagnoses. Chronic venous insufficiency (CVI) is the most common venous disease, which presents with a range of skin changes. Most people are familiar with venous eczema, lipodermatosclerosis and venous ulcers as manifestations of long-term venous insufficiency. The less familiar are changes such as acroangiodermatitis and pigmented purpuric dermatoses. Dilatation of venous structures is not always due to venous incompetence, and could be primary or secondary to systemic disease or to environmental influences such as actinic damage and radiation.

Common skin manifestations of venous insufficiency

CVI commonly presents with edema, corona phlebectasia paraplantaris (Figures 2.1 and 2.2), stasis dermatitis, pigmentory changes (hyper- and hypo-), atrophie blanche, lipodermatosclerosis and skin ulceration. Less common manifestations include pigmented purpuric dermatoses and acroangiodermatitis. Superficial thrombophlebitis can also occur in association with venous incompetence (Figure 2.3).

Venous hypertension is responsible for many manifestations of CVI, including edema, red cell extravasation, perivascular fibrin deposition, impaired arterial inflow, and other locally mediated disturbances. The local tissue sequelae of CVI are due to impaired clearance of cellular metabolites secondary to concurrent damage to the lymphatic system.

Corona phlebectatica paraplantaris (CPP)

This term describes the venulectasias and varicosties found along the paraplantar aspect of the foot (Figures 2.1 and 2.2). It is one of the earliest manifestations of

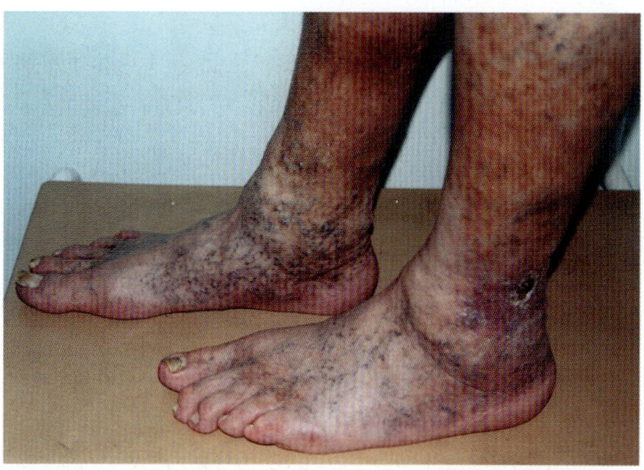

Figure 2.1 Corona phlebectatica paraplantaris

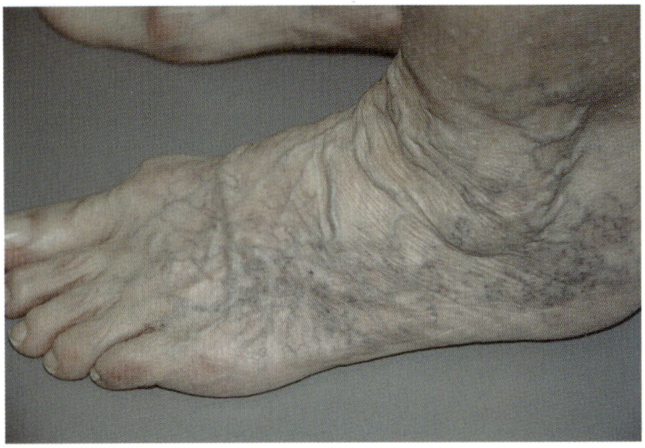

(a)

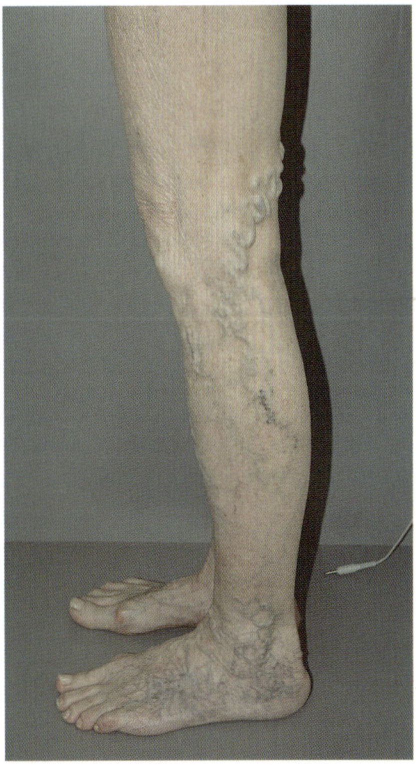

(b)

Figure 2.2 (a) Corona phlebectatica paraplantaris (CPP) affecting the left lateral foot. (b) Note the proximal varicosities of the lateral thigh system "feeding" the CPP of the lateral foot

venous hypertension and may be purely secondary to superficial venous incompetence. This finding should prompt the treating physician to look for underlying venous incompetence.

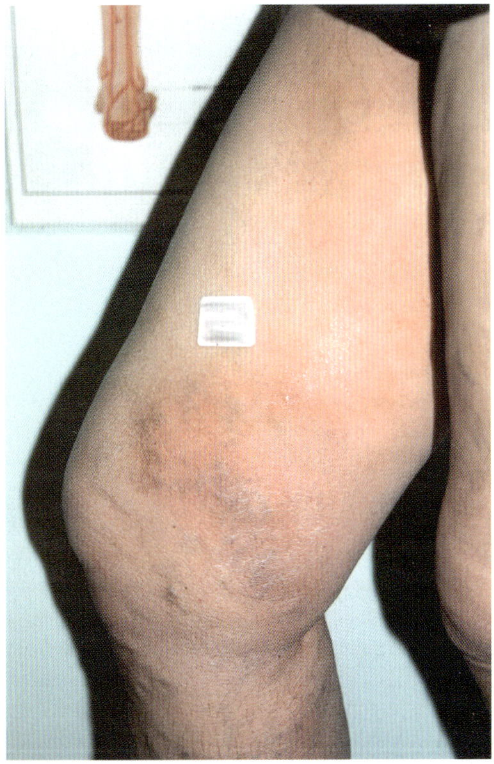

Figure 2.3 Superficial thrombophlebitis of a great saphenous vein tributary

Edema

Edema is defined as a clinically apparent increase in the interstitial fluid volume. Edema that retains an indentation when pressed with a finger is called pitting edema. Systemic causes of edema include congestive cardiac failure, hepatic insufficiency, renal failure, pretibial edema in myxedema, hypoproteinemia, and other systemic disorders.

A common manifestation of venous hypertension is lower limb edema. Usually, lower leg edema is symmetrical in patients with systemic disorders. Limb circumference should be measured at set landmarks and compared with the contralateral limb.

Lymphedema may be a sign of primary lymphatic outflow obstruction, or it may be secondary to the overproduction of lymph due to severe venous hypertension (so-called phlebolymphedema). Lymphoscintography or radiographic contrast lymphangiography may be required to confirm the diagnosis. The so-called

"Stemmer's sign," which is the inability to pinch and lift the skin between the first and second toes, is present in lymphedema. Presence of fat deposits of the so-called "lipedema" is the differential diagnosis of phlebolymphedema.

Eczematous eruptions

Venous eczema (Figures 2.4 and 2.5) is usually the earliest cutaneous manifestation of venous insufficiency, and is a precursor to hyperpigmentation and lipodermatosclerosis. The medial ankle is most frequently involved, revealing erythematous, scaling and sometimes exudative weeping patches and plaques (Figure 2.5).

Discoid eczema can also occur secondary to venous incompetence (Figure 2.6) and even a generalized eczematous eruption may occur as an idiosyncratic reaction to chronic venous eczema, termed an "id reaction." Secondary bacterial infection with *Staphylococcus aureus* can cause typical crusting. Pseudomonal colonization is a common complication. In long-standing cases, lichenification may occur as a consequence of chronic scratching and rubbing.

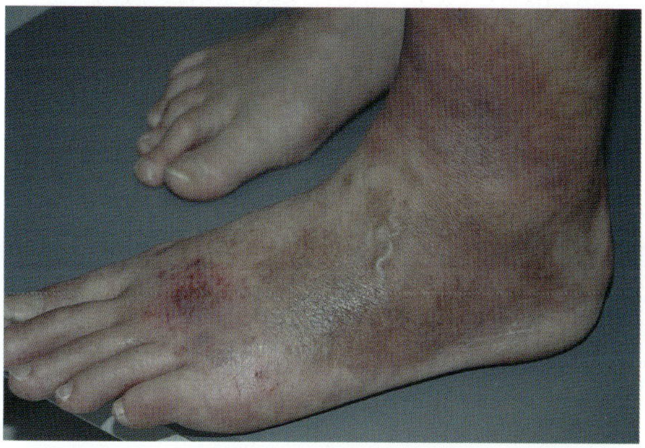

Figure 2.4 Venous eczema over the dorsum and hyperpigmentation over the lateral aspect of the foot

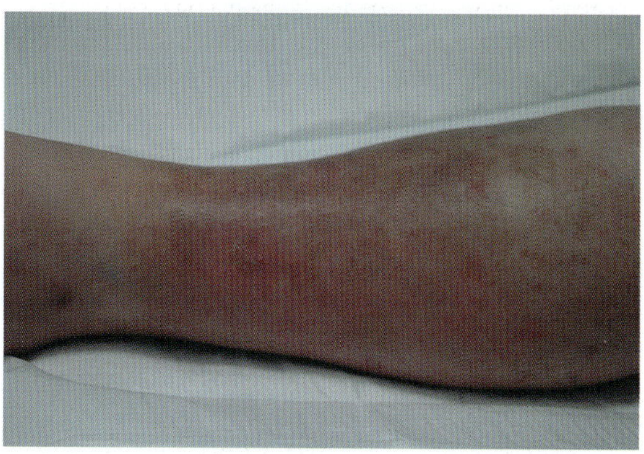

Figure 2.5 Venous eczema in an area of lipodermatosclerosis and venous hyperpigmentation

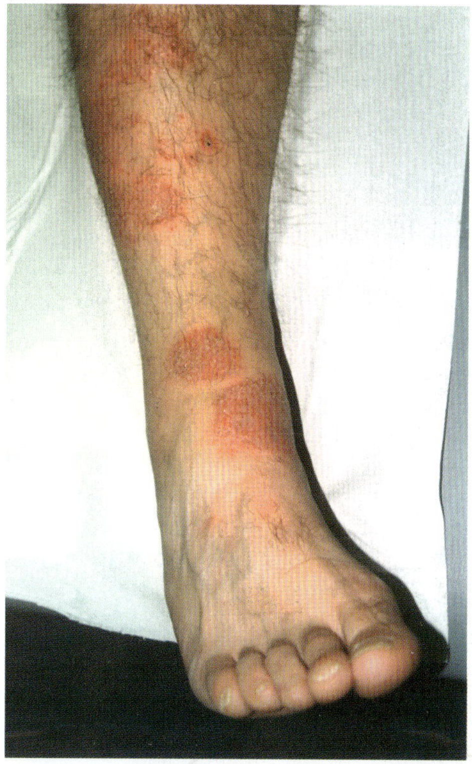

Figure 2.6 Discoid eczema associated with venous hypertension

Contact dermatitis is a common occurrence in patients with leg ulcers. Eighty percent of ulcer patients treated for more than 5 years are sensitive to at least one agent applied to their skin.[1] Allergic contact dermatitis to topical treatments – including neomycin, bacitracin, and some topical corticosteroids, adhesives, cream preservatives and stabilizers – has been reported.[2] Allergic contact dermatitis should be considered when venous eczema becomes clinically worse or does not improve despite appropriate topical treatment. These patients will require patch testing to identify the allergen. Topical antibiotics such as neomycin and popular preparations such as Kenocomb should never be used on open venous ulcers. Irritant contact dermatitis also occurs as a nonallergic reaction to soap-containing products, antiseptics, spirits and other irritants.

Pigmentary changes

Venous hypertension leads to red cell extravasation. Breakdown of red cells leads to hemosiderin deposition and cutaneous pigmentation (Figure 2.7). Hyperpigmentation secondary to red cell extravasation is difficult to treat and is not responsive to hydroquinone or other standard bleaching agents used to treat hypermelanosis. Treatment of the underlying venous hypertension can help in lightening the pigmentation, but in general, once hemosiderin pigmentation is present, it is mostly irreversible. Postinflammatory hypopigmentation may occur, which can even result in depigmentation. This should be differentiated from atrophie blanche.

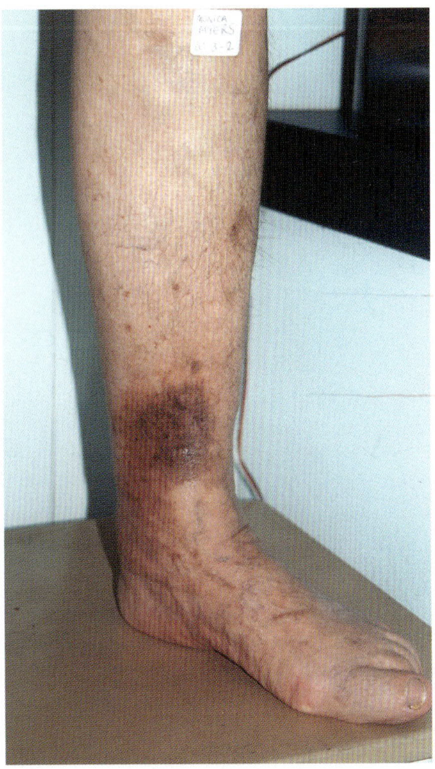

Figure 2.7 Typical venous hyperpigmentation of the medial gaiter area

Atrophie blanche

This is a specific type of dermal scarring, which usually presents as a small reticulated porcelain white patch. Dermoscopic examination of atrophie blanche demonstrates dilated capillary loops interspersed within the dermal scars. Atrophie blanche is caused by occlusion of dermal arterioles and infarction of the skin supplied by these vessels (Figures 2.8 and 2.9). This occurs secondary to venous hypertension or thrombo-occlusive vasculopathies involving dermal arterioles. Skin in this condition is avascular and prone to ulceration.

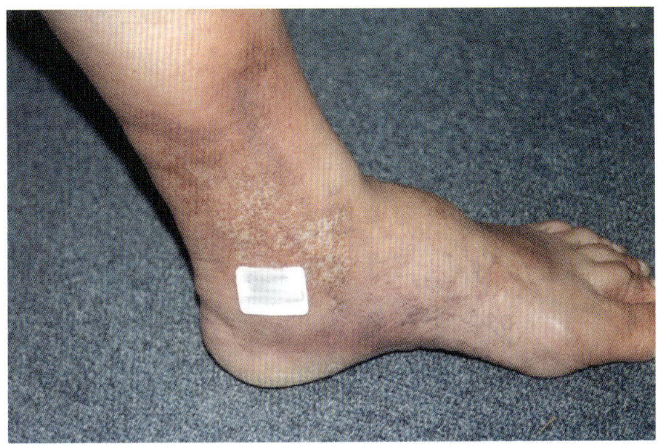

Figure 2.8 Porcelain white scars of atrophie blanche in an area of lipodermatosclerosis

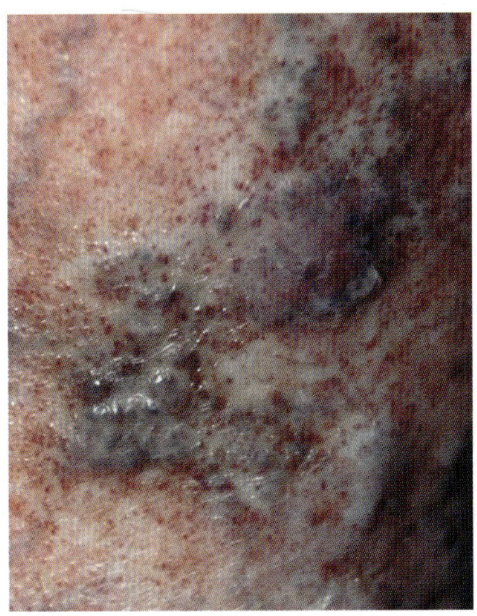

Figure 2.9 Close-up view of atrophie blanche, interspersed punctate telangiectasias and underlying varicose veins

Sclerotherapy in the affected areas should be performed with caution, as necrosis can occur readily.

Vasculitis involving the small and medium-sized vessels can also lead to identical white scars of atrophie blanche on the legs. Other systemic diseases, such as systemic lupus erythematosus (SLE), rheumatoid arthritis and Klinefelter's syndrome, can result in skin ulcerations that heal with atrophie blanche-like lesions.

Lipodermatosclerosis (LDS), ankylosis and equinus deformity of the ankle

Chronic LDS is a septal panniculitis that presents as induration of skin and the underlying fat in the gaiter area of lower legs (Figure 2.10). It usually extends from the ankles to the lower border of the calf muscle. Histologically, there is a chronic septal panniculitis and fibrosis involving the overlying dermis.[3] The differential diagnosis of LDS includes other septal panniculopathies and, in particular, erythema nodosum and necrobiosis lipoidica diabeticorum.

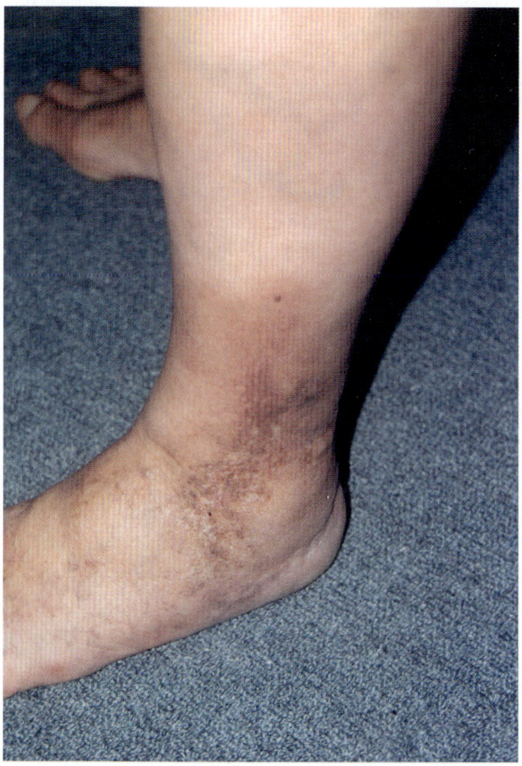

Figure 2.10 Lipodermatosclerosis associated with atrophie blanche

Further progression of disease and contraction of the fibrous tissue leads to the classic "inverted champagne bottle" appearance. In these patients, the tissue fibrosis of the gaiter area is so severe that there is a marked contrast with the normal calf and thigh tissue, hence creating the morphological description of an inverted champagne bottle. This interferes with ankle movement and causes edema of the foot. Further fibrosis can cause plantar flexion at the ankle (equinus deformity) and eventually a fibrous ankylosis in plantar flexion (Figure 2.11). This deformity is accelerated if the Achilles tendon is shortened due to fibrosis.

The induration and lack of perfusion of the tissue makes it prone to ulceration. Sclerotherapy of the underlying vessels should be performed with caution. Foam is quite often visualized on duplex imaging to ascend up to the dermis when the underlying vessels are injected. Given the lack of perfusion and scarring of the tissues, necrosis can occur readily. Also, given the induration of the skin and the subcutaneous tissue, it is very difficult to guide the needle to the target vessel. Other techniques such as catheter-guided sclerotherapy may be useful in this setting. The induration associated with LDS improves when the underlying venous hypertension is reversed, but may never reverse completely.

A lesser known form of LDS is the so-called "acute lipodermatosclerosis," which is primarily an acute panni-

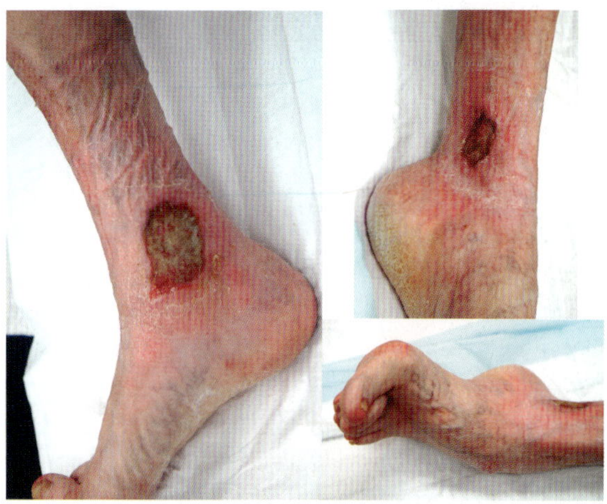

Figure 2.11 Advanced venous ulcers causing fixed foot deformity. This patient received ultrasound-guided sclerotherapy, and all ulcers healed. However, she eventually required a left below-knee amputation to facilitate mobility. Note the equinus deformity of the left foot

culitis. Acute lipodermatosclerosis can be confused with acute cellulitis or even acute venous eczema. Eventual induration of skin and the underlying adipose tissue leads to the more familiar clinical picture of chronic LDS.

Venous ulcers

Most chronic lower leg ulcers have a venous etiology.[4] Only a small number of venous ulcers are caused by deep vein incompetence or obstruction – the majority are caused by superficial venous incompetence.[5] Nonhealing ulcers of the medial ankle area are most likely due to underlying venous hypertension. The incompetent posterior tibial perforators (Cockett perforators) along the posterior accessory saphenous vein of the leg (the posterior arch vein) play an important role in the altered hemodynamics of this area. Once the higher sources of incompetence are treated, these incompetent perforators can be treated with ultrasound-guided foam sclerotherapy.

Venous ulcers are usually larger but shallower than other ulcers, and have a moist red granulating base and an irregular border (Figure 2.11). Calcification is a common finding. The tissue surrounding these ulcers may exhibit signs of venous eczema and other changes, such as atrophie blanche, hyperpigmentation and LDS.

Pain is characteristically mild in venous ulcers. The presence of severe pain in a typical venous ulcer may indicate infection, a concomitant arterial compromise or a wrong diagnosis. The complete absence of pain should suggest the possibility of a neuropathic ulcer or gumma.

Nonhealing, nodular areas of venous ulcers should be biopsied to exclude neoplastic change. The most common tumour is squamous cell carcinoma; however, rarely, basal cell carcinomas may develop too.[4] Malignant melanoma may present as a lower leg ulcer.

Other important differential diagnoses include ulcers of arterial, neuropathic or traumatic origin. Ischemic ulcers are often found on the feet and toes or on the inner or outer aspect of the heels. Traumatic ulcers are often surrounded by normal skin and in a site such as the anterior shin, which is frequently injured. Neuropathic ulcers commonly occur where there is pressure on the denervated skin. Typical locations include the sole of the foot, especially over the first metatarsophalangeal joint, and the base of the fifth metatarsals where shoes press and rub against the foot and the heel.

Pyoderma gangrenosum, vasculitis, self-induced artifact and infections can also mimic venous ulcers (Figure 2.12). Pyoderma gangrenosum (PG) begins as a small pustule or patch of necrotic skin and progresses rapidly to an ulcerated area with a necrotic base, cyanotic edge and surrounding erythema. PG is typically very painful. Minor trauma inducing new lesions is termed "pathergy" and is a feature of PG. PG is associated with Crohn's disease, ulcerative colitis, hematologic malignancies and arthritis, or could be idiopathic. PG responds to systemic steroids and immunosuppression.

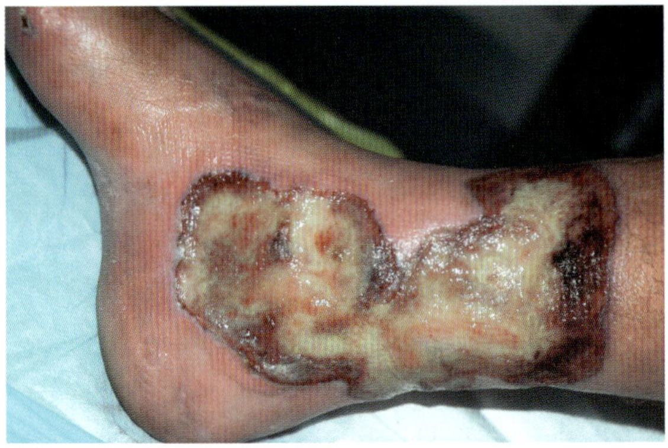

Figure 2.12 Pyoderma gangrenosum of the gaiter area can mimic venous ulcers. Note the cyanotic edge and erythermatous surrounding skin

Venous ulcers do not require biopsy, but in the case of a nonhealing ulcer not responding to conventional therapy, biopsy is indicated. Biopsies should be taken from the edge of the ulcer and not from its necrotic base. Multiple biopsies may be required for the diagnosis, and a wedge incisional biopsy to include the normal skin is the preferred method. Biopsy specimens should be sent for routine histology as well as direct immunofluorescence to exclude vasculitis and tissue culture to exclude bacterial, mycobacterial (typical and atypical) and deep fungal infections.

Compression should be used to prevent bleeding from the biopsy site.

If untreated, chronic ulcers can lead to fibrosis and contractures of the underlying tissues, and in some cases equinus deformity and restricted ankle mobility ensues. Fibrous ankylosis in plantar flexion severely restricts ankle mobility. Physiotherapy, compression, lengthening of the Achilles tendon and early intervention are essential to prevent further morbidity, which may even lead to amputation (Figure 2.11).

Uncommon manifestations of venous insufficiency

Acroangiodermatitis (pseudo-Kaposi's sarcoma)

Another manifestation of severe venous hypertension is the development of violaceous papules, plaques and nodules on the legs and dorsal aspects of the feet. Patients occasionally experience pruritus and pain. Bleeding may also occur. These lesions may undergo painful ulceration, and can be clinically indistinguishable from classic Kaposi's sarcoma (KS). This clinical appearance has led this entity to be called pseudo-KS or acroangiodermatitis (AAD).

AAD is a hyperplasia of pre-existing vasculature. In contrast, KS is a vascular tumour associated with human herpesvirus type 8. Vascular proliferation in KS is independent of the existing vessels.

Bilateral lesions are usually associated with CVI, whereas unilateral lesions suggest an underlying arteriovenous (AV) communication. AAD has been described in association with severe venous hypertension secondary to vascular malformations such as Klippel–Trenaunay syndrome. It can also occur distal to the site of surgically constructed AV fistulae for hemodialysis, congenital AV malformations or traumatic AV fistulae. In these patients, blood is shunted away from the peripheral vascular bed into the low-resistance pathways offered by the AV communication. In severe cases, it can result in distal tissue ischemia and necrosis. If fistula flow is great enough, there will be associated venous hypertension (Figures 2.13 and 2.14). In all cases, venous hypertension plays an essential role in the pathogenesis of AAD.

Lesions of AAD may resolve after closure, thrombosis or surgical elimination of the shunt or treatment of the underlying venous hypertension.

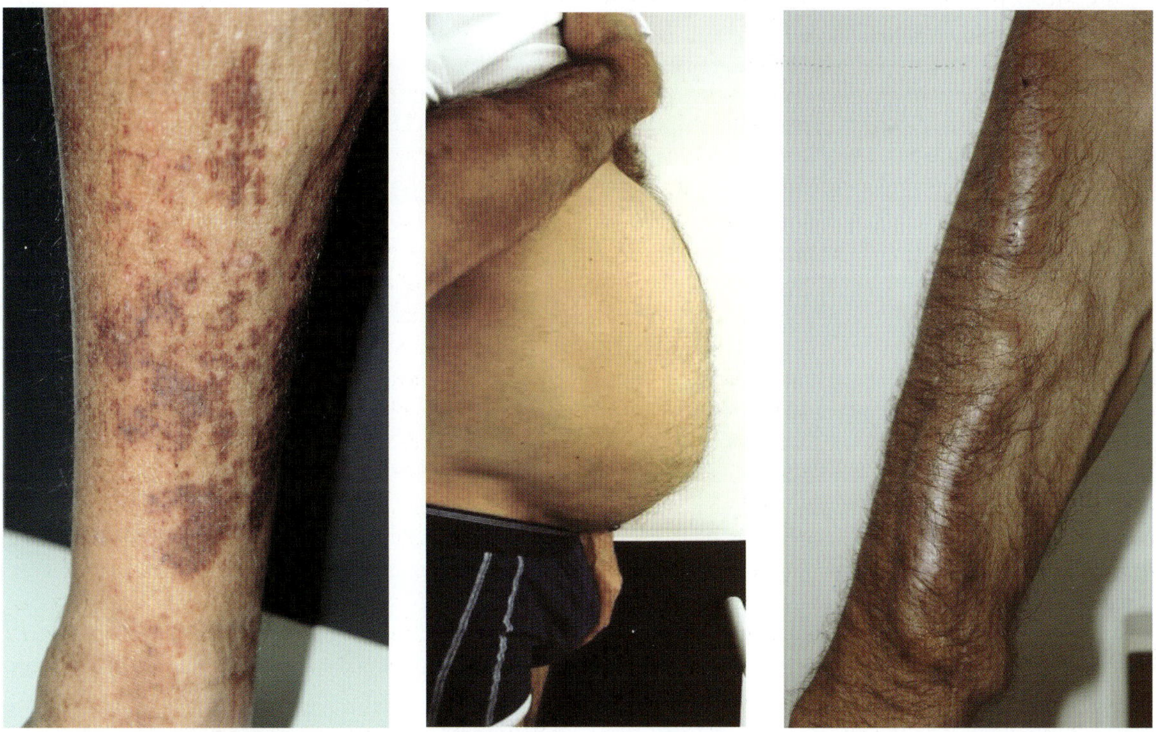

(a) (b) (c)

Figure 2.13 (a) Acroangiodermatitis in a patient with (b) polycystic kidney disease undergoing renal dialysis via (c) an arteriovenous fistula

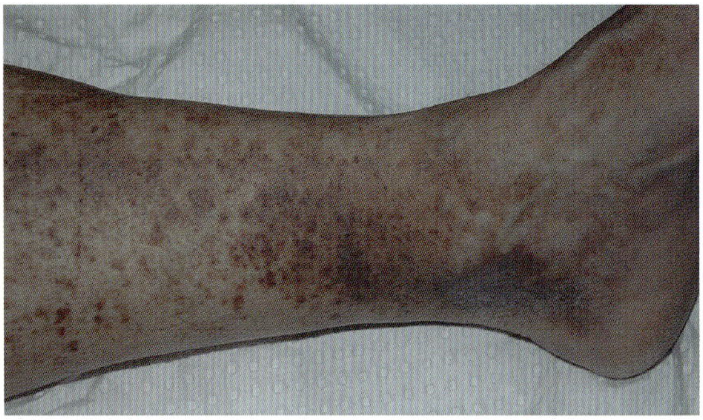

(a)

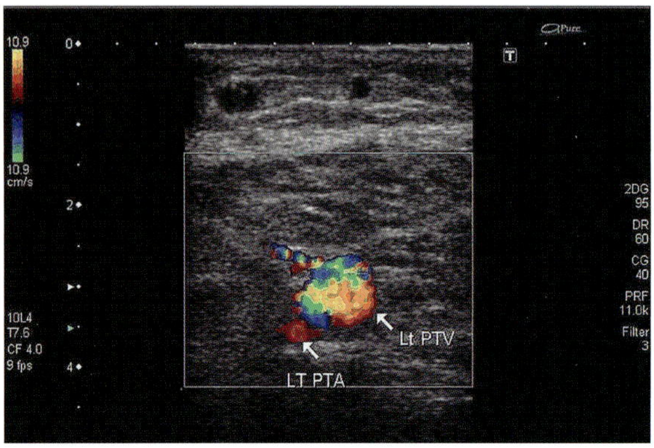

(b)

Figure 2.14 (a) Acroangiodermatitis of the medial ankle area secondary to (b) an arteriovenous communication between the posterior tibial artery and vein. Aliasing is evident secondary to turbulent flow

Pigmented purpuric dermatoses (PPDs)

These are a group of conditions characterized by extravasation of red cells and marked hemosiderin pigmentation of the skin. This condition has been wrongly called "capillaritis," although there is no evidence of a true vasculitis. The hallmark of a PPD is its characteristic orange–brown, speckled, cayenne pepper-like discoloration.

The etiology of PPDs is currently under investigation. Venous hypertension, contact dermatitis and certain drugs have been implicated in the pathogenesis of PPDs. Other associations are hypersensitivity to food dyes and preservatives such as tartrazine, and clothing dye dermatitis (especially khaki dyes). Drugs such as aspirin, glipizide, thiamine and interferon-α have been implicated.[6–9]

The author's recent research has discovered acquired coagulation abnormalities and in particular platelet function abnormalities in this group of patients. Coagulation factor deficiency such as von Willebrand's disease may be present.

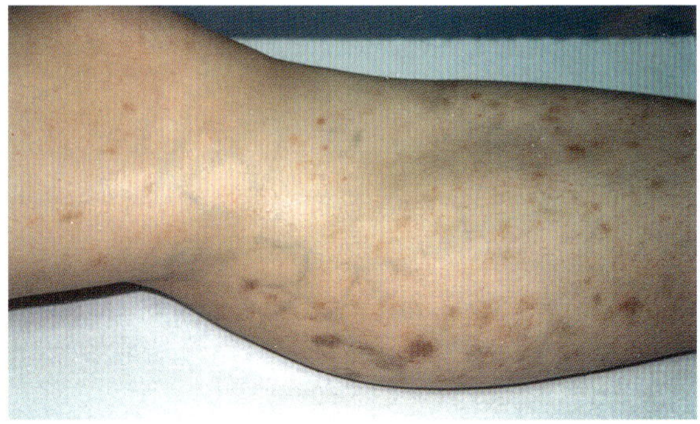

Figure 2.15 Itchy purpura

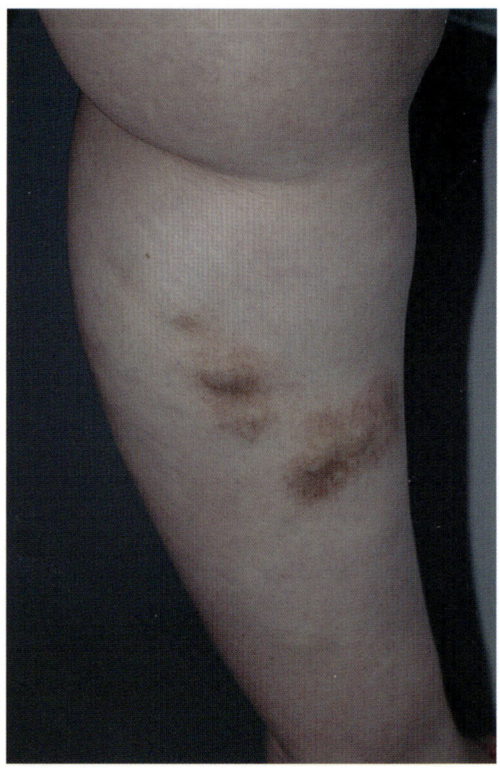

Figure 2.16 Lichen aureus overlying incompetent tributaries of the great saphenous vein

Differential diagnoses include angiocentric mycosis fungoides, venous hyperpigmentation, leukocytoclastic vasculitis, petechial hemorrhage and scurvy.

A number of clinical patterns are recognized. These include Schamberg's disease (progressive pigmented purpuric dermatosis), itchy purpura of Lowenthal (Figure 2.15), lichen aureus (Figures 2.16–2.18), purpura annularis telangiectodes (Majocchi's disease) (Figure 2.19), pigmented purpuric lichenoid dermatosis of Gougerot and Blum (Figure 2.20), unilateral PPD (Figures 2.21 and 2.22) and eczematoid-like purpura of Doucas and Kapetanakis. A granulomatous variant of PPD has also been reported.

These subclasses all share common histopathologic features of red cell extravasation, hemosiderin deposition and a lymphocytic infiltrate. A lichenoid inflammatory infiltrate is present in the Gougerot–Blum subtype. Spongiosis is present in the Doucas–Kapetankis subtype. Older lesions tend to be less inflamed, and extravasated red cells may no longer be present. In the author's experience, these subclassifications are somewhat arbitrary and one patient may exhibit multiple subtypes. Lichen aureus is commonly found in association with venous disease and sometimes directly over an underlying incompetent perforator. Treatment of the underlying localized venous hypertension can help in the resolution of lichen aureus. Ultrasound-guided foam sclerotherapy may be quite useful in resolution of these lesions (Figures 2.17 and 2.18). Topical steroids are possibly helpful only if pruritus is present, but otherwise have a limited role. The underlying condition – and in particular coagulation abnormalities – should be investigated and excluded. Patch testing, other forms of allergy testing and food elimination diets may be appropriate. Aspirin, vitamin E, fish oil and other forms of drugs and supplements interfering with platelet function should be stopped, if appropriate.

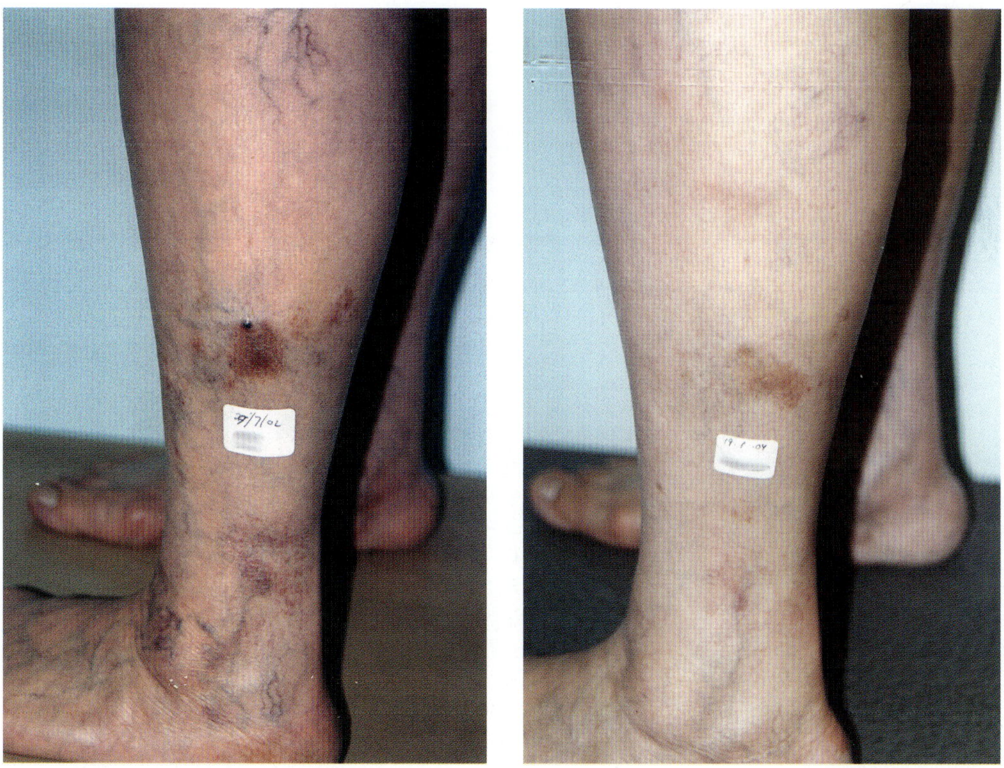

(a) (b)

Figure 2.17 (a) Lichen aureus of the left lateral calf. (b) Note resolution of the lesion after ultrasound-guided sclerotherapy of an incompetent lateral calf perforator

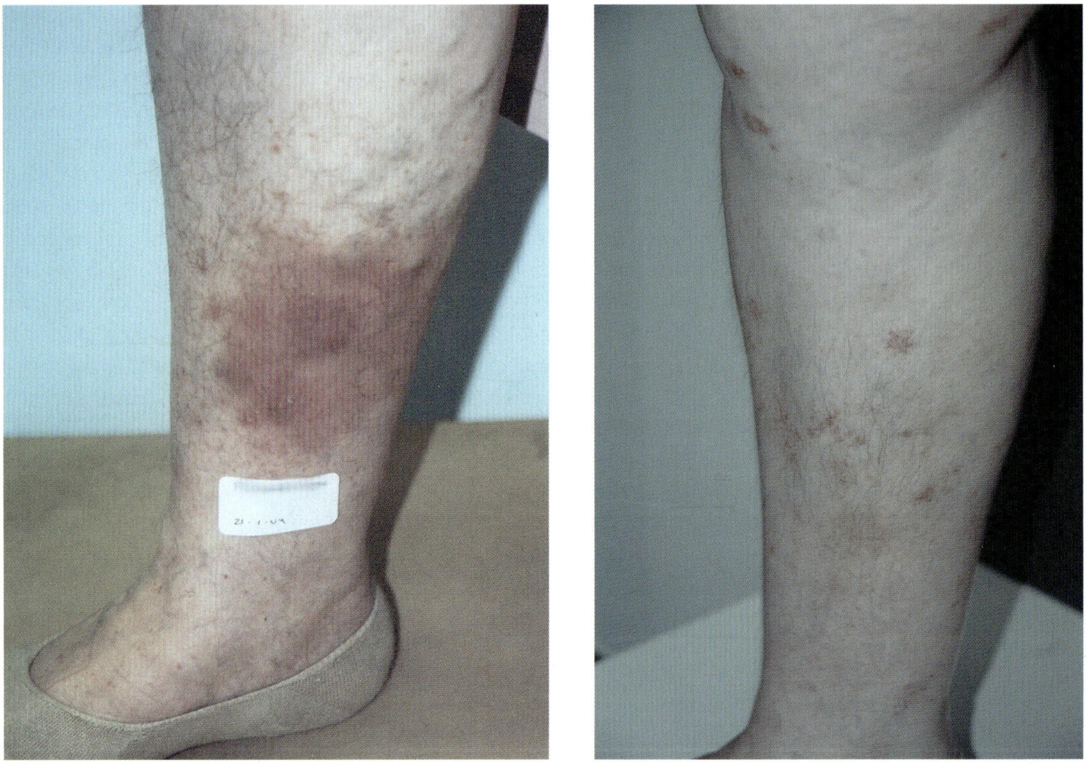

(a) (b)

Figure 2.18 Effect of sclerotherapy on pigmented purpuric dermatosis (PPD). (a) Large lesion of PPD over the right medial ankle area. (b) Resolution of the larger patch after ultrasound-guided sclerotherapy of the incompetent underlying vessels

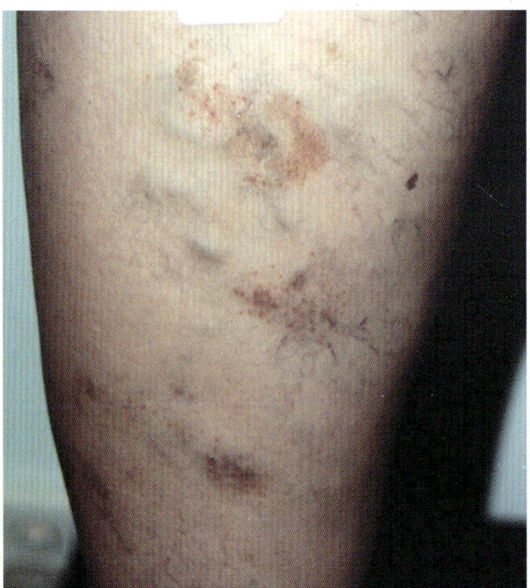

Figure 2.19 Majocchi's disease

Nodular vasculitis (erythema induratum)

This is a reactive inflammatory lobular panniculitis associated with vasculitis. It is an uncommon condition mainly affecting obese middle-aged females with CVI.[10] The most common cause is tuberculosis (TB), but cases without evidence of TB have been described in association with hepatitis C infection[11] and the use of propylthiouracil.[12] The main cutaneous manifestations of nodular vasculitis include recurrent bilateral painful erythematous subcutaneous nodules and plaques that commonly affect the lower limbs. Associated CVI and livedo reticularis may also be observed.

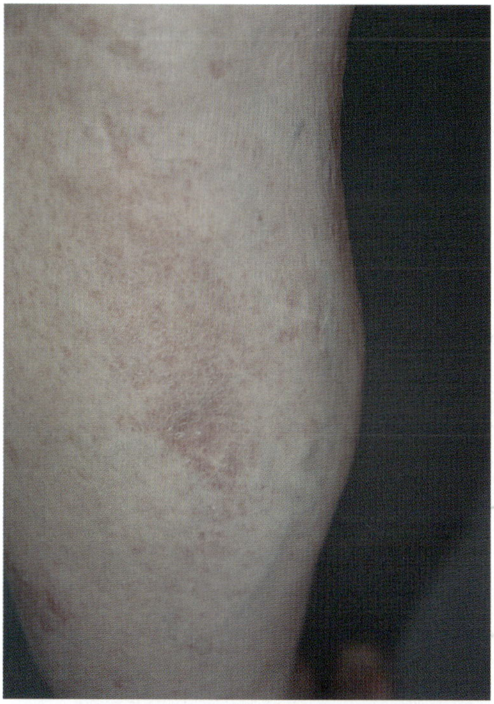

Figure 2.20 Pigmented purpuric lichenoid dermatosis of Gougerot and Blum

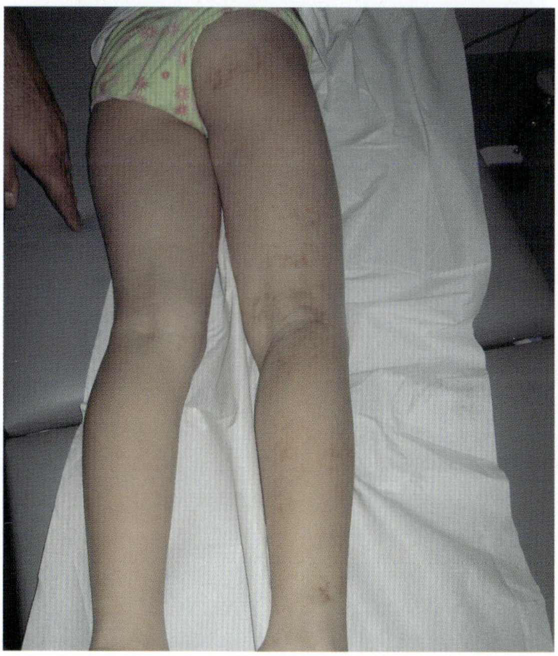

Figure 2.21 Unilateral pigmented purpuric dermatosis in a child

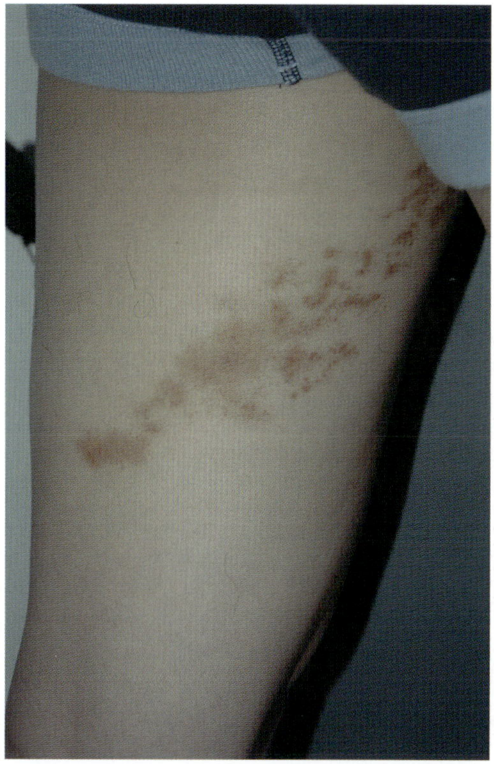

Figure 2.22 Unilateral pigmented purpuric dermatosis overlying the posteromedial vein of the thigh

Common skin manifestations of venous thromboembolism

Superficial thrombophlebitis (STP)

STP presents as a painful, warm, erythematous cord along the affected vein (Figure 2.3). It is very often confused with acute cellulitis. STP is inflammation and thrombosis of a superficial vein. It is usually an inflammatory response to thrombus, but it can also be due to primary vasculitis of medium- to large-size vessels. A granulomatous variety has been described,[13] and it occurs fairly commonly as a chemical or thermal phlebitis following sclerotherapy or endovenous laser therapy. A migratory variety is seen in malignancies and in thromboangiitis obliterans. Mondor's disease is STP of the chest veins extending from the breast to the axillary region.

STP is an inflammatory condition and in the majority of cases not an infection, and hence treatment with intravenous antibiotics is not required. Sclerotherapy-induced phlebitis settles with nonsteroidal anti-inflammatory drugs and compression. Concomitant intake of oral contraceptive pills and hormone replacement therapy during sclerotherapy can lead to an increased incidence of STP and even deep vein thrombosis, and hence should be avoided.

Superficial venous thrombosis (SVT) can occur without the associated inflammation. This also occurs commonly after sclerotherapy where vessels are not fully sclerosed. The coagulum is released transcutaneously by direct puncture or it can be evacuated via a syringe and under ultrasound guidance.

Deep vein thrombosis (DVT) and venous gangrene

DVT can be silent with no detectable signs or symptoms.[14] The occlusion of the vein by a thrombus can impede the venous return, which leads to an increase in the venous pressure and edema in the distal limb. DVT can therefore present with little or quite extensive edema. An inflammatory response to the thrombus will cause pain and tenderness. Prominent collateral veins appear early to bypass the obstruction and relieve the edema. Patients with antiphospholipid syndrome will exhibit livedo reticularis or, in advanced cases, reticulate purpura.

Calf vein thrombosis can be silent or can present with edema and pain of the affected limb. The calf muscle will be tender and there will be increased resistance to dorsiflexion of the foot (Homan's sign). A ruptured Baker's cyst is an important differential diagnosis of an acute DVT and presents with bruising and discoloration of the skin in the groove behind the medial malleolus.

Extensive DVT may present with a tensely swollen, warm, tender limb. With iliofemoral thrombosis, the limb is swollen from the foot to the inguinal region, with collateral veins forming from the thigh to the abdominal area. The limb may be pale (phlegmasia alba dolens), indicating arterial spasm. This is due to the so-called "veno-arteriolar axonal reflex," which controls the arterial inflow when there is an obstruction to the venous outflow.[15] A "white leg" is usually indicative of an iliofemoral thrombosis and the associated arterial spasm. Cold digits indicate a compromise in the arterial inflow. In comparison, a "blue leg" indicates venous congestion secondary to occlusion of the common iliac vein and outflow obstruction. This cyanotic appearance is termed "phlegmasia cerulea dolens" and may lead to venous gangrene if the outflow obstruction is not relieved. Venous gangrene presents with cyanosis of the toes. As against arterial gangrene, which normally affects one or two toes, venous gangrene affects all toes and may extend to the dorsal and ventral surfaces of the forefeet.

Post-thrombotic syndrome (PTS)

This is characterized by edema, pigmentary changes and ulceration of the lower limbs. The clinical manifestations may be indistinguishable from CVI. Pitting edema is often present but varicose veins are not always apparent. There is hypo- and hyperpigmentation present in an area of lipodermatosclerosis. Although cellulitis may occur, venous eczema is the cause of erythema and inflammation of the effected area. Venous ulcers occur in the medial ankle or lower calf area. The calf circumference of the affected leg may be larger than the nonaffected one (Figure 2.23).

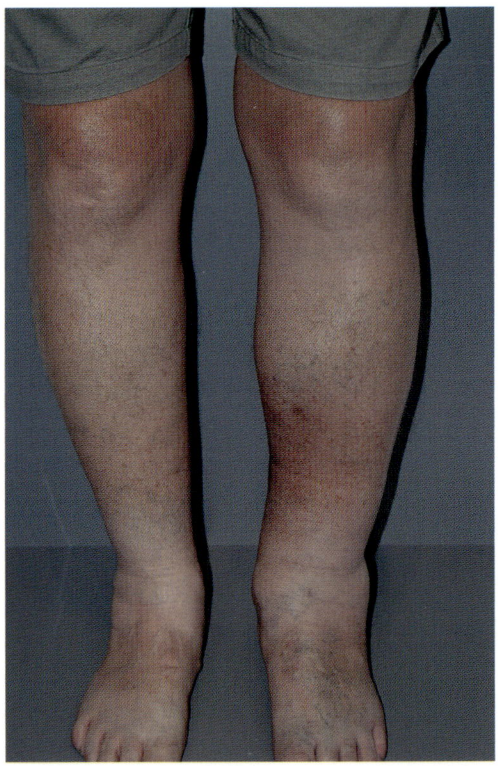

Figure 2.23 Post-thrombotic syndrome presenting with increased girth, pigmentation and lipodermatosclerosis of the left leg

Livedoid vasculopathy (LV)

Atrophie blanche is not always a manifestation of CVI, but can be a sign of LV. This condition is characterized by ulceration associated with a segmental pattern of reticulate purpura and atrophie blanche affecting the lower limbs (Figure 2.24). It has been falsely referred to as livedoid vasculitis, although true vasculitis is not a feature of this condition. It has also been described as "livedo reticularis with summer ulcerations." LV is a thrombo-occlusive process. Histologically, it shows fibrin deposition within both the wall and the lumen of affected vessels, but there is no evidence of a true vasculitis.[16] LV has been associated with Raynaud's phenomenon and acrocyanosis. Patients with LV may have a history of recurrent leg ulcerations. Such patients may have thrombophilic abnormalities such as factor V Leiden mutation, protein C or S deficiency, hyperhomocysteinemia, abnormalities in fibrinolysis, and increased platelet activation.[17]

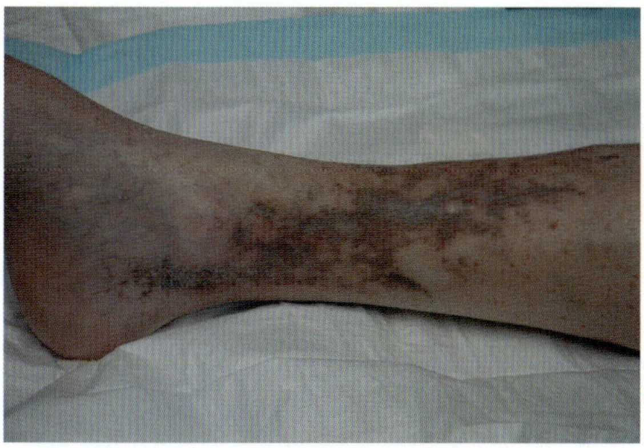

Figure 2.24 Livedoid vasculopathy secondary to protein S deficiency

Treatment of the underlying venous hypertension with foam sclerotherapy can help this condition by correcting the hemodynamics of the affected areas. The pigmentation improves and the ulcerations heal.

Vascular ectasias

Dilatation of blood vessels can be due to increased intravascular pressure or loss of elasticity of the vessel wall. Vascular ectasia could also be due to actinic damage and its associated elastolysis of the vessel wall.

Venous lake

Venous lakes are probably the most common vascular ectasias. These are dark blue phlebectasias that tend to occur on sun-exposed skin, especially on the lower lips or ears of elderly patients. Chronic actinic damage injures the vascular adventitia and the dermal elastic tissue, causing dilatation of normal venous structures. Treatment with sclerotherapy for larger lesions, and vascular laser therapy for smaller lesions, is usually successful. Malignant melanoma is a differential diagnosis and should be excluded. Venous lakes, as against melanomas, are compressible and empty with compression. Venous lakes are benign lesions but can bleed or thrombose causing pain.

Angiokeratomas

Angiokeratomas are a group of vascular ectasias that involve the papillary dermis. Angiokeratomas are not true angiomas but rather ectasias of pre-existing vessels. Overall, altered hemodynamics typically caused by trauma appear to produce telangiectatic vessels of the papillary dermis with an overlying reactive hyperkeratosis to the epidermis. These lesions may also produce papillomatosis, and acanthosis of the epidermis.[18]

Angiokeratoma of Fordyce

These are typically asymptomatic blue-red papules, 2–5 mm in size, with a scaly surface located on the scrotum, shaft of penis, labia majora, inner thigh, or lower abdomen. They are dilated ectatic capillaries in the superficial dermis with overlying epidermal hyperplasia. These lesions bleed easily. Angiokeratomas occur in the presence of varicoceles or vulvar varices, and venous hypertension has been implicated in their pathogenesis.[19] If treatment is needed, then locally destructive methods have been used. Light hyfrecation may not provide adequate hemostasis, and bleeding may occur. Vascular laser photocoagulation usually provides adequate treatment.

Angiokeratoma circumscriptum (AC)

This is a rare type of angiokeratoma with a unilateral distribution of discrete papules and nodules localized to a small area of the leg or trunk. Due to its unilateral and truncal distribution, AC has also been called angiokeratoma corporis neviform. AC has been classified as a combined capillary–lymphatic malformation. It has been reported to coexist with angiokeratoma of Fordyce and caviar spots (angiokeratomas of the tongue). It can be found in association with other vascular malformations and hemangiomas. Recurrent bleeding can occur. Women are affected more commonly than men, in a ratio of approximately 3 to 1.[18] These lesions respond well to vascular laser treatment.

Angiokeratoma corporis diffusum (Fabry's disease)

This is an X-linked disorder caused by a deficiency of the lysosomal enzyme α-galactosidase. This inborn error of metabolism results in deposition of neutral glycosphingolipids in the lysosomes of most cells. The most affected cell is the vascular endothelium.[20] Angiokeratomas form and tend to concentrate between the umbilicus and the knees, but usually spare the head. Lymphedema and varicose veins are present. Renal failure, cardiac failure and cerebrovascular disease are the major causes of death. Heterozygous females may develop angiokeratomas, but experience a milder clinical course.

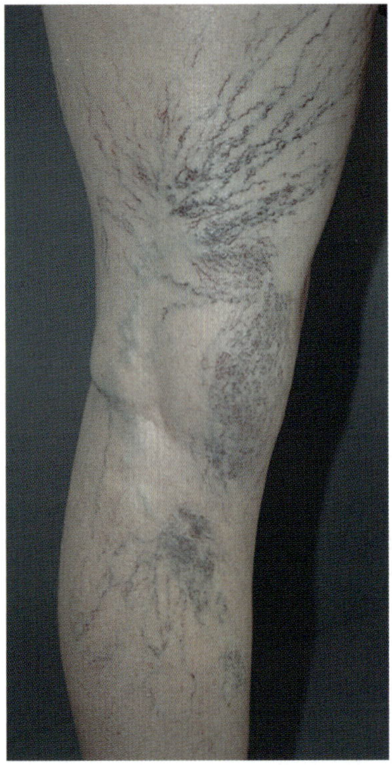

Figure 2.25 Leg telangiectasias and venulectasias associated with an incompetent lateral superficial venous system

Telangiectasia

Telangiectasias are dilated venules, arterioles or arteriovenous malformations visible on the skin or mucosal surfaces. Telangiectasias that develop in the absence of any preceding or coexisting cutaneous or systemic disease are considered to be primary or essential. Telangiectasias resulting from or in association with a known disease are classified as secondary.

Leg telangiectasias (spider veins)

These vessels are dilated, postcapillary venules demonstrating backflow from incompetent reticular (feeder) veins or directly from incompetent tributary or even truncal veins (Figure 2.25). Doppler examination may demonstrate reflux in even very small telangiectatic vessels. Telangiectasias associated with venous incompetence are usually dark red. Larger bluish vessels are termed venulectasias. Not all leg telangiectasias are secondary to venous incompetence, and essential telangiectasias are commonly found near the feet and ankles. The gold standard for treatment of leg telangiectasias is sclerotherapy. The underlying venous incompetence must be treated first, before any attempt is made at sclerosing the telangiectasias. Vascular laser therapy is unlikely to be effective if underlying venous incompetence is present.

Facial telangiectasias

Telangiectasias seen on the face and trunk are usually due to actinic damage. Facial telangiectasias may also be associated with flushing and vascular instability as seen in rosacea or carcinoid syndrome (Figure 2.26). The best treatment for these lesions is vascular laser therapy. Peri-alar telangiectasias usually demonstrate higher flow volumes and are more difficult to treat. They are more common in people suffering with sinus disease and chronic nasal congestion. This can lead to recurrent peri-alar telangiectasias despite adequate treatment. Vascular laser therapy may need to be repeated a number of times for larger peri-alar telangiectasias, or sclerotherapy can be attempted.

Postradiation telangiectasias

Radiotherapy can lead to appearance of telangiectasias up to 20 years after the procedure. The radiation damage

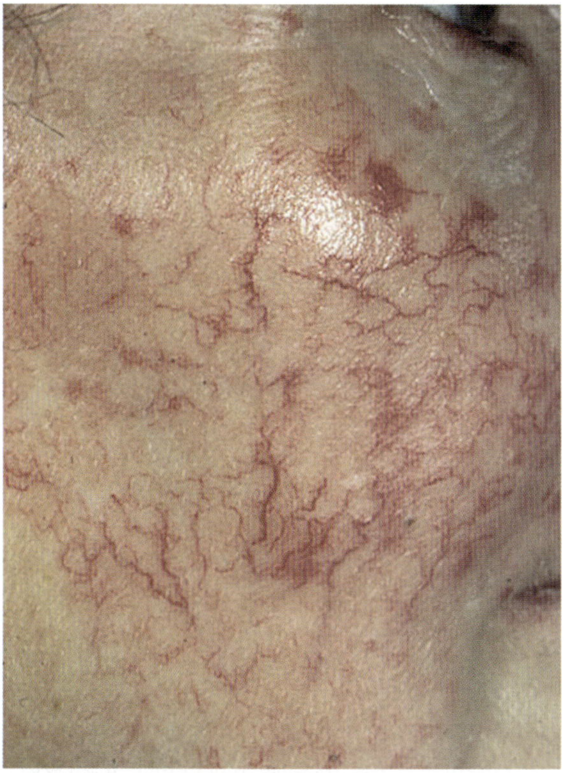

Figure 2.26 Fascial telangiectasias

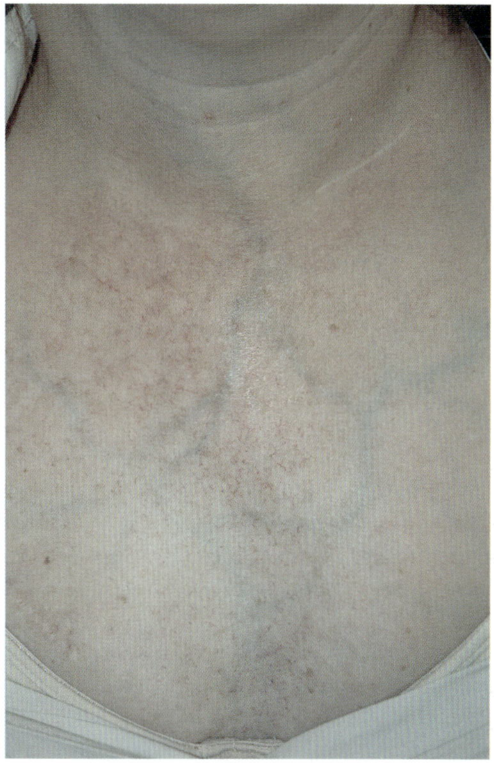

Figure 2.27 Postradiation telangiectasias

causes destruction of elastic fibers within vessels and leads to formation of the telangiectasias (Figure 2.27). Malignancy and in particular squamous cell carcinoma can develop in these areas.

Mat telangiectasias

These are patches of telangiectasias seen in patients with scleroderma and CREST syndrome (Figure 2.28). They present as flat and nonpulsatile vessels appearing as discrete mats. This should not be confused with telangiectatic matting, which is a complication of surgery and sclerotherapy.

Telangiectatic matting. This is a form of neovascularization that occurs as a complication of sclerotherapy or surgery (Figure 2.29). Patches of very small telangiectasias appear over the sites of recanalized vessels. Inflammation, especially inflammatory cytokines with angiogenic properties, seem to play an important role in the pathogenesis of this condition. Other associations include concurrent use of female hormonal supplements such as oral contraceptives and hormone replacement therapy. There are usually underlying small incompetence veins in direct association with these vessels.

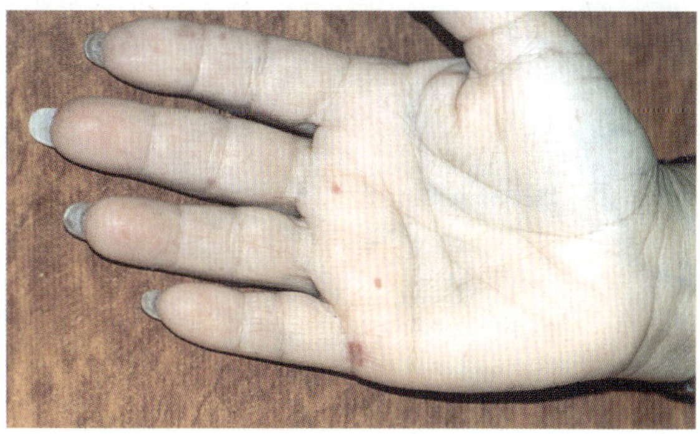

Figure 2.28 Mat telangiecasia of scleroderma

Poikiloderma of Civatte

Poikiloderma of Civatte refers to a reticulate erythematous pigmentation seen on the sides of the neck. Areas

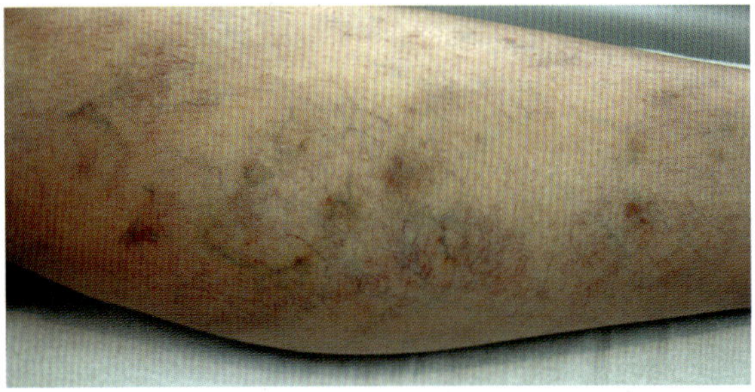

Figure 2.29 Telangiectatic matting, postsclerotherapy

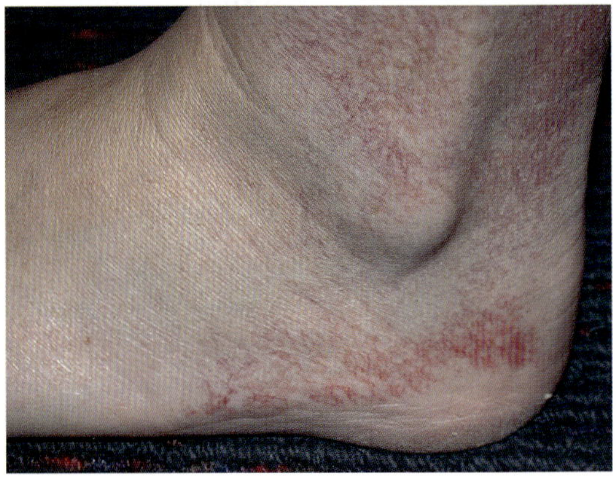

Figure 2.30 Essential telangiectasias starting near the feet

shaded by the chin are spared. The term poikiloderma refers to the combination of atrophy, telangiectasias and pigmentary changes (both hypo- and hyperpigmentation). It occurs most commonly in fair-skinned, middle-aged or elderly females. Chronic exposure to ultraviolet light appears to be a primary etiologic factor, but photosensitizing chemicals in perfumes or cosmetics have also been implicated.[21]

Periungual telangiectasias

These are telangiectasias along the proximal nailfold. They are visualized dermoscopically as dilated capillary loops. These are pathognomonic signs of connective tissue diseases, such as lupus, scleroderma, and dermatomyositis.[22]

Essential telangiectasia

This refers to the syndrome of widespread primary telangiectasias of unknown etiology. There is no reported association with venous disease or actinic damage. Familial cases have been reported with an autosomal dominant pattern of inheritance.[22,23]

The generalized form involves most of the trunk. However, it usually starts as light pink linear or punctuate telangiectasias on the feet, ankles and distal legs, and may gradually spread (Figure 2.30). When the lesions become confluent, the skin appears diffusely erythematous. Involvement of the oral mucosa and conjunctiva has been reported. This condition is usually asymptomatic, but tingling, burning or numbness is occasionally reported.[24] The age of onset is usually in the fourth or fifth decade, but it may be observed in younger adults.

Hereditary benign telangiectasia

This condition resembles essential telangiectasia. It commences in early childhood, and is usually present on sun-exposed skin.

Hereditary hemorrhagic telangiectasia (HHT–Osler–Rendu–Weber disease)

These lesions are arteriovenous malformations (AVMs) of the microvasculature. They usually appear as punctuate, dark red elevated lesions on mucous membranes, face and distal limbs. Lesions may involve the tongue, retina, lung and brain. HHT lesions appear during the third or fourth decade of life. Recurrent epistaxis is usually the presenting symptom. Coagulation factor deficiency such as von Willebrand's disease may be present. Pulmonary and cerebral AVMs may be present. Family screening is indicated.

Unilateral nevoid telangiectasia (UNT)

In this condition, patches of telangiectasia present in a unilateral linear distribution. The segmental pattern suggests a somatic mosaicism. Pregnancy, chronic liver disease and other states of estrogen excess are implicated in its pathogenesis. The third and fourth cervical dermatomes are the most common sites, but the thoracic dermatomes and scattered distant sites may also be involved.[3]

Telangiectasia macularis eruptiva perstans (TMEP)

This is the telangiectatic form of cutaneous mastocytosis. The lesions appear as brown telangiectatic macules that may be generalized in distribution. When a lesion of other forms of mastocytosis such as urticaria pigmentosa or mastocytoma is stroked, it typically urticates, becoming pruritic, edematous and erythematous. This change is referred to as Darier's sign, which can be explained on the basis of mast cell degranulation induced by physical stimulation. Darier's sign is usually negative in TMEP. This is because the lesions of TMEP are paucicellular, and, therefore, mast cells may not be present in sufficient numbers for significant degranulation to occur.[25] Diagnosis of TMEP is made on skin biopsy. Anesthetic should be injected without epinephrine adjacent to, and not directly into, the lesion to avoid mast cell degranulation, which would make histologic examination difficult.

Ataxia telangiectasia (AT)

This condition presents with ocular and cutaneous telangiectasias. Ocular telangiectasias extend from the lateral canthus in the equatorial region of the conjunctivae towards the corneal limb. Telangiectasias may also involve the ears, eyelids, and cubital and popliteal fossae. This is an autosomal recessive immunodeficiency characterized by progressive neurologic impairment and cerebellar ataxia. Patients are susceptible to sinopulmonary infections, impaired organ maturation and a predisposition to malignancy. Oculocutaneous telangiectasias have a later onset than ataxia. The telangiectases are predominantly of venous origin and are not AVMs.[26]

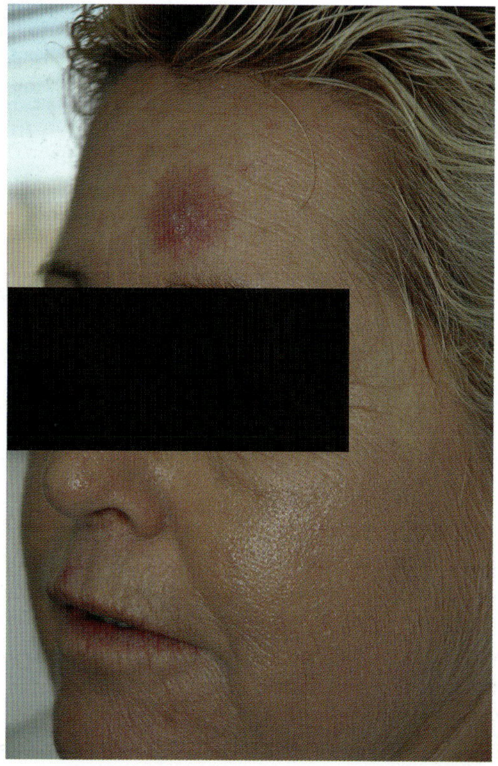

Figure 2.31 Spider nevus of the forehead in a patient with advanced liver disease

Spider nevi

Spider nevi are ectatic ascending arterioles. They usually exhibit radiating thin-walled vessels in association with a central ascending arteriole (Figure 2.31). These lesions are also referred to as spider angiomas and nevus araneus. Spider nevi are not vascular proliferations, but occur as a result of the dilation of pre-existing vessels. They demonstrate arterial flow on Doppler examination. Compression of the central arteriole produces blanching. When released, the lesion quickly refills from the central arteriole. Spider nevi are acquired lesions present in 10–15% of healthy adults and young children. Lesions are found most commonly on the face, neck, chest and arms. In young children, spider nevi are common on the backs of the hands and fingers. Hormonal changes play a role in pathogenesis of these lesions. Many women develop lesions during pregnancy or whilst taking oral contraceptives. The lesions usually resolve spontaneously from 6 to 9 months after delivery or after discontinuing oral contraceptives. Numerous lesions are seen in patients with significant hepatic disease such as advanced hepatitis C. Foam sclerotherapy is useful in treating the larger lesions. However, given the arterial nature of the nevus, necrosis can readily occur and the treatment should be performed with care.

References

1. Ryan T. The Management of Leg Ulcers. Oxford: Oxford Medical Publishers, 1983.
2. Paul C, Graeber M, Stuetz A. Ascomycins: promising agents for the treatment of inflammatory skin diseases. Expert Opin Investig Drugs 2000; 9: 69–77.
3. Weedon D, Strutton G. Skin Pathology. New York: Churchill Livingstone, 1997.
4. Mekkes JR, Loots MAM, Van Der Wal AC, Bos JD. Causes, investigations and treatment of leg ulceration. Br J Dermatol 2003; 148: 388–401.
5. Simon DA, Dix FP, McCollum CN. Management of venous ulcers. BMJ 2004; 328: 1358–62.

6. Dowd PM, Champion RH. Purpura, 6th edn. Oxford: Blackwell Science, 1998.
7. Newton RC, Raimer SS. Pigmented purpuric eruptions. Dermatol Clin 1985; 3: 165–9.
8. Taketuchi Y, Chinen T, Ichikawa Y, et al. Two cases of unilateral pigmented purpuric dermatosis. J Dermatol 2001; 28: 493–8.
9. Tristani-Firouzi P, Meadows KP, Vanderhooft S. Pigmented purpuric eruptions of childhood: a series of cases and review of literature. Pediatr Dermatol 2001; 18: 299–304.
10. Peters MS, Su WPD. Panniculitis. Dermatol Clin 1992; 10: 37–57.
11. Cardinali C, Gerlini G, Caproni M, et al. Hepatitis C virus: a common triggering factor for both nodular vasculitis and Sjögren's syndrome? Br J Dermatol 2000; 142: 187–9.
12. Wolf D, Ben-Yehuda A, Okon E, Naparstek Y. Nodular vasculitis associated with propylthiouracil therapy. Cutis 1992; 49: 253–5.
13. Saito R, Matsuoka Y. Granulomatous pigmented purpuric dermatosis. J Dermatol 1996; 23: 551–5.
14. Goldman MP, Bergan JJ, Guex J. Sclerotherapy: Treatment of Varicose and Telangiectatic Leg Veins, 4th edn: St Louis: Mosby/Elsevier, 2007.
15. Tran D, Parsi K. Veno-arteriolar reflex vasospasm of small saphenous artery complicating sclerotherapy of the small saphenous vein. Aust NZ J Phlebol 2007; 10: 29–32.
16. Freedberg IM, Eisen AZ, Wolff K, et al., eds. Fitzpatrick's Dermatology in General Medicine, 6th edn. New York: McGraw-Hill, 2003.
17. Leonard A, Pomeranz MK, Franks AG, Jr. A case of livedoid vasculopathy in a 22-year-old man. J Drugs Dermatol 2004; 3: 678–9.
18. Champion RH, Burton JL, Burns DA, Breathnach SM. Rook/Wilkinson/Ebling Textbook of Dermatology, 6th edn. Oxford: Blackwell Science, 1998: 592–5.
19. Leis-Dosil VM, Alijo-Serrano F, Aviles-Izquierdo JA, et al. Angiokeratoma of the glans penis: clinical, histopathological and dermoscopic correlation. Dermatol Online J 2007; 13(2): 19.
20. Spitz JL, ed. Genodermatoses: A Clinical Guide to Genetic Skin Disorders, 2nd edn. New York: Lippincott Williams & Wilkins, 2005.
21. Champion RH, Burton JL, Burns DA, Breathnach SM, eds. Rook/Wilkinson/Ebling Textbook of Dermatology. Oxford: Blackwell Science, 1998: 1790.
22. Weiss G, Confino Y, Shemer A, Trau H. Cutaneous manifestations in the cardiofaciocutaneous syndrome, a variant of the classical Noonan syndrome. Report of a case and review of the literature. J Eur Acad Dermatol Venereol 2004; 18: 324–7.
23. Long D, Marchman G. Generalised essential telangiectasia. Australas J Dermatol 2004; 45: 67–9.
24. Ali MM, Teimory M, Sarhan M. Generalized essential telangiectasia with conjunctival involvement. Clin Exp Dermatol 2006; 31: 781–2.
25. Sarkany RPE, Monk BE, Handfield-Jones SE. Telangiectasia macularis eruptiva perstans: a case report and review of the literature. Clin Exp Dermatol 1998; 23: 38–9.
26. Paller AS. Ataxia telangiectasia. In: Freedberg IM, Eisen AZ, Wolff K, Austen KF, Goldsmith LA, Katz S, eds. Fitzpatrick's Dermatology in General Medicine, 6th edn. New York: McGraw-Hill, 2003: 1833–6.

3 Sclerotherapy of varicose veins*– Guidelines of the German Society of Phlebology

Eberhard Rabe, Felizitas Pannier, Horst Gerlach, Franz Xaver Breu, Stefan Guggenbichler and Jan-Christoph GR Wollmann

Preamble

Guidelines are systematically elaborated recommendations designed to support the clinician and practitioner in his or her decisions about the appropriate care of patients in specific clinical situations.

Guidelines apply to "standard situations" and take into account the currently available scientific knowledge relating to the subject under consideration. Guidelines require ongoing review and possibly modification, in order to adapt to the most recent scientific findings and to practicability in daily routine. Guidelines are not intended to restrict the doctor's freedom to choose the most appropriate method of treatment. Compliance with the recommendations does not always guarantee diagnostic and therapeutic success. Guidelines make no claim to completeness. The decision about the appropriateness of any action to be taken is still the responsibility of the doctor in the light of the individual situation.

Definition

Sclerotherapy involves the injection of a sclerosant for the targeted elimination of intracutaneous, subcutaneous, and/or transfascial varicose veins (perforating veins), as well as the sclerosation of subfascial varicose vessels in the case of venous malformation. The various sclerosants induce marked damage of the vascular endothelium and possibly of the entire vascular wall. After successful sclerotherapy and in the long term, the veins are transformed into a fibrous cord, a process known as sclerosis.[1–3] The purpose of sclerotherapy is not merely to achieve thrombosis of the vessel, which per se may be amenable to recanalization, but definitive transformation into a fibrous cord. This cannot recanalize, and the functional result is equivalent to the surgical removal of a varicose vein.

Indications

The objectives of sclerotherapy are:

- treatment of varicosis and prevention of possible complications
- reduction or elimination of existing symptoms
- improvement of pathologically altered hemodynamics
- achievement of a good result that satisfies aesthetic and functional criteria.[4]

* These guidelines were drafted on behalf of the German Society of Phlebology (Deutsche Gesellschaft für Phlebologie, DGP), adopted by the Committee and Scientific Advisory Board of the DGP on 15.06.2001, and amended on 26.09.2007; the document replaces the previous version of 12.05.2003 (Rabe E, Pannier-Fischer F, Gerlach H, et al. Guidelines for sclerotherapy of varicose veins [ICD 10: I83.0, I83.1, I83.2, and I83.9]. Dermatol Surg 2004; 30: 687–93).

This document considers the present state of knowledge as reflected in the literature but not the licensing requirements for the various medicinal products, which are different in each case.

In principle all types of varicose veins are amenable to sclerotherapy, in particular:

- truncal veins – long saphenous vein (LSV) and short saphenous vein (SSV)
- collateral veins
- varicose veins associated with perforator incompetence
- reticular varicose veins
- spider veins
- residual and recurrent varicose veins after interventions to eliminate varicosities
- genital and perigenital varicose veins
- peri-ulcerous veins[5–7]
- venous malformations.[8]

Sclerotherapy is considered to be the method of choice for the treatment of small-caliber varicose veins (reticular varicose veins, spider veins).[4]

For the obliteration of varicose collateral veins and incompetent perforating veins, sclerotherapy competes with percutaneous phlebextraction and with ligation of perforating veins or endoscopic dissection of perforating veins.[9,10]

In the treatment of varicose truncal veins involving elimination of the proximal leakage point and of the incompetent venous portion, surgery is considered to be the method of choice. Nevertheless, treatment of truncal veins by sclerotherapy is also possible.[11–13] This applies in particular to foam sclerotherapy, as has been demonstrated by studies conducted in recent years.[14–18]

Contraindications

Absolute contraindications are[3,4,13]:

- known allergy to the sclerosant
- severe systemic disease
- acute deep vein thrombosis
- local infection in the area of sclerotherapy or severe generalized infection
- lasting immobility and confinement to bed
- advanced peripheral arterial occlusive disease (stage III or IV)
- hyperthyroidism (in the case of sclerosants containing iodine)
- pregnancy (unless a compelling medical reason exists).

For foam sclerotherapy:

- known symptomatic patent foramen ovale.

Relative contraindications are:[3,4,19]

- Leg edema, uncompensated
- Late complications of diabetes (e.g., polyneuropathy)
- Arterial occlusive disease, stage II
- poor general health
- bronchial asthma
- marked allergic diathesis
- known thrombophilia or hypercoagulable state with or without a history of deep vein thrombosis.[20–22]

For foam sclerotherapy:

- known asymptomatic patent foramen ovale[20]
- high risk of thromboembolic events
- visual disturbances or neurologic disturbances following previous foam sclerotherapy.

In addition, it is urgently recommended that due account be taken of the current prescribing information for the sclerosants used.[23]

Complications and risks

If performed properly, sclerotherapy is an efficient treatment method with a low incidence of complications. In the context of therapy, a number of adverse events may be encountered in principle.[2, 24–27] In particular, these are:

- allergic reaction[28–30]
- skin necroses[31–34]
- excessive sclerosing reaction (and thrombophlebitis)
- pigmentation[34–36]
- matting[34]
- nerve damage[37–39]
- scintillating scotomas[24]
- migraine-like symptoms[40–42]
- orthostatic collapse
- thromboembolism.[25,43,44]

In addition, it is urgently recommended that due account be taken of the current prescribing information for the sclerosants used.[23]

Allergic skin reactions occur occasionally in the form of allergic dermatitis, contact urticaria or erythema. Anaphylactic shock as well as inadvertent intra-arterial injection are extremely rare complications constituting an emergency situation.[28–30,45]

Transient migraine-like symptoms occur more commonly after foam sclerotherapy than after liquid sclerotherapy.[24] In this context, it has been speculated whether a patent foramen ovale (PFO), which is present in 15–25% of the population,[45a] might be a factor here, allowing foam bubbles to pass into the arterial circulation.[46–48]

Thromboembolic events (deep vein thrombosis, pulmonary embolism or stroke) occur in rare exceptional circumstances after sclerotherapy. A higher risk is present when larger volumes of sclerosant are used, particularly in the form of foam,[44,49,50] and in patients with a previous history of thromboembolism or known thrombophilia.[22] In patients with these risk factors, the indication for sclerotherapy must be established absolutely and additional precautionary measures must be observed.[20]

Skin necroses have been described both after paravascular injection of sclerosants in higher concentrations and, rarely, after properly performed intravascular injection with sclerosants in various concentrations, for example, 0.5% polidocanol in the treatment of spider veins.[33,34] In the latter case, a mechanism involving passage of the sclerosant into the arterial circulation via arteriovenous anastomoses has been suggested.[31] In individual cases, this has been described as embolia cutis medicamentosa.[51–53]

Extensive necroses occur after inadvertent intra-arterial injection.[33–35]

Instances of hyperpigmentation have been reported with frequencies ranging from 0.3% to 10%.[36,51] In general, this phenomenon regresses slowly. The incidence of pigmentation is likely to be higher after foam sclerotherapy.[24]

Matting – fine telangiectasias in the area of a sclerosed vein – is an unpredictable individual reaction of the patient, and can also occur after surgical removal of a varicose vein.[34]

Nerve damage has been reported experimentally after paravascular injection.[37–39] Local paresthesia after sclerotherapy is very rare.

Other transitory phenomena after sclerotherapy include intravascular clots, phlebitis, hematomas, disturbed sense of taste, feeling of tightness in the chest, pain at the injection site, swelling, induration, mild cardiovascular reactions and nausea. Additionally, complications may arise due to the compressive bandage, such as blister formation (e.g., blisters in the vicinity of an adhesive plaster).[2,3] Intravascular clots can be squeezed out after a stab incision to reduce the development of hyperpigmentation.

Sclerotherapy is an intervention that requires patients to be appropriately informed.

Diagnosis before sclerotherapy

Successful sclerotherapy requires thorough planning. Sclerotherapy is generally performed in the order of leakage points, proceeding from the larger to the smaller varicose veins. Therefore, a proper diagnostic evaluation should be performed prior to treatment.[2–4,19]

Diagnostic evaluation includes history-taking, clinical examination and Doppler ultrasound investigation.

Additionally, functional examinations (e.g., photoplethysmography, phlebodynamometry and venous occlusion plethysmography) and imaging modalities (e.g., duplex ultrasound and phlebography) may be considered.

Functional examinations make it possible to assess the improvement in venous function, which is to be expected for the elimination of varicosis.

Diagnostic imaging is especially suitable for identifying incompetent junctions with the deep venous system and for locating pathologic reflux, as well as for clarifying post-thrombotic changes[54,55] and for selecting the most appropriate treatment option.

Implementation of sclerotherapy of varicose veins

Aethoxysklerol®, which contains the active ingredient polidocanol in concentrations of 0.25/0.5/1/2/3 and 4%, is licensed in Germany for sclerotherapy of varicose veins:

The maximum daily dose of polidocanol is 2 mg/kg body weight.[23]

Sclerotherapy with sclerosant solutions (liquid sclerotherapy)

Table 3.1 provides guide values for concentration and volume per injection for liquid sclerotherapy.[23]

A smoothly functioning disposable or glass syringe is required for sclerotherapy, as well as a cannula with a small diameter. Cotton-wool rolls or pads and adhesive paper tapes are used for local compression. The different techniques vary considerably.[56] The following principles apply to liquid sclerotherapy proper:

Table 3.1 Guide values for concentration and volume per injection for sclerosants containing polidocanol used for liquid sclerotherapy

Sclerosants containing polidocanol		
Indications	**Volume per injection (mL)**	**Concentration (%)**
Spider veins	0.1–0.2	0.25–0.5
Central veins of spider veins	0.1–0.2	0.25–1
Reticular varicose veins	0.1–0.3	1
Small varicose veins	0.1–0.3	1
Medium-size varicose veins	0.5–2.0	2–3
Large varicose veins	1.0–2.0	3–4

- Puncture of the veins to be sclerosed can be performed with the patient standing or lying down.
- The injection is usually given with the patient lying down. After the vein has been punctured with the free cannula or with the syringe attached, the intravascular position is checked.
- Intravascular injection of the sclerosant is performed slowly, possibly in fractions, and checking that the cannula is positioned inside the vein. Severe pain during injection may be indicative of paravascular injection.
- Immediately after injection of the sclerosant and removal of the cannula, local compression is performed along the course of the sclerosed vein.[1,3,57,58]
- After sclerotherapy, compression is applied to the treated extremity. When sclerosing spider veins, compression is achieved in a variety of ways. Compression can be performed using both a compression stocking and a compression bandage.[1,59,60]
- Local compression can be removed the same evening or on the next day. Depending on the diameter and location of the varicose veins, compression is performed for hours up to several days and weeks after completion of sclerotherapy.[4,19,61]
- After a sclerotherapy session using the traditional technique, the patient should walk around for a while (physical thromboprophylaxis). A careful watch must be kept for any signs of allergic reactions.
- Intensive sports activity, hot baths, saunas and strong ultraviolet irradiation (solarium use) should be avoided in the initial days after sclerotherapy.

Sclerotherapy guided by duplex ultrasound

Duplex ultrasound-guided sclerotherapy has proved to be a useful addition to the range of methods for sclerosing saphenous junctions, truncal veins close to saphenous junctions, and perforating veins.[33,62–67] In this procedure, the vein to be sclerosed is visualized by duplex ultrasound with the patient lying down, and puncture is performed under visual control. The needle is visible on the ultrasound image, and intravascular injection can be monitored. Some authors recommend intermittent compression using the ultrasound transducer after injection.[66,67] This enables contraction of the injected venous segment and the length of the sclerosed portion to be assessed. The purpose of this method is to achieve a more controlled procedure with fewer complications and increased efficacy.

Sclerotherapy with foam sclerosants (foam sclerotherapy)

The literature has long contained reports of sclerotherapy with foamed sclerosants.[54,55,68–71] In recent years, as the technology has improved, foam sclerotherapy has become established particularly for the treatment of larger varicose veins.[65,72,73] Detergent-type sclerosants such as polidocanol can be transformed into fine-bubbled foam by special techniques.

In the Monfreux technique[73] negative pressure is generated by drawing back the plunger of a glass syringe, the tip of which is tightly closed. The resulting influx of air produces a large-bubbled, fairly fluid foam.[71] In the Tessari technique, the foam generated is fine-bubbled and fluid at low concentrations and rather viscous at high concentrations; it is produced by the turbulent mixture of liquid and air in two syringes connected via a three-way stopcock. The mixing ratio for sclerosant plus air is 1 + 3 to 1 + 4.[74] The DSS (double-syringe system) technique involves the turbulent mixing of polidocanol with an air in a sclerosant plus air ratio of 1 + 4 in two syringes linked via a connector. The resulting product is a fine-bubbled, viscous foam.[71,75]

The standardized transformation of a licensed liquid sclerosant into a foam sclerosantare permissible provided that the patient has been adequately informed about the procedure and about the benefits and risks of the method, and consents to its use. Even if foam is used off-label, the published evidence and data document the use as a standard procedure.

The Second European Consensus Conference on Foam Sclerotherapy took place at Tegernsee in April 2006. On the basis of the experts' own experience and the available literature, the following recommendations on foam sclerotherapy were given,[20] partially modified for this guideline.

Puncture and injection:

- When treating the long saphenous vein (LSV) by direct puncture, it is recommended that venous puncture be performed in the proximal thigh area. If long catheters are used, it is recommended to make the access to the LSV below the knee.
- When treating the short saphenous vein (SSV) by direct puncture, it is recommended that venous puncture be performed in the proximal or middle part of the lower leg.
- When treating the perforating veins, it is recommended that the injection should not be made directly into the affected vein.

Foam generation, concentrations and volumes:

- The Tessari and Tessari/DSS methods are recommended for the generation of foam sclerosant for all indications.
- Air is accepted and/or proposed as the gas component for the generation of foam sclerosant for all indications. A mixture of carbon dioxide and oxygen may also be used.
- The preferred ratio of liquid sclerosant and gas for the generation of a foam sclerosant is 1 + 4 (1 part liquid plus 4 parts gas). Ratios between 1 + 1 and 1 + 5 are used for reticular varicose veins and spider veins, but the 1 + 4 ratio is also used by the majority.
- The preferred foam volumes per venous puncture are shown in Table 3.2 and the preferred concentrations are outlined in Table 3.3.

Table 3.2 Foam volume per venous puncture

	Mean foam volume per puncture (mL)	Maximum foam volume per puncture (mL)
LSV	2–4	Up to 6
SSV	2–4	Up to 4
Collateral veins	Up to 4	Up to 6
Recurrent varicose veins	Up to 4	Up to 8
Perforating veins	Up to 2	Up to 4
Reticular varicose veins	<0.5	<1
Spider veins	<0.5 mL	<0.5
Venous malformations	2–6	<8

- The recommended maximum foam volume per leg and session (given in a single injection or in several injections) is 10 mL.
- When treating large-caliber varicose veins, the foam sclerosant should be as viscous as possible.

Safety measures:

- Safety during foam sclerotherapy of the GSV and SSV can be improved by:
  - Avoiding immediate compression of the injected areas
  - Using ultrasound to monitor foam distribution
  - Injecting a highly viscous foam
  - Ensuring that there is no patient or leg movement for 2–5 minutes, and no Valsalva maneuver or other muscle movement
  - Encouraging active muscle movement, e.g., repeated foot flexion, if a larger volume of foam is detected in the deep venous system.
- The known presence of a PFO is a relative contraindication for foam sclerotherapy. In such patients, the following is recommended:
  - The patient should remain lying down for longer (8–30 minutes)

Table 3.3 Polidocanol concentrations / indication[a]

	Liquid	0.25%	0.5%	1%	2%	3%	4%
LSV	–	–	–	+	++	++	–
SSV	–	–	–	+	++	+	–
Collateral veins	–	–	–	++	–	–	–
Recurrent varicose veins	–	–	(+)	++	++	+	–
Perforating veins	–	–	(+)	++	+	(+)	–
Reticular varicose veins	(+)	(+)	++	+	–	–	–
Spider veins[b]	++	(+)	(+)	–	–	–	–
Venous malformations	–	–	+	++	+	–	–

[a]The stated concentrations refer to the liquid polidocanol solution from which foam is generated.
[b]Foam sclerotherapy is not the treatment of choice for vessels less than 1 mm in diameter. For sclerotherapy of spider veins, the recommendation is first to use polidocanol in liquid form. Where foam is used, small volumes of a 0.25% foam (possibly even of a 0.5% foam) should be given.

  - Use only small volumes of foam (2 mL) or liquid sclerotherapy
  - Avoid Valsalva maneuvers
  - Elevate the patient's leg by about 30 cm.
- Prior to foam sclerotherapy, it is not necessary to perform specific investigations for PFO.
- A high risk of thromboembolism in the patient's history and known thrombophilia (especially in combination with a high risk of thromboembolism) is a relative contraindication for foam sclerotherapy. In such patients, the following is recommended:
  - Institute adequate low-molecular-weight heparin prophylaxis (in line with relevant guidelines/recommendations)
  - Implement physical prophylaxis
  - Use low sclerosant concentrations for foam generation
  - Use small volumes of foam
  - Decide on a case-by-case basis (perform a benefit–risk assessment based on the particular indication).
- Prior to foam sclerotherapy it is not necessary to perform specific investigations for thrombophilia.

Patient information:

- Before foam sclerotherapy, patients should be informed about risks and possible adverse effects in the same way as before liquid sclerotherapy. In addition, they should be told that:
  - There is a slightly higher risk of hyperpigmentation and inflammation
  - There is a risk of developing (transient) neurologic symptoms
  - There is a risk of developing (transient) visual disturbances
  - There is a risk of triggering migraine.
- As before liquid sclerotherapy, patients should be informed about the expected treatment outcome. In addition, they should be told that:
  - Short-term outcomes are highly satisfactory
  - Further therapy is possible and may be necessary in some cases, especially in treatment for large varicose veins
  - Foam sclerotherapy is more effective than liquid sclerotherapy.

Duplex ultrasound in foam sclerotherapy :

- The therapeutic effect of foam sclerotherapy on the patient and on the patient's leg should be assessed clinically and on the basis of symptoms.
- The therapeutic effect of foam sclerotherapy on the LSV, SSV, collateral branches, recurrent varicose veins, perforating veins and venous malformations can be assessed additionally using duplex ultrasound.
- In terms of puncturing non-visible varicose veins, duplex-guided ultrasound is an important instrument that enables puncture errors to be avoided. Ultrasound visualization (preferably duplex-guided) is necessary for the direct puncture of nonvisible LSV, SSV and perforating veins, as well as of nonvisible varicose veins in the groin and popliteal fossa.
- Duplex guidance is recommended for other nonvisible varicose veins.

Criteria for assessing the therapeutic effect of foam sclerotherapy are presented in Table 3.4.

Table 3.4 Assessment of treatment outcome following foam sclerotherapy

Grade/name	Duplex criteria		Clinical criteria	Symptoms
2 Successful	No Reflux	(a) • Complete disappearance of treated vein *or* • "Fibrous cord" (noncompressible, echogenic cord at the site of the treated vein) (b) • Complete occlusion (noncompressibility) of the treated venous segment (c) • Patency of the treated venous segment with reduced diameter and *antegrade* blood flow	Normalized (i.e., no visible varicose veins)	Absent or improved
1 Partially successful	Reflux <1 s	• Partial noncompressibility and • Partial occlusion of the treated venous segment and • Diameter reduction	Normalized or improved (i.e., varicose veins less visible)	Absent or improved
0 Unsuccessful	Reflux >1 s or unchanged	• Complete (or incomplete) patency and/or • Diameter unchanged	No change or worse (i.e., larger varicose veins or deterioration in terms of CEAP)	No change or worse

Further information:

- Duplex ultrasound is performed with the patient standing.
- The length of the occluded venous segment must be compared with the length of the incompetent venous segment that was to be occluded by sclerotherapy injection (the segment to be treated must therefore be defined before injection). This is important for establishing after sclerotherapy whether the "whole vein" is occluded.
- Reflux is assessed during a Valsalva maneuver or during distal compression/decompression.
- In terms of symptom assessment, where appropriate, more sophisticated and standardized symptom scores such as the VCSS may be used; otherwise visual analog scales (VAS) from 1 to 10 are helpful and simple to use.
- In terms of clinical assessment, where appropriate, more sophisticated and standardized classifications such as in the CEAP classification may be used.
- When treatment is being given simultaneously for medical and aesthetic reasons, two separate assessment forms should be used.
- This classification is applicable for all endovenous treatment methods (laser, radiofrequency and sclerotherapy techniques) and should facilitate comparability.
- Details of the number of treatments (injections and sessions) and the type of treatment should be recorded.

Efficacy

A wealth of published clinical series (e.g., Refs 7, 35, 49 and 76–87) and controlled clinical trials[14–18,88–90] provide undoubted evidence to corroborate the elimination of intracutaneous and subcutaneous varicose veins by sclerotherapy. The success rates of sclerotherapy vary depending on technique, sclerosant (liquid or foam) and venous calibre.

Sclerotherapy is considered to be the standard treatment for intracutaneous varicose veins (spider veins and reticular veins), allowing improvement of up to 90% to be achieved.[31,91–95]

Compression treatment with medical compression

stockings may improve the result of sclerotherapy for spider veins.[36,96–98] The incidence of pigmentation decreases significantly.[36,60]

Local eccentric compression significantly increases local pressure in the sclerosed area and improves the efficacy of sclerotherapy.[57]

In older studies with liquid sclerotherapy, surgery was significantly more effective in the treatment of truncal varices.[9] In the sclerosis of truncal varicose veins, foam sclerotherapy is significantly more effective than liquid sclerotherapy.[15,17,18]

References

1. Drake LA, Dinehart SM, Goltz RW, et al. Guidelines of care for sclerotherapy treatment of varicose and teleangiectatic leg veins. J Am Acad Dermatol 1996; 34: 523–8.
2. Goldmann PM, Bergan JJ, Guex JJ. Sclerotherapy: Treatment of Varicose Veins and Telangiectatic Leg Veins, 4th edn. St Louis, Mo: Mosby/Elsevier, 2007.
3. Rabe E, ed. Grundlagen der Phlebologie. 3. Erweiterte und vollständig überarbeitete Neuauflage, Viavital, Köln 2003.
4. Baccaglini U, Spreafico G, Castoro C, Sorrentino P: Consensus Conference on Sclerotherapy or Varicose Veins of the Lower Limbs. Phlebology 1997; 12: 2–16.
5. De Waard MM, Der Kinderen DJ. Duplex ultrasonography-guided foam sclerotherapy of incompetent perforator veins in a patient with bilateral venous leg ulcers. Dermatol Surg 2005; 31: 580–3.
6. Hertzman PA, Owens R. Rapid healing of chronic venous ulcers following ultrasound-guided foam sclerotherapy. Phlebology 2007; 22: 34–9.
7. Stücker M, Reich S, Hermes N, et al. Safety and efficiency of perilesional sclerotherapy in leg ulcer patients with postthrombotic syndrome and/or oral anticoagulation with Phenprocoumon. JDDG 2006; 4: 734–8.
8. Yamaki T, Nozaki M, Sasaki K. Color duplex-guided sclerotherapy for the treatment of venous malformations. Dermatol Surg 2000; 26: 323–8.
9. Einarsson E, Eklöf B, Neglén P. Sclerotherapy or surgery as treatment for varicose veins: a prospective randomized study. Phlebology 1993; 8: 22–6.
10. Malouf GM. Ambulatory venous surgery versus sclerotherapy. Hawaii Med J 2000; 59: 248–9.
11. Bullens-Goessens YIJM, Mentink LF, Nelemans PJ, Van Geest AJ, Veraart JCJM. Ultrasound-guided sclerotherapy of the insufficient short saphenous vein. Phlebologie Germany 2004; 33: 89–91.
12. Schultz-Ehrenburg U, Tourbier H. Doppler-kontrollierte Verödungsbehandlung der Vena saphena magna. Phlebol Proktol 1984; 13: 117–22.
13. Vin F. Principes de la sclérothéraphie des troncs saphènes internes. Phlebologie 1997; 50: 229–34.
14. Ceulen RPM, Bullens-Goessens YIJM, Pi-Van De Venne SJA. Outcomes and side effects of duplex-guided sclerotherapy in the treatment of great saphenous veins with 1% versus 3% polidocanol foam: results of a randomized controlled trial with 1-year follow-up. Dermatol Surg 2007; 33: 276–81.
15. Hamel-Desnos C, Desnos P, Wollmann JC, et al. Evaluation of the efficacy of polidocanol in the form of foam compared with liquid form in sclerotherapy of the long saphenous vein: initial results. Dermatol Surg 2003; 29: 1170–5.
16. Hamel-Desnos C, Ouvry P, Benigni JP, et al. Comparison of 1% and 3% polidocanol foam in ultrasound guided sclerotherapy of the great saphenous vein: a randomised, double-blind trial with 2 year-follow-up. "The 3/1 Study." Eur J Vasc Endovasc Surg 2007; 34: 723–9.
17. Rabe E, Otto J, Schliephake D, Pannier F. Efficacy and safety of great saphenous vein sclerotherapy using standardised polidocanol foam (ESAF): a randomised controlled multicentre clinical trial. Eur J Endovasc Vasc Surg 2008; 35: 238–45.
18. Yamaki T, Nozaki M, Iwasaka S. Comparative study of duplex-guided foam sclerotherapy and duplex-guided liquid sclerotherapy for the treatment of superficial venous insufficiency. Dermatol Surg 2004; 30: 718–22.
19. Villavicencio J., Pfeifer J, Lohr J, et al. Sclerotherapy for varicose veins: practice guidelines and sclerotherapy procedures. In: Glovicki P, Yao J, eds. Handbook of Venous Disorders. London: Chapman & Hall Medical, 1996: 337–54.
20. Breu FX, Guggenbichler, Wollmann JC. Duplex ultrasound and efficacy criteria in foam sclerotherapy from the 2nd European Consensus Meeting on Foam Sclerotherapy 2006, Tegernsee, Germany. Vasa 2008; 37(Suppl 1): 3–29.
21. Feied CF. Deep vein thrombosis: the risks of sclerotherapy in hypercoagulable states. Sem Dermatol 1993; 12: 135–49.
22. Hamel-Desnos C, Ouvry P, Desnos P, et al. Sclérothérapie et thrombophilie: démarche pour un consensus dans la sclérothérapie chez les thrombophiles, Phlebologie 2003; 56: 165–9.
23. Kreussler: Fachinformationen Aethoxysklerol 0,25%/0,5%/1%/2% Stand 06/2005, Aethoxysklerol 3%/4%, Stand 09/2005, Chemische Fabrik Kreussler & Co. GmbH.
24. Guex JJ, Allaert F-A, Gillet J-L. Immediate and

midterm complications of sclerotherapy: report of a prospective multicenter registry of 12 173 sclerotherapy sessions. Dermatol Surg 2005; 31: 123–8.
25. Hohlbaum G. Über iatrogene Schäden bei der Varizensklerosierung. In: Staubesand J, E Schöpf E, eds. Neuere Aspekte der Sklerosierungstherapie. Berlin: Springer Verlag, 1990: 70–81.
26. Munavalli GS, Weiss RA. Complications of sclerotherapy. Semin Cutan Med Surg 2007; 26: 22–8.
27. Weiss RA, Weiss MA. Incidence of side effects in the treatment of telangiectasias by compression sclerotherapy: hypertonics saline vs. polidocanol. J Dermatol Surg Oncol 1990; 16: 800–4.
28. Feied CF, Jackson JJ, Bren TS, et al. allergic reactions to polidocanol for vein sclerosis. J Dermatol Surg Oncol 1994; 20: 466–8.
29. Feuerstein W: Schwere anaphylaktische Reaktion auf Hydroxypolyaethoxydodecan. Vasa 1973; 3: 292–4.
30. Pradalier A, Vincent D, Hentschel V, et al. Allergie aux sclérosants des varices. Rev Fr Allergol 1995; 35: 440–3.
31. Bergan JJ, Weiss RA, Goldman MP. Extensive tissue necrosis following high concentration sclerotherapy for varicose veins. Dermatol Surg 2000; 26: 535–42.
32. Duffy DM. Cutaneous necrosis following sclerotherapy. J Aesthet Dermatol Cosmet Surg 1999; 1: 157–68.
33. Fisher DA. Regarding extensive tissue necrosis following high concentration sclerotherapy for varicose veins. Dermatol Surg 2000; 26: 1081.
34. Goldman MP, Sadick NS, Weiss RA. Cutaneous necrosis, telangiectatic matting and hyperpigmentation following sclerotherapy. Dermatol Surg 1995; 21: 19–29.
35. Conrad P, Malouf GM, Stacey MC. The Australian polidocanol (Aethoxysklerol) study. Results at 2 years. Dermatol Surg 1995; 21: 334–6.
36. Weiss RA, Sadick NS, Goldman MP, Weiss MA. Postsclerotherapy compression: controlled comparative study of duration of compression and its effects on clinical outcome. Dermatol Surg 1999; 25: 105–8.
37. Seydewitz V, Staubesand J. Das ultrastrukturelle Substrat der Wirkung paravasal und intraarteriell applizierter Sklerosierungsmittel: Ein experimenteller Beitrag zum Problem iatrogener Schäden nach Sklerotherapie. In: Staubesand J, Schöpf E, eds. Neuere Aspekte der Sklerosierungstherapie. Heidelberg: Springer-Verlag, 1990: 40–65.
38. Van der Plas JPL, Lambers JC, van Wersch JW, Koehler PJ. Reversible ischaemic neurological deficit after sclerotherapy of varicose veins. Lancet 1994; 343: 428.
39. Zipper SG. Nervus peronäus-Schaden nach Varizensklerosierung mit Aethoxysklerol. Versicherungsmedizin 2000; 4: 185–7.
40. Benigni JP. Sclérothérapie à la mousse et migraines à aura. Phlebologie 2005; 58: 323–4.
41. Künzelberger B, Pieck C, Altmeyer P, Stücker M. Migraine ophthalmique with reversible scotomas after sclerotherapy with liquid 1% polidocanol. Dermatol Surg 2006; 32: 1410–13.
42. Ratanahirana H, Benigni JP, Bousser MG. Injection of polidocanol foam (PF) in varicose veins as a trigger for attacks of migraine with visual aura. Cephalalgia 2003; 23: 850–1.
43. Breu FX, Partsch B. Reversible neurologische Komplikationen bei der Schaum-Sklerotherapie. Phlebologie 2006; 3: 115–16.
44. Forlee MV, Grouden M, Moore DJ, et al. Stroke after varicose vein foam injection sclerotherapy. J Vasc Surg 2006; 43: 162–4.
45. Oesch A, Stirnemann P, Mahler F. The acute ischemic syndrome of the foot after sclerotherapy of varicose veins. Schweiz Med Wochenschr 1984; 114: 1155–8.
45a. Fisher DC, Fisher EA, Budd JH, et al. The incidence of patent foramen ovale in 1000 consecutive patients. Chest 1995; 107(6): 1504–9.
46. Morrison N, Cavezzi A, Bergan J, Partsch H. Regarding "Stroke after varicose vein foam injection sclerotherapy." J Vasc Surg 2006; 44: 224–5.
47. Passariello F. Sclerosing foam and patent foramen ovale. The final report. In: World Congress of the International Union of Phlebology; 2007, June 18–20; Kyoto, Japan. Int Angiol 2007; 26(2 Suppl 1): 87.
48. Wagdi P. Migräne und offenes Foramen Ovale: nur ein vorübergehender Hoffnungsschimmer? Kardiovasc Med 2006; 9: 32–6.
49. Breu FX, Marshall M. Sklerotherapie mit Polidocanol in einer angiologisch–phlebologischen Spezialpraxis. Prospektive und retrospektive Erhebung über Ergebnisse und Komplikationen. Phlebologie 2003; 32: 76–80.
50. Wright D, Gobin JP, Bradbury AW, et al. Varisolve European Phase III Investigators Group. Varisolve® polidocanol microfoam compared with surgery or sclerotherapy in the management of varicose veins in the presence of trunk vein incompetence: European randomized controlled trial. Phlebology 2006; 21: 180–90.
51. Georgiev M. Postsclerotherapy Hyperpigmentations. J Dermatol Surg Oncol 1993; 19: 649–52.
52. Kersting E, Hornschuh B, Bröcker E-B: Embolia cutis medicamentosa nach Varizensklerosierung mit Polidocanol. Phlebologie 1998; 27: 55–7.
53. Remy W, Vogt H-J, Borelli S. Embolia cutis medicamentosa – artige Hautnekrosen nach Sklerosierungsbehandlung. Phlebol Proktol 1978; 7: 67–72.
54. Frullini A, Cavezzi A. Sclerosing foam in the treatment

of varicose veins and telangiectasases: history and analysis of safety and complications. Dermatol Surg 2002; 28: 11–15.
55. Sigg K: Neuere Gesichtspunkte zur Technik der Varizenbehandlung. Ther Umschau 1949; 6: 127–34.
56. Baccaglini U, Stemmer R, Partsch U: Internationale Fragebogenaktion zur Praxis der Verödungsbehandlung. Phlebologie 1997; 26: 129–42.
57. Stanley PRW, Bickerton DR, Campbell WB. Injection sclerotherapy for varicose veins – a comparison of materials for applying local compression. Phlebology 1991; 16: 37–9.
58. Tazelaar DJ, HAM Neumann, KP de Roos. Long cotton wool rolls as compression enhancers in macrosclerotherapy for varicose veins. Dermatol Surg 1999; 25: 38–40.
59. Fegan WG. Continous compression technique of infecting varicose veins. Lancet 1963; ii: 109–12.
60. Goldman PM, Beaudoing D, Marley W, et al. Compression in the treatment of leg teleangiectasia: a preliminary report. J Dermatol Surg Oncol 1990; 16: 322–5.
61. Reddy P, Wickers J, Terry T, et al. What is the correct period of bandaging following sclerotherapy? Phlebology 1986; 217–20.
62. Frullini A, Cavezzi A. Ultrasound guided sclerotherapy in the treatment of long saphenaous vein insufficiency. Vasomed 1999; 11(Suppl 1): 8.
63. Grondin L, R Young, L Wouters. Sclérothérapie èchoguidée et sécurité: Comparison des techniques. Phlebologie 1997; 50: 241–5.
64. Guex JJ. Ultrasound guided sclerotherapy (USGS) for perforating veins. Hawaii Med J 2000; 59: 261–2.
65. Sadoun S, Benigni JP, Sica M. Étude prospective de l'efficacité de la mousse de sclérosant dans le traitement des varices tronculaires des membres inférieurs. Phlébologie 2002; 55(3): 259–62.
66. Schadeck M. Duplex-kontrollierte Sklerosierungsbehandlung der Vena saphena magna. Phlebologie 1996; 25: 78–82.
67. Schadeck M, Allaert FA: Résultats à long terme de la sclérothérapie des saphènes internes. Phlebologie 1997; 50: 257–62.
68. Cabrera J, Redondo P, Becerra A, et al. Ultrasound-guided injection of polidocanol microfoam in the management of venous leg ulcers. Arch Dermatol 2004; 140: 667–73.
69. Flückiger P. Nicht-operative retrograde Varicenverödung mit Varisylschaum. Schweiz Med Wochenschr. 1956; 48: 1368–137.
70. Mayer H, Brücke H. Zur Ätiologie und Behandlung der Varizen der unteren Extremität. Chir Praxis 1957; 4: 521–8.
71. Wollmann JC. Schaum – zwischen Vergangenheit und Zukunft. Vasomed 2002; 16: 34–8.
72. Henriet JP. One year experience with sclerotherapy of reticular veins and telangiectases using polidocanol foam in daily routine: feasibility results, complications. Phlébologie 1997; 50: 355–60.
73. Monfreux A. Traitement sclérosant des troncs saphèniens et leurs collatèrales de gros calibre par la méthode mus. Phlebologie 1997; 50: 351–3.
74. Tessari L, Cavezzi A, Frullini A. Preliminary experience with a new sclerosing foam in the treatment of varicose veins. Dermatol Surg 2001; 27: 58–60.
75. Breu FX, Guggenbichler S. European consensus meeting on foam sclerotherapy. April 4–6, 2003, Tegernsee, Germany. Dermatol Surg 2004; 30: 709–17.
76. Barrett J M, Allen B, Ockelford A, Goldman M P. Microfoam ultrasound-guided sclerotherapy of varicose veins in 100 legs. Dermatol Surg 2004; 20: 6–12.
77. Bergan JJ, Pascarella L, Mekenas L. Venous disorders: treatment with sclerosant foam. J Cardiovasc Surg 2006; 47: 9–18.
78. Brodersen JP. Catheter-assisted vein sclerotherapy: a new approach for sclerotherapy of the greater saphenous vein with a double-lumen balloon catheter. Dermatol Surg 2007; 33: 469–75.
79. Cavezzi A, Frullini A, Ricci S, Tessari L. Treatment of varicose veins by foam sclerotherapy: two clinical series. Phlebology 2002; 17: 13–18.
80. Coleridge Smith PD. Chronic venous disease treated by ultrasound guided foam sclerotherapy. Eur J Vasc Endovasc Surg 2006; 32: 577–83.
81. Darke SG, Baker SJ. Ultrasound-guided foam sclerotherapy for the treatment of varicose veins. Br J Surg 2006; 8: 969–74.
82. Hübner K. Ambulante Therapie der Stammvarikose mittels Krossektomie und Sklerotherapie – ein Beitrag aus der Praxis des niedergelassenen Phlebologen. Phlebologie 1991; 20: 104–8.
83. Kakkos SK, Bountouroglou DG, Azzam M, et al. Effectiveness and safety of ultrasound-guided foam sclerotherapy for recurrent varicose veins: immediate results. J Endovasc Ther 2006; 13: 357–64.
84. Milleret R, Garandeau C. Sclérose des grandes veines saphénes à la mousse délivrée par cathéter écho-guidé sur veine vide: alpha-technique – Bilan des 1000 treatments. Phlébologie 2006; 59: 53–8.
85. Myers KA, Jolley D, Clough A, et al. Outcome of ultrasound-guided sclerotherapy for varicose veins: medium-term results assessed by ultrasound surveillance. Eur J Vasc Endovasc Surg 2007; 33: 116–21.
86. Schadeck M. Sclérose de la petite veine saphéne éviter les mauvais résultats? Phlebologie 2004; 57: 165–9.

87. Wildenhues B. Endovenöse kathetergestützte Schaumsklerosierung. Phlebologie Germany 2005; 34: 165–70.
88. Alòs J, Carreño P, López JA, et al. Efficacy and safety of sclerotherapy using polidocanol foam: a controlled clinical trial. Eur J Vasc Endovasc Surg 2006; 31: 101–7.
89. Kahle B, Leng K. Efficacy of sclerotherapy in varicose veins – a prospective, blinded placebocontrolled study. Dermatol Surg 2004; 30: 723–8.
90. Rao J, Wildemore JK, Goldmann MP. Double-blind prospective comparative trial between foamed and liquid polidocanol and sodium tetradecyl sulfate in the treatment of varicose and telangiectatic leg veins. Dermatol Surg 2005; 31: 631–5.
91. Dover J, Sadick N, Goldman MP. The role of lasers and light sources in thetreatment of leg veins. Dermatol Surg 1999; 25: 328–36.
92. Kahle B. Effizienz der Sklerosierungstherapie von Besenreisern. Eine prospektive, randomisierte, doppelblinde, placebokontroliierte Studie. Vasomed 2006; 18: 148.
93. Kern P, Ramelet AA, Wütschert R, et al. Single-blind, randomized study comparing chromated glycerin, polidocanol solution and polidocanol foam for treatment of telangiectatic leg veins. Dermatol Surg 2004; 3: 367–72.
94. McCoy S, Evans A, Spurrier N. Sclerotherapy for leg telangiectasia – a blinded comparative trial of polidocanol and hypertonic saline. Dermatol Surg 1999; 25: 381–6.
95. Norris MJ, Carlin MC, Ratz JL. Treatment of essential telangiectasia: effects of increasing concentrations of polidocanol. J Am Acad of Dermatol 1989; 20: 643–9.
96. Kern P, Ramelet AA, Wütschert R, Hayoz D. Compression after sclerotherapy for telangiectasias and reticular leg veins. A randomized controlled study. J Vasc Surg 2007; 45: 1212–16.
97. Massay RA. Regarding the use of compression stockings after sclerotherapy. Dermatol Surg 1999; 25: 105–8.
98. Mc Donagh B. Comments on the use of post-sclerotherapy compression. Dermatol Surg 1999; 25: 519–21.

4 Legal guidelines for use of polidocanol and sodium tetradecyl sulfate for sclerotherapy

Lowell S Kabnick

Introduction

Sclerotherapy for the treatment of lower extremity varicosities has existed as a treatment option since the 1930s. Since its conception, a multitude of sclerosing agents have been studied and utilized in the endeavor to achieve successful sclerotherapy results. Present-day sclerosing agents include three different classes: osmotic, chemical, and detergent. While each class offers individual advantages, detergent sclerosing agents such as sodium tetradecyl sulfate (STS) and polidocanol (POL) have long been recognized as a preferred class of agents due to their relatively low side-effect profile and proven efficacy.

Recently, legal issues involving the use of these agents have come to the forefront, leaving several clinicians unsure about what is or is not legal regarding their use. This chapter addresses the current legal guidelines for using STS and POL in the United States, including:

- legal history of sclerosing agents
- the Food and Drug Administration (FDA) and sclerosants
- legal status of STS
- legal status of POL
- compounding guidelines for sclerosing agents
- foam sclerotherapy legality
- physician liability.

While this chapter contains legal guidelines, the author is not a lawyer and the legal interpretations contained in this text are not intended to serve as legal advice. Clinicians should consult a lawyer, state board of medical examiners or malpractice insurance carrier for validation and substantiation.

Legal history of sclerosing agents

The Food, Drug and Cosmetic Act of 1938 was the first law requiring new drugs to be tested for safety before marketing.[1] Adequate labeling for safe use, as well as a new drug application (NDA) was obligatory by the FDA to gain approval.[1] This was a significant milestone in the regulation of pharmaceuticals, since prior to 1938 the responsibility of drug safety was deferred almost entirely to the consumer.[2]

A second advancement in the FDA's supervision over pharmaceuticals occurred in 1951 with the Durham–Humphrey Amendment, which provided clarification between prescription and nonprescription drugs.[1] The law specifically stated that dangerous drugs, defined by various parameters, could not be dispensed without a prescription.[1] In 1962, Congress passed a monumental amendment for drug regulation; the Food, Drug and Cosmetic Act of 1938 was revised requiring a new drug also be proven *effective*, as well as safe, to obtain FDA approval.[3] During 1938 to 1962, once a drug received approval, similar drugs were included within the same approval parameters.[3] Additionally, many manufacturers, based on their own safety testing, introduced drugs into the market during this same time frame.[3]

Recognizing the need for regulation, the amendment in 1962 also required that the FDA conduct a retrospective evaluation between 1938 and 1962 regarding the effectiveness of the drug products that had been approved as safe during that time.[3] Over 3400 drugs were evaluated, and the reports were submitted to the FDA in the late 1960s and early 1970s.[3] The FDA mandated that manufacturers withdraw from the market products that were not found to be effective.

STS, sodium morrhuate (SM), and ethanolamine oleate (EO) were all approved before 1962; these still remain the only drugs approved in the United States for use as sclerosing agents. The 1962 amendment did allow a "grandfather" clause, which exempted a drug from efficacy testing if the drug's composition and labeling had not changed since 1962.[3] However, the FDA "believes that there are very few drugs on the market that are actually entitled to grandfather status because the drugs currently on the market likely differ from the previous versions in some respect, such as formulation, dosage or strength, dosage form, route of administration, indications, or intended patient population."[3]

STS was first approved for marketing in the United States in 1946 and manufactured by Elkins Sinn under the trade name of Sotradecol®. Due to the favorable safety and efficacy profiles of STS, it became the preferred agent in the United States for sclerotherapy. In accordance with the 1962 amendment of the Food, Drug and Cosmetic Act, Sotradecol® was reviewed and approved for *efficacy* in 1972 when Elkins Sinn was granted approval on a new drug application.[4]

Elkins Sinn submitted five subsequent new drug applications in 1975, 1977, 1985, 1988 and 1991 to update items such as labeling, dosage recommendations and adverse reactions. It is highly likely that SM and EO were also approved and validated for efficacy under the 1962 amendment; however, these agents were not required (at that time) to undergo the complete modern-day drug regulatory process. This is evidenced by the significant extravasation and allergic reactions associated with SM and EO since their approval. Following the 1962 amendment, a program known as the *Prescription Drug Wrap-Up* was instated in 1984. This program addressed marketed, nonapproved drugs, prior to 1962, that had not been previously tested for safety and/or efficacy.[3]

As the popularity of Sotradecol® increased, manufacturers from other countries began advertising a less expensive version of STS to physicians in the United States. Although STS was FDA-approved, Sotradecol® was the only form of it that was approved for use in the United States. According to the laws of the Food, Drug and Cosmetic Act, other brands of STS were illegal to import and use.

In 1991, the FDA took steps to stop this illegal activity by issuing an *Import Alert,* which was classified as an "Automatic Detention."[5] The alert charged STD Pharmaceutical (Hereford, United Kingdom) and Omega Laboratories (Montreal, Canada) as having "a new drug without an approved new drug application (NDA)."[5] The alert went on to explain that the "referenced firms are illegally exporting STS injection into the United States," and that the "foreign firms may be mailing the product directly to physicians in small quantities to avoid Customs/FDA intervention."[5] The alert instructed Customs officials to automatically detain all entries of the products.

Six years later, the Food and Drug Administration Modernization Act of 1997 was passed to further improve the regulation of drugs. Section 127 of the Modernization Act added section 503A to the Food, Drug and Cosmetic Act to specifically clarify the status of pharmacy compounding under Federal law.[6] This Act was in response to an increasing number of pharmacies that were compounding drugs outside the bounds of traditional pharmacy practice, such as mass production of commercially available drugs.

In 2000, Elkins Sinn (a division of Wyeth-Ayerst at the time) discontinued the manufacturing and marketing of Sotradecol® as the company was unable to maintain the integrity of the active pharmaceutical ingredient (API) of Sotradecol® to comply with FDA standards.[7] Since an industrial cleaning chemical was being used to make the active pharmaceutical ingredient, the FDA expressed concerns about the presence of contaminants.

Therefore, after 2000, a shortage of STS quickly developed and physicians were forced to seek alternative means in order to perform sclerotherapy.[8] Since Sotradecol® was an FDA-approved drug, but no longer commercially available in the United States, compounding pharmacies could legally manufacture the sclerosing agent. In addition to compounding Sotradecol®, pharmacies obtained the active pharmaceutical ingredient for POL and compounded the drug for physicians.

In 2002, a court decision (Supreme Court in Thompson vs Western States Medical Center, No. 01-344) declared Section 503A of the Food, Drug and Cosmetic Act invalid, as it contained unconstitutional restrictions on commercial speech.[6] Compounding pharmacies argued that they had a constitutional right to advertise compounded drugs. This Supreme Court ruling eliminated several federal laws addressing the practice of compounding, which in turn propagated illegal compounding activity.[9]

Additionally, illegal drug importation increased. Other versions of STS, as well as POL, were routinely shipped to individual physicians within the United States. The STS shortage also proliferated off-label usage of non-sclerotherapeutic FDA-approved drugs for indications other than their intended use: sclerotherapy of leg veins. Two such agents commonly used off-label were hypertonic saline and 72% glycerin.

Hypertonic saline (23.4% sodium chloride injection) is indicated as a source of water and electrolytes and voluntary interruption of pregnancy. Glycerin, used intravenously, is approved for treatment of acute ischemic cerebral infarct. Both have historically been utilized off-label primarily for the treatment of small telangiectasias (<1 mm in diameter).

Clearly, the need for a regulated sclerosant became widely acknowledged. In order to answer this need, the Drug Price Competition and Patent Term Restoration Act of 1984, which authorizes the approval of duplicate versions of drug products approved under an abbreviated new drug application (ANDA) procedure, was utilized.[10] A company filing an ANDA is required to show that the drug for which they are seeking approval contains the same active pharmaceutical ingredient in the same strength and dosage form as the "listed drug."[10] The drug presented in the ANDA must also be a version of the drug that was previously approved under a new drug application.[10]

In 2004, under the terms of this Act, Bioniche Pharma USA, Inc. (Belleville, Ontario, Canada), submitted to, and received approval from, the FDA to market 1% and 3% STS in the United States. At present, Sotradecol® is the only preferred sclerosing agent that is approved in the United States for vein sclerotherapy (Table 4.1). In 2005, Bioniche licensed exclusive distribution rights to AngioDynamics®, Inc., Queensbury, New York.

Table 4.1 Summary of the legal history of sclerosants

Event	Date	Market impact
Food, Drug and Cosmetic Act of 1938	1938	Drugs required to be tested for safety before marketing
Sotradecol® approved by FDA	1946	Sclerosant available that was tested for safety
Durham–Humphrey Amendment	1951	Provided clarification between prescription and nonprescription drugs
Food, Drug and Cosmetic Act of 1962	1962	Drugs required to be tested for efficacy before marketing; drugs approved after 1938 required to be tested
Sotradecol® receives FDA-approval for efficacy	1972	Sotradecol® complies with 1962 FDCA and is approved for safety and efficacy
Prescription Drug Wrap-Up	1984	Required safety and efficacy testing of drugs approved before 1962 that had not been previously tested
Drug Price Competition and Patent Term Restoration Act of 1984	1984	Authorizes the approval of duplicate versions of drug products approved under an ANDA procedure
FDA initiates Important Alert calling for "Automatic Detention" of STS illegally obtained from other countries	1991	One of the first enforcement actions by the FDA pertaining to illegal sclerosants
FDA Modernization Act of 1997	1997	Section 127 adds section 503A to the FDCA and defines pharmacy compounding under the Federal law
Elkins-Sinn withdraws Sotradecol® from the market	2000	Shortage of legal STS in the United States
Supreme Court decision No. 01-344 invalidates Section 503A of FDCA	2002	Virtually all federal laws addressing compounding are eliminated
Bioniche receives approval to market Sotradecol® with an ANDA	2004	Legal, pharmaceutical grade STS available in the United States
FDA initiates Important Alert calling for "Detention Without Physical Examination" of all polidocanol products	2007	FDA takes a firmer stance on the regulation of illegal sclerosant importation and usage

The FDA and sclerosants

The current process for FDA approval of a drug is stringent; it is designed to analyze parameters ranging from efficacy and safety to the conditions under which a drug is manufactured.[11] The steps required to bring a drug to market within this process are extensive and take several years to complete (Table 4.2).

The first step, or preclinical research, establishes data that indicate if the drug is reasonably safe for small-scale clinical studies. The next step includes clinical trials, containing three phases to establish side-effects, safety and efficacy in humans: Phase 1 studies are typically conducted on healthy volunteers (20–80 people) to determine the drug's safety; Phase 2 focuses on efficacy, targeting people who have a certain disease or condition; Phase 3 entails large-scale studies encompassing several thousand people to gather more information about safety and effectiveness.[12] Lastly, an NDA is filed and the FDA reviews the application and renders a decision.

Lack of a desirable alternative for an FDA-approved sclerosing agent other than Sotradecol® has been debated for several years. Several physicians have advocated the approval of POL, given its worldwide proven track record of efficacy and safety. However, a deterrent for many drug manufacturers has been the cost associated with bringing a drug to market in the United States. The time, cost, and complexity of the FDA drug regulatory process have escalated over the past 50 years. In the 1950s, it took 7 months to approve a new drug application, compared with an average of 2½ years in the 1990s.[2]

According to the Pharmaceutical Research and Manufacturers of America (PhRMA), United States drug companies spent $39.4 billion on research and development in 2005.[13] DiMasi et al evaluated data from the Tufts Center for the Study of Drug Development; they concluded that an average of 90.3 months elapsed from the start of Phase 1 clinical trials to FDA marketing approval.[14] In addition, the authors estimated that taking a drug from Phase 1 to approval, when the expenses of failed drugs are included, costs $802 million.[14] A majority of these costs are tied into the expense of providing the clinical data that is required by the FDA to approve the drug. A large expense, $896 200, is also associated with the current fee that the FDA charges for submitting a new drug application.[15] This is strictly an application fee, and does not include other expenditures a manufacturer accrues from the required clinical trials.

Market research data from the Millennium Research Group (Toronto, Ontario, Canada) revealed that in 2005 sclerotherapy procedures for treating varicose veins (not including telangiectasia) were valued at $510 000.[16] The report predicts a steep growth curve for this sector of the sclerotherapy market, reaching nearly $12 million by the year 2010.[16] Although these data do not include sclerotherapy treatment of telangiectasia, the overall value of the market is relatively small considering the immense costs involved in gaining FDA approval.

AngioDynamics®, Inc. (Queensbury, New York) estimates the current United States sclerotherapy market potential (including cosmetic procedures) to be worth over $70 million per annum; this figure is based on 1.7 million patients per year receiving sclerotherapy treatment of lower extremity veins.[8,17] Drug manufacturers evaluate the potential return on investment when considering the feasibility of bringing a drug to market. Comparatively, a $70 million potential may not present a large enough financial opportunity for other drug manufacturers seeking to enter the United States sclerotherapy market.

Similarly, agents such as hypertonic saline and glycerin that have been used off-label for sclerotherapy

Table 4.2 FDA drug review steps[11]

1. Preclinical (animal) testing
2. An investigational new drug application (INDA) outlines what the sponsor of a new drug proposes for human testing in clinical trials
3. Phase 1 studies (typically involve 20–80 people)
4. Phase 2 studies (typically involve a few dozen to about 300 people)
5. Phase 3 studies (typically involve several hundred to about 3000 people)
6. The pre-NDA period prior to a new drug application (NDA) submission. A common time for the FDA and drug sponsors to meet
7. Submission of an NDA is the formal step asking the FDA to consider a drug for marketing approval
8. After an NDA is received, the FDA has 60 days to decide whether to file it, so it can be reviewed
9. If the FDA files the NDA, an FDA review team is assigned to evaluate the sponsor's research on the drug's safety and effectiveness
10. The FDA reviews information that goes on a drug's professional labeling
11. The FDA inspects the facilities where the drug will be manufactured as part of the approval process
12. FDA reviewers will approve the application or find it either "approvable" or "not approvable"

would require a large amount of data to obtain additional FDA approval. This extensive data collection translates into substantial costs that may not be recouped by the respective companies seeking further indications. Additionally, in recent years, the enhanced regulatory oversight of the FDA has resulted in long lead times and high costs for overall drug development, including sclerosing agents.

Sodium tetradecyl sulfate

STS has a long history of safety, efficacy, and use in the United States and is currently the only FDA-approved, preferred sclerosing agent. The Sotradecol® active pharmaceutical ingredient developed by Bioniche was established under the present rigorous FDA standards; it does not contain contaminants, thereby making it distinctly different from the previous and unregulated versions of STS. Testing of STS produced from nonapproved manufacturers has demonstrated a failure to meet all of the FDA standards for STS (Table 4.3). According to the Sotradecol® submission to the FDA, specifications for impurities during STS stability studies are as follows:

Impurity	Specification
7-Ethyl-2-methyl-undec-3-ene/7-ethyl-2-methyl-undec-4-ene	0.5%
Benzaldehyde	0.3%
7-Ethyl-2-methyl-4-undecanol (tetradecanol)	0.7%
Largest single unknown	0.2%
Carbitol (considered as unknown)	0.2%
Total impurities	1.4%[18]

Unlike other versions of STS, Sotradecol® is subject to the standards of the Current Good Manufacturing Practice for Finished Pharmaceuticals. These standards contain a lengthy list of validations, which the FDA inspects before a drug is allowed to be manufactured. Examples of the validations include:

- organization/personnel responsible for quality control
- facility design, amenities and maintenance
- equipment cleaning and maintenance
- control of components and drug product containers and closures
- production and process controls
- packaging and labeling control
- warehousing and distribution
- laboratory controls (stability, contamination testing)
- records and reports (laboratory records, control records, complaint files)
- returned and salvaged drug products.[19]

One of the FDA's primary concerns is the pharmaceutical companies' ability to uphold quality control during mass production of the drug.[11] Unregulated versions of STS are not evaluated for any of these parameters, leaving uncertainty of the drug's concentration, impurities and overall quality control. As an FDA-approved drug, Sotradecol® is subject to regular inspections by the FDA, ensuring that the drug continues to meet the standards of the Current Good Manufacturing Practices. Versions of STS that are available from other countries or compounding pharmacies are not subject to these validations.

The FDA has an evident enforcement policy regarding the importation and use of nonapproved agents, as demonstrated by the previously mentioned "Automatic Detention" alert issued in 1991. In 2005, the FDA's Office of Criminal Investigations sentenced a physician to 1-year's probation and a $150 000 fine for importing and using Fibrovein®, a version of STS manufactured by

Table 4.3 Comparison of sodium tetradecyl sulfate (STS) products to the FDA standards[7,18,40]

Product	Company	pH	3% concentration	Carbitol
FDA specifications	FDA	7.8–8.1	2.85–3.15%	<0.02%
Sotradecol®	Bioniche Pharma	7.9	3.01%	0.000%
Fibrovein®	STD Pharmaceuticals	7.5	3.0%	0.045%
Compounded STS	Central Avenue Pharmacy	7.89	2.59%	1.79%
Compounded STS	McGuff	8.01	3.39%	4.18%
Compounded STS	Kronos	7.99	3.21%	0.33%

STD Pharmaceutical in the United Kingdom.[20] The physician was convicted of "violating one count of 21 U.S.C. §§ 331(d) and 333(a)(1) – Introduction into Interstate Commerce of an Unapproved Drug."[20] From a legal perspective, Sotradecol® provides a lawful, effective sclerosing agent that eliminates the risks involved in obtaining illegal sclerosants.

Polidocanol

POL is manufactured by several companies outside the United States, including Kreussler Pharma (Germany) and Omega Laboratories (Canada). These companies actively market to physicians in the United States and have routinely shipped product into the United States in the past. Not currently FDA-approved for any indication in the United States, POL's use is considered illegal. POL was first introduced in 1936 in Germany as an anesthetic agent and was recognized as a sclerosing agent in 1967.[21] POL is currently the only approved agent in Germany for sclerotherapy, and has been utilized there as well as other European countries for several years. While POL is recognized in the international community as a safe and effective sclerosant, no pharmaceutical manufacturer to date has attained FDA approval.

Several companies have investigated submitting an NDA to the FDA in recent years. One such company is BioForm Medical, Inc. (San Mateo, California). This medical aesthetics company has licensed a distribution agreement with Kreussler Pharma (Wiesbaden, Germany) for the development and commercialization of Aethoxysklerol®.[22] Kreussler is currently conducting Phase 3 clinical trials pursuant to a Special Protocol Assessment (SPA) that was submitted to the FDA.[22]

An SPA is a unique FDA evaluation of clinical trial protocols, which helps ensure that the parameters will meet the FDA requirements for submission of an NDA. It is reserved for drugs that are being tested primarily for efficacy and it must be submitted at least 90 days before clinical trials commence.[23] If the clinical trials are successful, Kreussler plans to submit an NDA in 2008. Given that the average time for the FDA to approve an NDA is 2½ years, a 2008 filing may not see approval until 2010 or later. Additionally, as discussed earlier, an NDA is very costly, with the return on investment being less than optimal for a new drug entering the sclerosing agent market.

The FDA has recently increased its enforcement over illegal importation and use of POL. In January of 2007, the government issued an *Import Alert* (IA) called a "Detain Without Physical Examination" pertaining to POL.[24] The *Import Alert* states the following: "Detention without physical examination of all polidocanol finished dosage form products and active pharmaceutical ingredients from all sources under all brand names including Aetoxisclerol, Aethoxysklerol, and Sclerovein."[24] The alert specifically references items entering customs at the United States border. It goes on to explain that drugs containing POL are brought into the United States by private physicians for the treatment of spider veins and that, currently, no products containing POL are approved for marketing in the United States.[24] Despite POL's worldwide use, there are significant legal risks involved in illegally importing the drug or its active pharmaceutical ingredient for use in the United States.

Compounding of sclerosing agents

Compounding pharmacies have long been recognized as a valuable source to create medication tailored to meet the needs of an individual patient per the prescription of a physician. The FDA regards traditional compounding as the combining, mixing or altering of ingredients; all compounded prescription drugs by definition are "new drugs" within the meaning of the Food, Drug and Cosmetic Act.[25] Under Federal law, a compounded product is *not* "generally recognized, among experts … as safe and effective."[25] Although pharmacies and/or compounded drugs are not exempt from the laws of the Food, Drug and Cosmetic Act, the FDA has not historically brought legal action against pharmacies that practice traditional compounding.[25]

According to the FDA Compliance Policy Guide for Pharmacy Compounding, the FDA is primarily concerned with compounding pharmacies that engage in activities that more closely resemble a drug manufacturer or violate the Food, Drug and Cosmetic Act.[6] The Policy Guide lists the following acts as grounds to initiate legal action against a pharmacy:

1. Compounding of drugs in anticipation of receiving prescriptions, except in very limited quantities in relation to the amounts of drugs compounded after receiving valid prescriptions.
2. Compounding drugs that were withdrawn or removed from the market for safety reasons.

3. Compounding finished drugs from bulk active ingredients that are not components of FDA-approved drugs without an FDA sanctioned investigational new drug application (INDA).
4. Receiving, storing, or using drug substances without first obtaining written assurance from the supplier that each lot of the drug substance has been made in an FDA-registered facility.
5. Receiving, storing or using drug components not guaranteed or otherwise determined to meet official compendia requirements.
6. Using commercial-scale manufacturing or testing equipment for compounding drug products.
7. Compounding drugs for third parties who resell to individual patients or offering compounded drugs at wholesale to other state-licensed persons or commercial entities for resale.
8. Compounding drug products that are commercially available in the marketplace or that are essentially copies of commercially available FDA-approved drug products. In certain circumstances, it may be appropriate for a pharmacist to compound a small quantity of a drug that is only slightly different than an FDA-approved drug that is commercially available. In these circumstances, the FDA will consider whether there is documentation of the medical need for that particular variation of the compound for that particular patient.
9. Failing to operate in conformance with applicable state law regulating the practice of pharmacy.[6]

When Elkins Sinn discontinued the manufacturing and marketing of Sotradecol®, compounding pharmacies began supplying compounded STS, using the same industrial-grade active pharmaceutical ingredient with which the FDA had original concerns. Since Sotradecol® was no longer commercially available, the compounding of STS served as a legal, practical alternative.

However, if an FDA-approved drug is commercially available, a pharmacy cannot compound copies of the drug product regularly or in inordinate amounts.[26] Additionally, according to the FDA Compliance Guide and the FDA Modernization Act of 1997, it is illegal to distribute and use a compounded drug that is a copy of an FDA-approved drug.[6,27] A compounding pharmacy has the right to manufacture a drug that is a *modification* of an FDA-approved drug on an individual patient basis. The purpose for the drug compound must be medically necessary; for example, a patient allergic to an ingredient of a mass-produced, commercially available product. Since the approval of Sotradecol® in 2004, several compounding pharmacies have violated this law by receiving and using large quantities of bulk drug substances to manufacture sizeable amounts of STS.

To enforce the established laws, the FDA has recently initiated regulatory action against compounding pharmacies producing STS in mass quantities. Several *Warning Letters* have been sent to various compounding pharmacies, informing them to immediately discontinue the production of STS.

A warning letter is the first step in a very serious FDA enforcement action; the FDA may take further action without additional notice.[28] In a letter to Wedgewood Village Pharmacy concerning STS 3%, the FDA states that the pharmacy "... produces finished drug products that are essentially copies of commercially available products, and ... does not document a medical need for particular patients for these versions of otherwise commercially available products."[29] The warning letter goes on to explain that the pharmacy engages in the large-scale manufacturing of nonapproved drugs, including copies of commercially available FDA-approved drugs, which raises safety concerns and poses a significant threat to the drug approval process of the Federal Food, Drug and Cosmetic Act.[29]

As with illegally imported STS, the FDA has concerns regarding a compounded drug's concentration and impurities. These performance measures were evaluated in a 2007 study by Almeida and Raines comparing compounded STS with Sotradecol® (Bioniche Pharma USA, Inc., Belleville, Ontario, Canada) for venous sclerotherapy.[30] The results revealed that the compounded STS contained numerous impurities, a significant variation in concentration, and a higher incidence of incomplete ablation ($p = 0.02$); whereas, Sotradecol® did not have any impurities or concentration variations.[30] While the levels of impurities necessary to elicit an adverse event have not been documented, impurities in other drugs are known to cause adverse effects, and therefore are cause for concern.[30] The findings reinforce the FDA's position and desire for a more strict regulation of STS compounding.

In addition, it is illegal for a pharmacy to compound a drug that has never received FDA approval. When the STS shortage ensued, compounding pharmacies also began manufacturing POL in mass quantities despite its lack of FDA approval. Although POL is a detergent agent, it has a different active pharmaceutical ingredient (hydroxypolyethoxydodecane) than Sotradecol® (7-ethyl-2-methyl-4-undecanol sulfate sodium salt).

It is not only illegal to import POL; it is also illegal to compound the drug from raw chemicals. In response to the growing number of compounders manufacturing POL, the FDA has initiated the confiscation of this agent from chemical suppliers throughout the United States.[31] Numerous *Warning Letters* have been sent, informing suppliers to cease and immediately discontinue the manufacturing and supply of POL as it is illegal.

Pharmacies typically obtain the active pharmaceutical ingredient for a drug from a chemical supplier and compound the intended drug by adding other inactive ingredients. One such supplier is Spectrum Chemicals and Laboratory Products, Inc., which received a *Warning Letter* from the FDA Department of Health and Human Services (DHHS) in November 2005. The letter explains that the FDA does not sanction the repacking and distribution of the POL API for use in pharmacy compounding, and that the FDA may use its enforcement discretion to rectify the violation.[32]

The FDA has targeted pharmacies that are obtaining the POL active pharmaceutical ingredient and compounding the drug. For instance, the following is an excerpt from a *Warning Letter* to Hopewell Pharmacy from the DHHS: "We … note that your firm is compounding drug products containing POL. This is not an active ingredient contained in any FDA-approved drug product, and FDA will not sanction its use in pharmacy compounding."[33]

In another letter to Custom Scripts Pharmacy, the DHHS goes on to explain that "the agency is seriously concerned about the public health risks associated with the compounding of POL injection. Known adverse events include deep venous thromboses, necrosis, and ulceration at the treated site."[34] Language from several *Warning Letters* states the same message regarding potential FDA action: "You should take prompt action to correct these deviations. Failure to promptly correct these deviations may result in additional regulatory action without further notice. These actions include, but are not limited to, seizure of your products or injunction against you and your firm."[28,34,35]

Even as the compounding of drugs serves a vital purpose for medically necessary situations, the FDA is clearly dedicated to eliminating the illegal mass production of commercially available, non-FDA-approved drugs.

Foam sclerotherapy

The use of foamed sclerosing agents is documented as early as 1939; several methods and techniques have developed since that time.[36] While foam sclerotherapy has been established by many researchers and physicians as a safe and effective method of treatment, its legal use is currently questioned in the United States. In essence, the addition of a substance to make foam from an FDA-approved drug is a substantial change, altering the biological behavior. This alteration requires an FDA NDA, which is markedly different from drug compounding. Compounding of a drug does not change the biological behavior of the drug. Since foamed STS has not been evaluated or approved by the FDA, any foamed drug used for sclerotherapy currently falls into the same category as other non-FDA-approved agents such as POL.

Provensis (London, United Kingdom) is the manufacturer of Varisolve®, proprietary POL microfoam. The manufacturer received approval from the FDA in 2002 to commence a pilot study for Varisolve®. At present, Varisolve® is in Phase 2 clinical trials in the United States.[37] The question remains as to whether the manufacturer will submit an NDA to the FDA. Currently, the FDA has not approved any foamed sclerotherapeutic drug.

Physician liability

The liability for physicians using a nonapproved or illegally compounded drug is considerable, with several negative and significant consequences. A major liability for a physician who uses a nonapproved drug is the possible invalidation of malpractice insurance. Malpractice insurance typically excludes coverage of procedures that involve the use of illegal drugs.[8] Unlike pharmaceutical companies, compounders do not carry liability insurance that is sufficient to protect physicians from catastrophic damages.[8] The use of an illegally compounded or imported drug could leave a physician with tremendous personal liability and possible criminal prosecution.

Additionally, the FDA and Medicare can impose criminal charges and significant fines against a physician who is convicted of using illegally imported or illegally compounded drugs. Medicare Part B will pay for compounded drugs when they meet the criteria for coverage.[38] However, it is considered Medicare fraud to bill for a drug that is nonapproved or illegal.

The Centers for Medicare and Medicaid Services have taken an aggressive position in recent years to prevent fraud. Under the Federal False Claims Act, any person who knowingly submits a false or fraudulent claim to Medicare or Medicaid is liable to the Federal Government for three times the amount of the Federal Government's damages plus penalties of $5000–10 000 for each claim.[39] This is evidenced by the aforementioned 2005 case, where the penalized physician was mandated to pay $150 000 restitution under the False Claims Act. In the case, the physician billed Medicare for 62 procedures, all of which Medicare refused payment because the drug utilized was nonapproved.[20]

Under the Federal False Claims Act, persons who report fraudulent claims to the United States Government are entitled to a reward equal to 15–25% of the recovery of Federal damages.[39] This provides tremendous incentive to persons who have exposure to Medicare or Medicaid billing to report any activity that may be deemed as false. A fraud conviction can be very costly for a physician, as the penalties are paid out of pocket unless the physician has supplemental insurance specifically for Medicare fraud.

Conclusions

- Currently, Sotradecol® is the only legal, preferred, FDA-approved sclerosing agent available in the United States.
- The importation and use of STS or POL from manufacturers outside the United States is illegal.
- Mass production of STS by compounding pharmacies is a direct violation of the Food, Drug and Cosmetics Act.
- Pharmacy compounding of POL is illegal because it is not an FDA-approved drug.
- Foaming of any sclerosing agent is a chemical alteration and creates a new drug, which is considered illegal.
- Use of a nonapproved or illegally compounded sclerosant can create tremendous liability for physicians, including invalidation of malpractice insurance and Medicare legal action.

References

1. Hamilton D. 1997. A Brief History of the Center for Drug Evaluation and Research. Available online at www.fda.gov/cder/about/history/Histext.htm.
2. Williams P. The Right Balance: Issues in Drug Regulation. The Harvard Mahoney Neuroscience Institute Letter. On the Brain 1995; 4: 1.
3. US Food and Drug Administration. 2006. Chapter 4: Compliance Policy Guide, Subchapter 440: Marketed Unapproved Drugs, Section 440.100: Marketed New Drugs Without Approved NDAs or ANDAs. Available online at www.fda.gov/cder/guidance/6911fnl.pdf.
4. Center for Drug Evaluation and Research. 1972. NDA 5970/S13: Sotradecol® Chemistry Review. Available online at www.fda.gov/cder/foi/nda/pre96/5970-S013_SOTRADECOL%203%25_CHEMR.PDF.
5. US Food and Drug Administration. 1991. Import Alert IA6653: Automatic detention of STD Injection or Thromboject 1% Injection and 3% Injection. Available online at www.fda.gov/ora/fiarsora_import_ia6653.html.
6. US Food and Drug Administration. 2002. Chapter 4: Compliancy Policy Guide, Subchapter 460: Compliance Policy Guidance for FDA Staff and Industry, Section 460.200: Pharmacy Compounding. Available online at www.fda.gov/ohrms/dockets/98fr/02D-0242_gdl0001.pdf.
7. Goldman MP. Sodium tetradecyl sulfate for sclerotherapy treatment of veins: Is compounding pharmacy solution safe? Dermatol Surg 2004; 30: 1454–56.
8. Hobbs EP. 2006. The saga of Sotradecol: why it wasn't available and why it is now. Presented at the AIM Conference, 15 November 2006, New York, NY.
9. Shimron Y, Gardner A. Cream's safety wasn't tested. The Sunday News and Observer 2005 January 30.
10. US Food and Drug Administration. 2002. Determination that sodium tetradecyl sulfate injection was not withdrawn from sale for reasons of safety or effectiveness. Available online at www.fda.gov/ohrms/dockets/98fr/110702b.htm.
11. US Food and Drug Administration. 2002. The FDA's drug review process: ensuring drugs are safe and effective. FDA Consumer Magazine July–August 2002; FDA05-3242.
12. US Food and Drug Administration. 2007. The New Drug Development Process: Steps from Test Tube to New Drug Application Review. Available online at www.fda.gov/cder/handbook/develop.htm.
13. Healthcare Economist. 2006. Cost to bring drug to market: $802m. Available online at healthcare-economist.com/2006/04/29/802m.
14. DiMasi JA, Hansen RW, Grabowski HG. The price of innovation: new estimates of drug development costs. J Health Econo 2003; 22: 151–85.
15. Colangelo K. 2007. Planning for Successful, Efficient Pharmaceutical Product Development. April 25. Available online at www.fda.gov/cder/meeting/SBA_presentations/Colangelo_2007.pdf.

16. Millennium Research Group. US Markets for Varicose Vein Treatment Devices 2006. Toronto: Millennium Research Group, Inc., 2006.
17. AngioDynamics, Inc. 2007. Data on file.
18. Bioniche Pharma Group. 2004. FDA Submission: Sotradecol® (Sodium tetradecyl sulfate injection 1%, 3%). Bioniche Pharma Group, Belleville.
19. US Food and Drug Administration. 2007. 21 Code of Federal Regulations; Parts 210 and 211. Available online at www.fda.gov/cder/dmpq/cgmpregs.htm.
20. FDA Office of Criminal Investigations. 2005. Physician Found Using Unapproved Drug in Treatment of Varicose Veins. Available online at www.fda.gov/ora/about/enf_story2005_archive/ch6/default.pdf.
21. Weiss RA, Feied CF, Weiss MA. Vein Diagnosis and Treatment: a Comprehensive Approach. New York: McGraw Hill; 2001: 126.
22. BioForm Medical, Inc. 2007. BioForm Licenses US Rights to Leading European Varicose Vein Treatment. August 9. Available online at files.shareholder.com/downloads/BFRM/262994784x0x140089/0583e7ad-3cf0-458e-bc7b-eba3d69940df/140089.pdf.
23. Department of Health and Human Services. 2002. Guidance for Industry: Special Protocol Assessment. Available online at www.fda.gov/cber/gdlns/protocol.pdf.
24. US Food and Drug Administration. 2007. Import Alert IA6649: Detention without physical examination of all polidocanol finished dosage form products and active pharmaceutical ingredients (APIs) from all sources under all brand names including Aetoxisclerol, Aethoxysklerol, and Sclerovein. Available online at www.fda.gov/ora/fiars/ora_import_ia6649.html.
25. Department of Health and Human Services. 2006. FDA Warning Letter to Rotech Healthcare, Inc. Sent August 9, 2006. [CIN-06-27353-15].
26. US Food and Drug Administration. 2007. Federal Food, Drug and Cosmetic Act. Chapter V-Drugs and Devices, Subchapter A-Drugs and Devices, Section 503A-Pharmacy Compounding. Available online at www.fda.gov/opacom/laws/fdcact/fdcact5a.htm.
27. US Food and Drug Administration. 1997. FDA Modernization Act of 1997. Section 127: Application of Federal Law to Practice of Pharmacy Compounding. November 21, 1997.
28. Department of Health and Human Service. 2006. FDA Warning Letter to CCS Medical. Sent August 9, 2006. [FLA-06-30].
29. Department of Health and Human Services. 2006. FDA Warning Letter to Wedgewood Village Pharmacy. Sent October 31, 2006. [06-NWJ-07].
30. Almeida JI, Raines JK. FDA-approved sodium tetradecyl sulfate (STS) versus compounded STS for venous sclerotherapy. Dermatol Surg 2007; 33: 1037–44.
31. Isaacs MN. 2007. From the Editor's Desk: Polidocanol Paradox. Available online at www.phlebology.org.
32. Department of Health and Human Services. 2005. FDA Warning Letter to Spectrum Chemicals and Laboratory Products, Inc. Sent 28 November 2005. [06-NWJ-05].
33. Department of Health and Human Service. 2004. FDA Warning Letter to Hopewell Pharmacy. Sent 4 June 2004. [04-NWJ-14].
34. Department of Health and Human Services. 2006. FDA Warning Letter to Custom Script Pharmacy. Sent 4 December 2006. [*FLA-07-05*].
35. Department of Health and Human Services. 2006. FDA Warning Letter to Triangle Compounding Pharmacy. Sent 4 December 2006. [07-ATL-04].
36. Wollmann JC. The history of sclerosing foams. Dermatol Surg 2004; 30: 694–703.
37. BTG International LTG. 2007. Product pipeline: Varisolve®. Available online at www.btgplc.com/BTGDevelopmentProgrammes/228/Varisolvesupregsup.html.
38. Department of Health and Human Services. 2006. Letter to Charles E. Grassley, United States Senate. Sent 22 August 2006.
39. Federal False Claims Act. 1986. Title 31: Money and Finance; Subtitle III: Financial Management; Chapter 37: Claims; Subchapter III: Claims against the United States Government; 3729: False Claims. Available online at www.taf.org/federalfca.htm.
40. Bioniche Pharma USA, Inc. 2004. Abbreviated New Drug Application (ANDA) for Sotradecol. Department of Health and Human Services. 12 November 2004 (ANDA 40-541).

PRACTICE

5 The science of producing extemporary foam and its clinical results

Alessandro Frullini

The use of sclerosing foam, as described elsewhere in this book, may become an established treatment for a variety of conditions. In the treatment of varicose veins, the most common condition encountered, the technique has a high success rate, low cost and few major complications. Sclerosant foam is a mixture of one or several gasses and a liquid solution with tensioactive properties. The gasses must be well tolerated or physiological, and the foam bubble size should preferably be under 100 μm.

The behavior of injected sclerosing foam is different from the action of its liquid component. It forms a coherent bolus inside the vein that prevents any dilution of the drug with the blood into which it is injected. Thus, its effects in sclerotherapy are vastly amplified.

Sclerotherapy has experienced different phases following the initial enthusiasm of Raymond Tournay, Carl Sigg and George Fegan.[1,2] Despite the efforts of those pioneers, surgery has been considered to be the gold standard for varicose vein treatment; that is, until now, when the effects of foam sclerotherapy have manifested.[3] Sclerosing foam allows us to have full control of the drug concentration inside a vein and its contact time (dwell time) with the endothelium. Our perspective on varicose vein treatment has been entirely changed now that we can achieve closure of the saphenous vein with its tributary varicosities with a single injection at a low cost, without hospitalization or anesthesia, and a virtually painless treatment.

The idea of using air and a drug in combination is quite old. Orbach described an "air block" technique in 1944, over 60 years ago.[4] He used sodium tetradecyl sulfate (STS) which is still is use today, especially in America. Although this publication is erroneously referred to as the seminal work on foam sclerotherapy, the technique was neither employed nor suggested in this work. The publication did, however, report observations that were prescient and had the potential to revolutionize phlebology.

The situation changed entirely in 1993 when Juan Cabrera proposed the use of therapeutic foam consisting of STS or the detergent polidocanol in the treatment of varicose veins. This represented a revolutionary step forward in the stagnant world of sclerotherapy, and, of course, it was a step forward in the treatment of superficial venous insufficiency.[5]

Many authors have reported different methods for producing sclerofoam. In 1997, Alain Monfreux reported a technique utilizing a glass syringe and a sterile plug to produce weak foam.[6] Two years later, Patrick Benigni and Symon Sadoun presented their personal technique for producing polidocanol foam with a disposable syringe and a tap.[7] In 1999, Mingo-Garcia reported another technique using helium and a specially designed device.[8] As the century changed in the year 2000, a turning point occurred in foam sclerotherapy when Lorenzo Tessari presented his three-way tap technique, which was capable of preparing a very good foam at an extremely low cost.[9] To produce Tessari's foam with STS, a three-way stopcock is needed, coupled to a 2.5 mL syringe filled with 1 mL of drug, and a 5 mL syringe containing 4–5 mL of atmospheric air. Twenty quick passages of the solution are made, and after the first 10 passages the tap is narrowed as much as possible. This procedure forms a foam of high quality and consistency (Figure 5.1).

Tessari popularized his method using a long catheter for his injections, but this may interfere with the structure of the sclerosing foam, altering its characteristics.

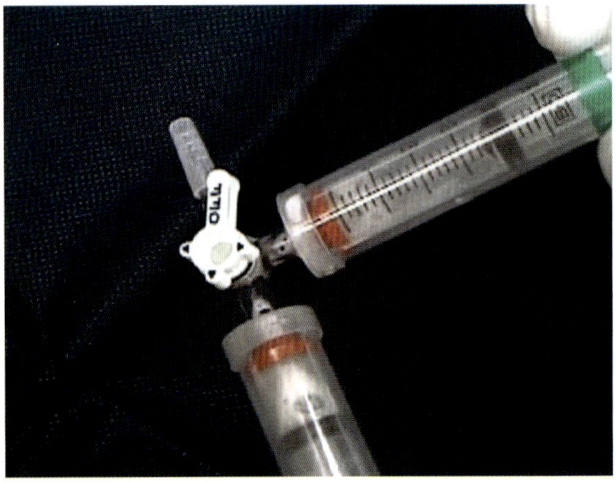

Figure 5.1 The Tessari 3-way tap technique, which is capable of preparing a very good foam. This photograph shows the 3-way stopcock with a 2.5 mL syringe filled with 1 mL of drug, and a 5 mL syringe containing 4–5 mL of atmospheric air. Twenty quick passages of the solution are made, and after the first 10 passages the tap is narrowed as much as possible. This will form a high-quality foam very quickly

The polar macromolecules of the sclerosant are linked together in order to form bubbles. The silicone that is usually present in catheters and syringes breaks down those links, altering the half-life of the foam. For this reason, the shorter the exposure of sclerosant to such surfaces, the better the quality and duration of the foam. Small cannulae and steel needles are particularly active in this regard. Moreover, with the use of foam, the delivery site is not important, as sclerosant foam forms a coherent bolus, which migrates into the vein under total ultrasound control even for long segments of the veins.

We presented our own method of making foam in the year 2000.[10] Our technique generates foam in a vial of sclerosing solution, provided that the vial has a rubber cap. Foam generation is due to the Venturi effect that occurs when there is forceful passage of a fluid into a narrow opening. In the original description of this method, a small connector was used to couple the syringe and the vial. At least five passages are generally necessary to create a good foam similar to Tessari's. It is necessary to choose the size of the vial and the syringe carefully, as a small syringe cannot be coupled to a large vial.

In the meantime, the pharmaceutical companies have started to be interested in foam, and currently the British company Provensis is developing a highly standardized industrial-grade microfoam called Varisolve. This may represent the ultimate foam for varicose vein treatments.

Foam and sclerotherapy

Sclerotherapy is the "art" of transforming the wall of a varicose vein into a fibrotic cord. The most desirable end-point of sclerotherapy is permanent occlusion, but this does not always occur with liquid sclerosant. The main cause of incomplete sclerotherapy is the volume of blood in which the drug will be diluted. With liquid sclerosant, the injection in a vein segment properly raises the drug concentration in the location of the injection to a peak followed by a quite rapid decrease in concentration, as the sclerosant is diluted by blood. The shape of the curve is determined by the speed of injection, the ratio of injected volume to the size of the vessel, and the blood flow. Sclerosis is triggered only if a threshold level of drug concentration develops or if there is a minimum effective concentration for a sufficient period.

In telangiectasias, we can expect an abrupt rise in concentration and a relatively long-lasting plateau of drug inside the vessel. In contrast, in a large great saphenous vein, the peak concentration is reached more slowly, which is related to the size of the needle and the fluidity of the sclerosant. The maximum concentration of the agent in this situation is related to the volume of blood into which it is diluted.

This explains why sclerotherapy has never been a problem in terms of drug concentration for telangiectasias and why saphenous sclerotherapy has always been unsatisfactory in the long term. The introduction of sclerofoam has completely changed this perspective. When foam is injected, it forms a coherent bolus inside the vein. Due to its properties, this bolus has uniform activity and can be expected to be in situ for a definite time. This leads to optimal and – for the first time – controlled sclerosis (Figure 5.2).

Foam is a nonequilibrium dispersion of gas bubbles in a relatively small volume of liquid that contains surface-active macromolecules (surfactants). These preferentially absorb at the gas–liquid interface and are responsible both for the tendency of a liquid to convert to a foam and for its stability.

Sclerosing foam is a mixture of gas and a liquid solution with tensioactive properties. As indicated above, the behavior of sclerosing foam after injection is different from that of a liquid solution.

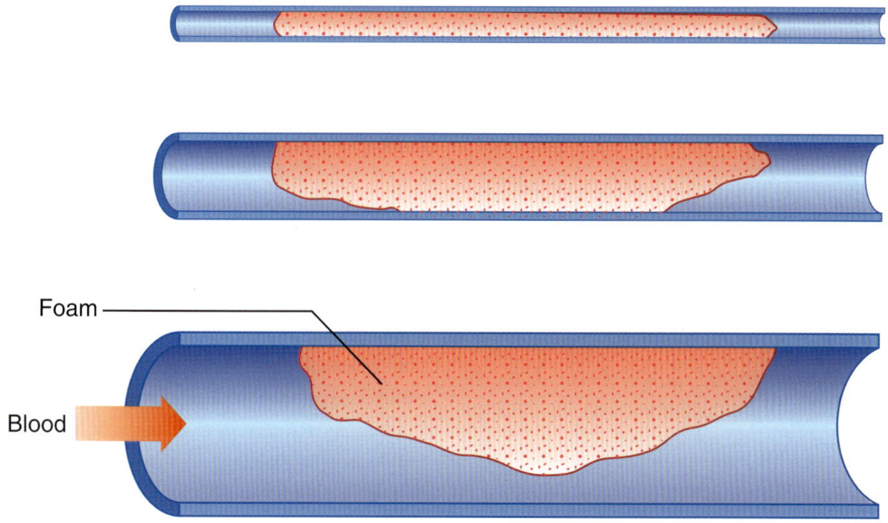

Figure 5.2 In these three drawings, viewing from the bottom upward, we see the coherent bolus of foam floating on liquid blood. As the foam initiates spasm, the vessel fills and ultimately proceeds into tight spasm, dispersing the foam proximally and distally. Thus a small quantity of foam can fill the entire venous arborization. This shows why calculating the therapeutic foam treatment volume from the vein diameter and length is useless

It is a common mistake to consider foam as a single entity. In fact, it varies according to the method of manufacture. It is possible to produce very different foams with different characteristics, complication rates and therapeutic indications. We can classify foams by bubble diameter (froth foam, mini-foam and micro-foam) or by the relative quantity of liquid. The bubble shape is the result of the competition between surface tension and interface forces.

Wet foam produces nearly spherical bubbles. Wetness of the volume fraction of liquid is over 5% in such foams. Dry foam produces polyhedral bubbles, and the volume fraction of liquid is under 5%. Wet foam has maximum stability because, when the bubble is polyhedral, as in dry foam, there is greater competition between surface tension and interface forces. Uniform diameters also mean more stability since smaller bubbles empty into larger ones according to the law of LaPlace, because their smaller diameters cause a higher internal pressure. Extemporary sclerosing foams such as Monfreux's foam often display two-stage behavior, firstly acting as dry foam with polyhedral bubbles, then with dissolution into larger spherical bubbles creating a wet environment. More standardized sclerosing foams such as Tessari's appear to be wet even in the initial stages, which produces more stability and uniformity.

Another way to classify foam is to consider the standard of production. It can be of low grade or medium grade for extemporary foam, but is maximal only for the industrial high standard foam. Even when it seems very stable, foam is always evolving. Three factors introduce disorder: (1) drainage, the changing into liquid from foam; (2) disproportion, the change in bubble-size distribution and coalescence; and (3) the fusion of bubbles. These three factors will in time lead to complete dissolution. This process can be slowed down in several ways, such as by freezing, but for clinical use this is not necessary, as the therapeutic properties are more important then the duration of the foam.

Another aspect of foam is its response to forces of flow. Foam can exhibit features of different basic states of matter, acting as a solid, a liquid or a gas. In fact, sclerosant foam exhibits striking mechanical properties because, as a semi-solid, it resists being pushed gently as it is maneuvered inside a vein. But it reacts as a liquid if pushed forcefully as in a syringe; bubble disruption ultimately converts the entire foam into a liquid and a gas.

Properties of foam

Sclerosing foam shows some advantageous properties such as adhesiveness and compactness. These allow manipulation of the foam after injection, thus displacing the dilution effect of blood. Syringeability is another property that allows foam injection through a small needle without loss of its characteristics. With foam, it is possible to produce a greater volume of agent for the same quantity of liquid, and this allows long segments of veins to be treated. When foam has long duration, this guarantees therapeutic action. Also, foam has an enhanced spasm generation that causes less blood dilution inside the affected vein. Other properties of foam include echo visibility and enhancement of sclerosing power, with reduced drug dose and reduced drug concentration. Selective action of foam on endothelium causes less risk of tissue damage on extravasation. It must be stressed that each type of foam has different properties and characteristics, as indicated elsewhere in this book.

Clinical application of foam sclerosants

Foam can be used in every kind of classical sclerotherapy. New and exciting indications have been tried with success. In our experience, neovascularization after saphenous vein surgery is just as good an indication for foam as is a refluxing saphenous vein. Midterm results of such therapy for both indications are very encouraging.

The first series of foam sclerotherapy treatments of the saphenous vein was published in 1997 as a report of 261 great saphenous veins treated with ultrasound-guided injection of a standardized Cabrera microfoam.[11] Our first paper in the English literature on foam sclerotherapy was published in 1999.[12] In 2000, we presented our results with 167 large veins treated with foam sclerotherapy. The results were very good.[13] Treatment with STS or polidocanol foam was generally performed in the great saphenous vein with ultrasound-guided Doppler assistance. In that experience, STS was used as a 1% or 1.5% solution. Polidocanol was used in 2% or 3% concentrations, and usually a thick foam was prepared with the Tessari or Frullini method. A volume of 3 mL of this foam was enough to treat most great saphenous veins less than 9 mm in diameter. Larger veins occasionally needed more concentrated liquid or a greater quantity of foam. In any case, a maximum of 5 mL of extemporary foam was recommended in order to keep the treatment safe.

Further experience was then gained with a higher concentration and greater volumes. I presently use polidocanol or STS at 3% in most great saphenous veins, with a maximum volume of 10 mL. The Varisolve foam can be used safely in larger volumes, but the coalescence rate of extemporary foam has not yet been controlled enough to perform injections exceeding 5 mL of foam.

We feel that telangiectasias are the poorest indication for sclerosant foam, and liquid sclerosants such as polidocanol are used for standard telangiectasias. Polidocanol foam is reserved for resistant cases or for telangiectatic matting. That condition is a good indication for sclerosant foam with polidocanol at 0.1–0.25% concentration.

Due to its lower compactness, Monfreux foam is more suitable for telangiectasias. Thicker foams such as Tessari or Frullini foams are difficult to push into the small vessels. Minor complications have been reported with foam as with liquid sclerosant in treating telangiectasias. Even experienced physicians have reported pigmentation and skin necrosis. This is due to the greater sclerosing power of foam. Among major complications, deep venous thrombosis (DVT) has been reported, and in every case this was asymptomatic without sequelae at 3 months.[14] A similar rate of DVT has been reported for surgery of varicose veins. Unfortunately, such patients treated with classical sclerotherapy or surgery are rarely routinely studied with duplex ultrasound immediately after treatment. This is different from the patients who are treated with ultrasound-guided sclerosant foam, who are regularly studied with duplex ultrasound after treatment.

Lowering the concentration of the sclerosing drug used for foam generation and avoiding large-volume injections such as in the small saphenous vein are extremely important in lessening the chances of DVT, which is considered to be a rare and generally limiting complication of sclerotherapy, but the need for routine ultrasound evaluation after treatment must be stressed.

Discussion

Nowadays, three new options are offered to patients with varicose veins and to their physicians: endovenous laser, radiofrequency closure and foam sclerotherapy. In my opinion, a treatment is needed that is capable of achieving good results safely and less invasively than surgery. The technique should be capable of treating tributary varicosities at the same time as the main saphenous trunk, and it should be cheap and repeatable in cases of recurrent or persistent varicose veins.

Laser or radiofrequency techniques are only a different way to treat the saphenous trunk during interventions that are similar to surgery. A sterile field is necessary and anesthesia must be given. In my opinion, inversion stripping of the greater saphenous vein is possible under local anesthesia, and is less traumatic than standard stripping, laser ablation or radiofrequency closure. Considering that at least 60% of great saphenous vein insufficiency is due to terminal valve incompetence, proper treatment that does not include saphenofemoral junction ligation will be found only in a minority of cases.

A different treatment for saphenous insufficiency is a necessity. At present, only foam sclerotherapy has the ideal requisites: it is cheap, time-saving, and easy for a trained doctor to perform. Varicose tributaries are treated at the same time as the saphenous trunk, and return to daily activity is resumed immediately. No anesthesia is required and post-treatment pain is completely absent. The volume of air or physiological gas injected with foam is far less than the uncontrolled and unknown volume of smoke and vapor produced by laser in the venous system. An ultimate study with Level I evidence and a comparison of the various methods is still lacking. The few studies currently available do not compare homogenous cases or properly done treatments.

It must be stressed that an alternative treatment to surgery must not complicate the work of the physician or the life of the patient. If, in a large clinical experience, foam sclerotherapy demonstrates that it is capable of achieving results similar to or better than surgery, then we will have made a huge step forward in the control of venous insufficiency.

Conclusions

Extemporary sclerosant foam in its short history has shown the capability of dominating the treatment of venous insufficiency in its most common form, varicose veins. It has demonstrated its ability to lower healthcare costs, and experience has taught physicians how to minimize adverse events. The future looks bright for this simple, inexpensive and universally available method of treatment.

References

1. Tournay R. Terapia sclerosant delle varici. Milan: Rallaello Cordina Editore, 1984: 65–72.
2. Fegan WG. Continuous compression technique of injecting varicose veins. Lancet 1963; 20: 108–12.
3. Cabrera Garrido JR, Cabrera Garrido-Olmedo JR, Garcia-Olmedo Dominguez MA. Enlargissement des limites de la sclerotherapy: noveaux produits sclerosants. Phlebologie 1997; 50: 181–8.
4. Orbach EJ. Sclerotherapy of varicose veins: utilization of intravenous air block. Am J Surg1944; 56: 362–6.
5. Cabrera Garrido JR, Cabrera Garrido-Olmedo JR, Garcia-Olmedo Dominguez MA. Nuevo metodo de esclerosis en las varices truncular es. Pathol Vasculares 1993; 1: 55–72.
6. Monfreux A. Traitment sclérosant des troncs saphènies et leurs collaterals de gros caliber par la méthode MUS. Phlebologie 1997; 50: 351–3.
7. Benigni, JP, Sadoun, S, Thirion, V, et al. Télangectasies et varices réticulaires. Traitement par la mousse d'Aetoxisclérol a 0.25%. Présentation d'un etude pilote. Phlebologie 1999; 3: 283–90.
8. Mingo-garcia J. Esclerosis venos con espuma: Foam Medical System. Rev Esp Med Cirug Cosmet 1999; 7: 29–31.
9. Tessari L. Nouvelle technique d'obtention de la scleromousse. Phlebologie 2000; 53: 129.
10. Frullini. A. new technique in producing a sclerosing foam in a disposable syringe: the Frullini method. Dermatol Surg 2000; 26: 705–6.
11. Cabrera Garrido JR, Cabrera Garrido-Olmedo JR, Garcia-Olmedo Dominguez MA. Treatment of varicose long saphenous veins with sclerosant in microfoam form: long term outcomes. Phlebology 2000; 15: 19–23.
12. Cavezzi A, Frullini A. The role of sclerosing foam in ultrasound guided sclerotherapy of the saphenous vein and of recurrent varicose veins: our personal experience. Aust NZ J Phlebol 1999; 3: 49–50.
13. Frullini A, Cavezzi A. Echosclérose por mousse de Tétradécylsulfate de sodium et de polidocanol: deux années d'expérience. Phlebologie 2000; 53: 431–5.
14. Frullini A, Cavezzi A. Sclerosing foam in the treatment of varicose veins and telangiectases: history and analysis of safety and complications. Dermatol Surg 2002; 28: 11–15.

6 Ultrasound guidance for therapeutic interventions

John Bergan and Van Le Cheng

Introduction

Duplex ultrasound sonography is the best choice for evaluation of venous reflux in the lower extremities.[1] It is inexpensive, noninvasive, and generally acceptable to the patient.[2] It provides direct visualization, localization and quantitation of venous reflux with a surprisingly high sensitivity (95%) and specificity (100%).[3] Duplex ultrasound findings have been confirmed by angioscopic observation of incompetent vein valves in advanced chronic venous insufficiency.[4] Yamaki has demonstrated that high peak reflux velocities (>30 cm/s), reflux duration greater than 3 s and an enlarged valve annulus measured by duplex ultrasonography at the saphenofemoral junction are all closely related to angioscopically deformed and incompetent terminal valves (types III and IV of Hoshino).

Foam sclerotherapy actually began before the development of ultrasound imaging. Phlebologists of the 1950s developed ways of producing foamed sclerosants and observed the distribution of therapeutic foam by sensing crepitus.[5] However, all credit for the origination of foam sclerotherapy, as we know it today, goes to Juan Cabrera of Granada, Spain. It was he who combined the manufacture of fine foam with administration of the agent under ultrasound guidance.[6,7]

Pretreatment assessment

The evaluation should always begin with confirmation of the medical history. A family and personal venous history are of great importance. In the personal history, the reasons for the treatment should be confirmed. The patient's view of the objectives of the procedure should be recorded. Symptoms such as aching heaviness, limb fatigue, itching and burning pain are typically present and these should be recorded. Similarly, a detailed recording of previous treatments and their failure will be of importance in seeking insurance coverage for the intervention. History of pregnancies and their number, as well as the number of deliveries and abortions, are of importance. Any limb trauma, fractures and confining illnesses should be recorded. A history of deep venous thrombosis and treatment must be paired with its method of diagnosis. A detailed description of previous venous treatments must be a part of the treatment record. Comorbidities, allergies and pharmacologic history must be documented. The body mass index is calculated from the patient's height and weight and should be recorded.

If a proper, standing, duplex reflux examination has not been done or is not part of the patient's record, it should be accomplished before treatment is initiated. The patient should be examined in a standing position for procedural planning, identification of the venous access site, and its relation to perforating veins, varicosities, and areas of tortuosity, stenosis or dilation.

In this preparatory phase, some anatomic landmarks should be clearly recognizable, including the femoral vein, saphenofemoral junction, saphenous compartment, great saphenous vein (GSV) and the variable small saphenous junction anatomy. This should be supplemented by cold light transillumination of the skin with a bright white light such as the "vein light," to identify reticular veins. A hand-held Doppler can serve to perform a confirmatory screening examination if a proper pretreatment reflux examination is part of the record.

Three levels of pathologic veins are evaluated using the methods just mentioned. Telangiectasias in the skin are visually inspected, reticular veins are transilluminated with the vein light, and varicosities and the saphenous veins with ultrasound. Clinical data should be integrated into the CEAP classification.[8,9.]

Equipment

The duplex ultrasound scanner should be able to detect blood flow rates as low as 6 cm/s. Dedicated high-resolution vascular scanners with color and/or power Doppler functions as well as the continuous-wave Doppler are available. Linear transducers in the range of 4–7 MHz are used for the pretreatment as well as the definitive examination.[10] The inferior vena cava, pelvic veins and deep veins of the limbs in obese patients may be imaged with lower-frequency, 3 MHz transducers. Linear hockey-stick transducers in the range of 5–12 MHz will provide detailed imaging of smaller veins and perforating veins.

After the year 2000, advances in technology allowed duplex ultrsound scanners to become smaller, more transportable, and more operator friendly.[10] These miniaturized devices feature transducers designed with advanced architecture that allow a single probe to image across a greater range of depths within an application and across applications. Thus, in many ways, the portable ultrasound instrument supplements the stethoscope in patient evaluation. The transducer for peripheral vascular examinations operates from 5 to 10 MHz and provides resolution from the skin surface to 7 cm in depth. The technology incorporates power Doppler sonography, tissue harmonic imaging and direct connectivity to a personal computer (Figure 6.1). The overall performance of miniaturized ultrasound devices is comparable to that of the more traditional and much larger ultrasound equipment that allowed establishment and growth of the vascular laboratory.

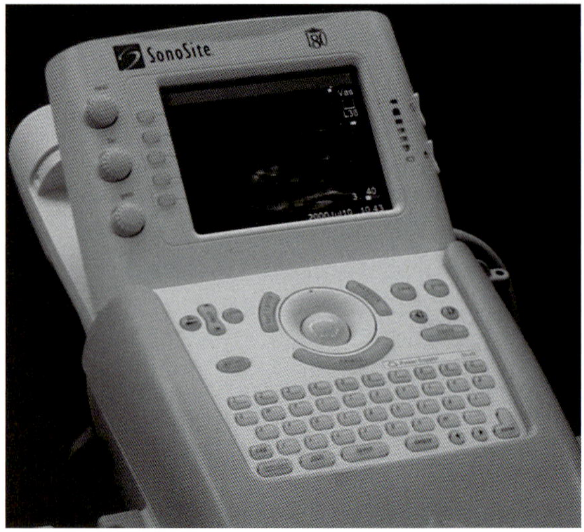

Figure 6.1 This portable ultrasound instrument operates from 5 to 10 MHz and incorporates power Doppler sonography with tissue harmonic imaging. This is useful for preprocedural, intraprocedural and postprocedural monitoring

Venous testing and mapping

Not only is a detailed duplex ultrasound study of the normal and pathologic venous anatomy essential, but a map should be created to guide therapy. A detailed verbal description of the examination and its findings is useful for record purposes, but the map is most useful during therapy. A clear and illustrative graphic notation of significant vein diameters, anomalous anatomy, superficial venous aneurysms, perforating veins, and presence and extent of reflux should always be recorded during the examination.

As mentioned, the ultrasound examination is conducted with the patient standing.[11,12] This position has been found to maximally dilate leg veins, and challenges vein valves. Sensitivity and specificity in detecting reflux are increased in examinations performed with patient standing rather than when the patient is supine. Supine examinations for reflux are unacceptable.

The veins are scanned by moving the probe vertically up and down along their course. Transverse scans are most informative, but a mental reconstruction must be created to record the venous map. Duplicated segments, sites of tributary confluence, large perforating veins and their deep venous connections are identified, as well as the very common superficial venous aneurysms. Location of abnormalities as measured in "centimeters from the floor" assists in preparing a therapeutic guide. Measurements from the medial malleolus are commonly recorded, but are not as precise. Transverse and longitudinal scans combined with continuous scanning provide a clear mapping of the venous system.

Patency of peripheral veins is usually assessed by compression of the vein with the transducer. Residual ancient thrombus, partial patency and extrinsic compression should all be noted in the verbal description of findings. Reflux is detected by flow augmentation with compression and release maneuvers of the thigh and calf. The Valsalva maneuver is used only at the saphenofemoral junction, because presence of a competent proximal valve negates the value of the examination.

Automated rapid inflation and deflation cuffs have been used, but are cumbersome. However, they do offer the advantage of a standardized stimulus,[13,14] which allows timing of reflux. Although reflux greater than 500 ms is considered pathologic,[15] this is only precisely accurate when a standard stimulus is applied.

The diameter of the saphenofemoral junction and femoral vein are recorded in preparation for radiofrequency VNUS Closure® and endovenous laser ablation.[16] Important information is also gained from diameters of the GSV at mid-thigh and distal thigh (Figure 6.2a). Radiofrequency ablation is commonly used to treat veins from 2 to 12 mm in diameter, although diameters recorded with the patient standing do not apply when treatment is given with the patient supine (Figure 6.2a, b).

The supragenicular, infragenicular or immediate subgenicular GSVs are often the access point for introduction of sclerosant foam.[17] Therefore the depth of the GSV in these regions should be recorded.

Accessory saphenous veins by definition run parallel to the GSV in the thigh.[18] It is imperative to map their course accurately and to note their communication with varices and eventual communication with GSVs, as well as their presence or absence of reflux with relationship to varicosities (Figure 6.3). The accessory veins are easily confused with the GSV during continuous longitudinal scanning when the saphenous vein appears to leave the saphenous compartment. This error is avoided when transverse scans are done. The GSV is scanned throughout the leg and the thigh so that its tributaries are identified.

The diameters of the popliteal vein and the small saphenous vein (SSV) are recorded at the junction, as well as diameters of the SSV along its course in the leg. Intersaphenous veins should be identified and the extreme variability of the SSV termination carefully recorded.

The pretreatment venous reflux examination also includes the mapping of exit and re-entry perforating veins (PVs), wherever they are identified.[19] PV reflux is detected as outward flow duration greater than 350 ms during the release phase of the flow augmentation maneuver (distal compression has higher sensitivity in detecting PV reflux; Figure 6.4). PVs should be accu-

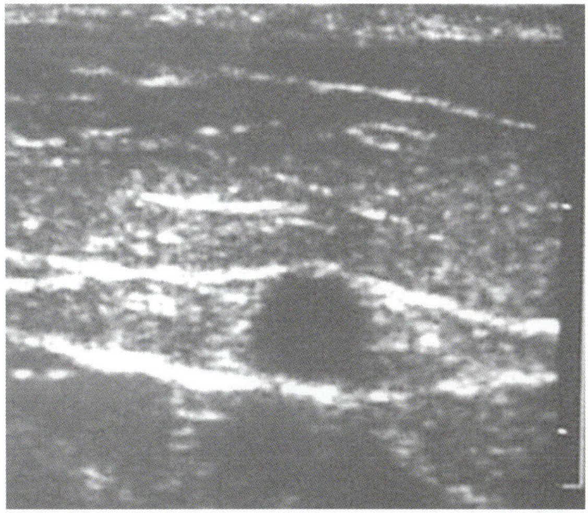

(a)

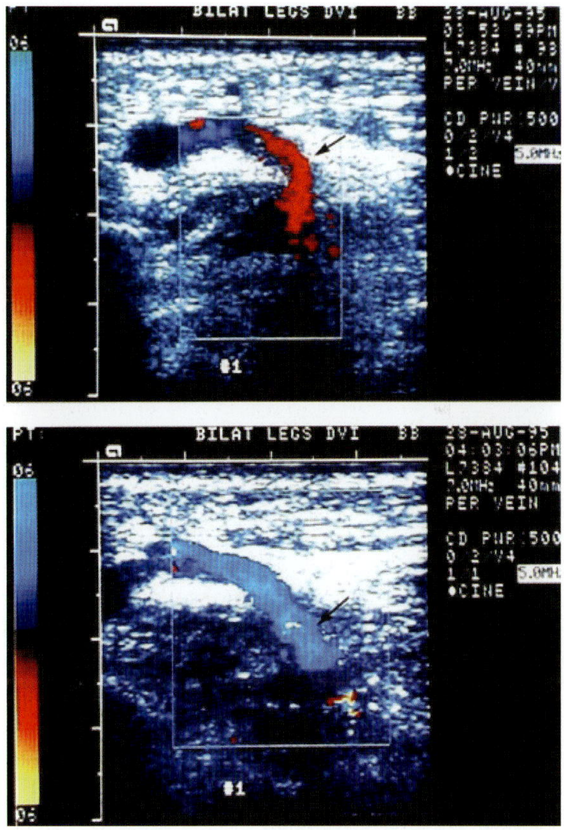

(b)

Figure 6.2 (a) Transverse view of the saphenous vein was introduced and popularized by ultrasound scanning. It was never a part of the teaching of gross anatomy. (b) Typical configuration of perforating veins and their response to compression and release maneuvers. Direction of flow is best perceived in real time

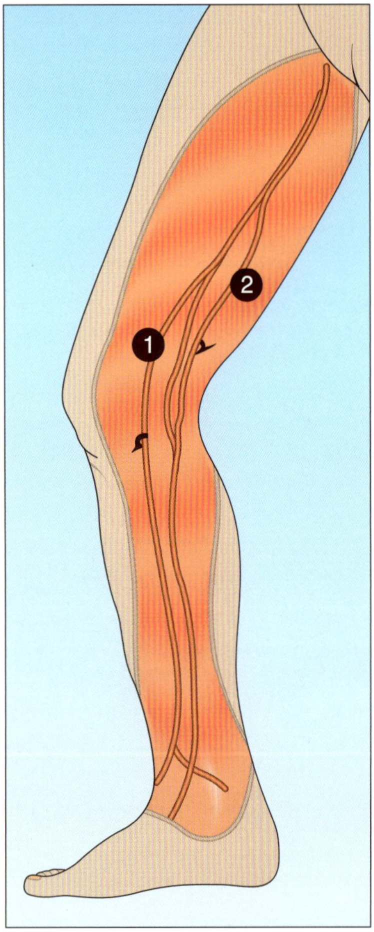

Figure 6.3 Common superficial venous pattern: (1) great saphenous vein, (2) accessory saphenous vein, which is commonly the source of reflux of calf varicosities. Note that it is not a branch of the saphenous vein but is a tributary to it

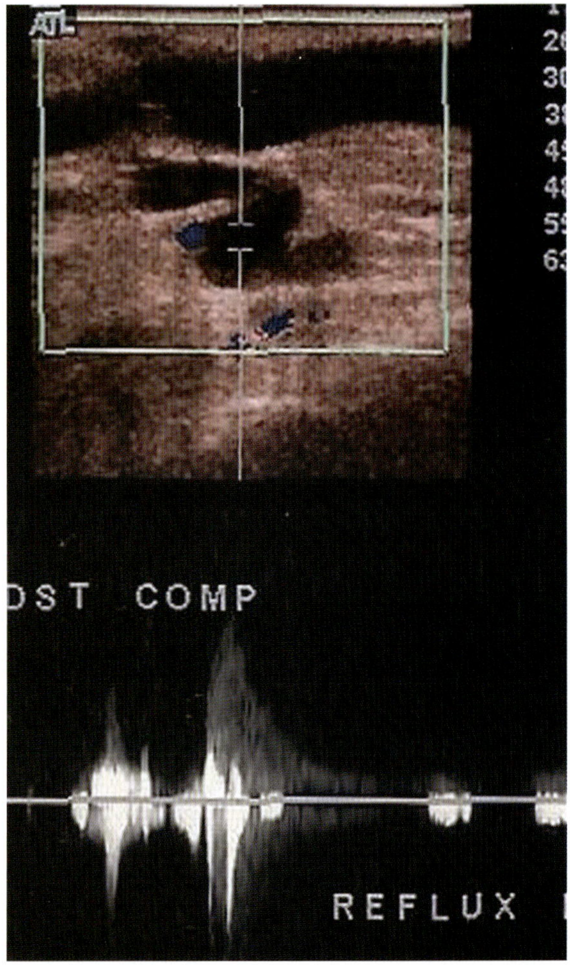

Figure 6.4 Judging between normal and pathologic perforating veins by ultrasound criteria is still imperfect. However, if during compression the flow (in red) is outward and the overlying skin is atrophic and hyperpigmented, the visualized perforating vein should probably be interrupted. Augmentation maneuver

rately mapped in their different locations in the leg, and their positions should be measured as distances (cm) from the floor.[20]

Ultrasound monitoring during sclerofoam treatment

The advent of foam sclerotherapy has added a powerful tool for treatment of chronic venous insufficiency. Endothermic coagulation is caused by the generation of heat, which is applied to the endothelial surface of targeted veins. Sclerosant foam has a similar end result: stripping off the endothelium. Foam agents provoke endothelial damage by several mechanisms.[21] They change the surface tension of the plasma membrane (detergents) and/or the intravascular pH and osmolarity. The final result is a chemical fibrosis of the treated vessel.

The endovenous techniques accomplish this by heat. It is been suggested that the coagulation process is related to the intravascular vaporization of blood (steam) during laser therapy, with intimal denudation and collagen fiber contraction. Vein wall thickening and rapid reorganization of the vessel to form a fibrotic cord follows. If the endothelium is destroyed, the targeted vein is closed permanently. Venous occlusion is usually visualized within 10–20 s of the electromagnetic or chemical stimulus. Both thermal and the chemical techniques have been proven to be safe and effective.[22] Percutaneous introduction of foam, laser fiber and the RF catheter have made surgical intervention obsolete because of elimination of post-treatment pain, absence of cutaneous incisions and prevention of postprocedural disability (Figure 6.5).

Sclerosing foams, as described elsewhere in the book, are mixtures of gas and a liquid solution with surfactant properties. One of the intrinsic limits of liquid sclerosants in treatment of varicose veins is their dilution by blood, with reduction of their efficacy. Also, they are rapidly cleared by the moving blood stream. Sclerosing foams do not mix with blood, and instead remain in the vessel, where they strip off the endothelium. Persistence of the agent in the vessel causes an increased contact time with the intimal surface. Foam preparation is remarkably simple. The Tessari method is the most commonly used,[23] but there is an increasing use of physiological gases as a substitute for room air.

As with endovenous ablation, the treatment starts with clear ultrasound mapping as described above. The GSV or the SSV can then be directly cannulated with an angiocath, an echogenic Cook® needle or a butterfly needle.[24] Nearly all descriptions of the technique explain direct ultrasound-guided access to the saphenous vein. In contrast, many experienced operators achieve a satisfactory and rapid obliteration of the GSV and SSV by cannulating a peripheral varicosity.[24] Although the saphenous vein cannot be cannulated with a catheter by way of a varicosity, because of its angle of connection, there is no such obstacle to the flow of foam.

Foam functions as an efficient ultrasound contrast medium because of its air content. Its injection is easily monitored. Its ultrasound appearance is that of a solid hyperechogenic core with an accompanying acoustic shadow.

Foam is introduced into a varix or the saphenous vein with the patient supine. As the foam reaches the saphenofemoral junction as monitored by ultrasound, compression of the saphenofemoral or the saphenopopliteal junctions may be done in order to preserve foam in the limb. Such a maneuver does not prevent foam from reaching the systemic circulation, however.

Vasoconstriction and vasospasm in foam-filled veins can be induced by intermittent compression of the veins by the ultrasound transducer and by elevating the limb. This minimizes the blood content of the treated veins. Foam will be seen by ultrasound to flow distally in the elevated limb. As mentioned, it flows selectively through incompetent valves and is blocked by competent valves. Femoral vein compression and leg elevation have the

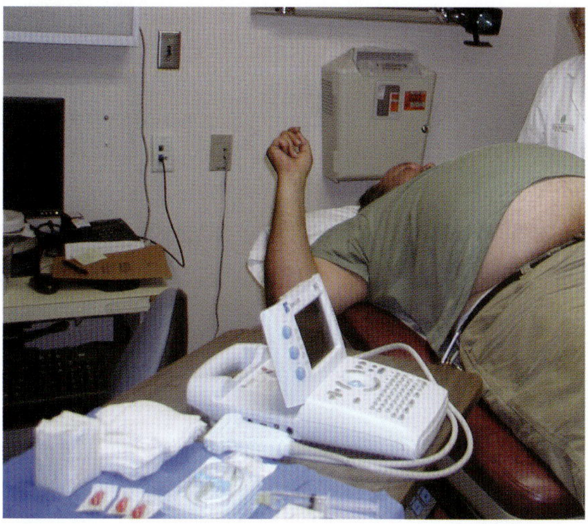

Figure 6.5 Advent of foam sclerotherapy has allowed treatment of some patients who would have been refused general, regional and even local anesthesia. Note the simple layout of equipment for foam sclerotherapy

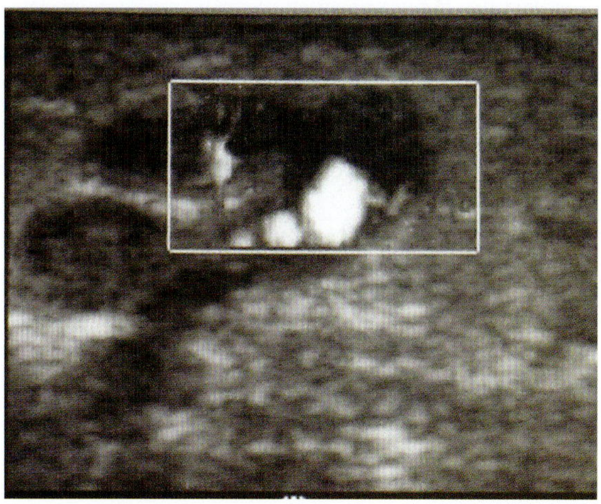

Figure 6.6 As other adverse events have been eliminated, skin discoloration remains a major deterrent to acceptance of foam sclerotherapy. It is usually accompanied by patent venous channels as shown here. These should be closed by repeat injections under ultrasound guidance

effect of prolonging the action of the foamed sclerosant on the distal intima, improving the efficacy of the entire treatment. In addition, leg elevation for 5–10 minutes allows the foam to revert to its liquid state, so that foam particles will not reach the right atrium or a patent foramen ovale.

The femoral, popliteal and deep veins of the leg are scanned intermittently throughout the entire procedure. Foam particles are washed out of deep veins such as the gastrocnemius or tibial veins by flexion–extension maneuvers of the foot. Repetitive dorsiflexion of the foot completely clears the deep veins of any foam particles.

Despite much consternation, major thrombotic events have rarely been described with the use of sclerofoam. In a study of over 12 000 sclerotherapy sessions by Guex, over half of which involved foam, only a single femoral vein thrombus was encountered.[25] Thromboses of the gastrocnemius, tibial and peroneal veins have been reported occasionally, and intra-arterial injections are even rarer.[26]

Ultrasound sonography has confirmed the presence of the tangled network of small varicose veins, reticular varices and incompetent perforating veins under lipodermatosclerotic plaques and under venous ulcers. Ultrasound monitoring should confirm the fact that these vessels are filled with foam during treatment.

Ultrasound guidance is also used in treatment of incompetent perforating veins. Direct cannulation and controlled injection can be done easily if the primary treatment has failed to heal an ulcer or improve the condition of lipodermatosclerosis.[6] Often, superficial peripheral veins can be directly injected with the objective of obliterating the attached perforator and its network of the incompetent veins.

Post-treatment assessment

Early post-treatment duplex scanning should be performed. This is best done at 1 and 7 days postprocedure, looking for deep venous thrombosis. Many have eliminated the 1-day examination because deep venous thrombosis is uncommon. Successful obliteration of the saphenous vein is confirmed by its contraction to a residual diameter of <2 mm. Patencies of the common femoral artery and vein are confirmed by ultrasound. Any thrombus generated by the manipulations can be seen as a hyperechogenic core. Even though thrombus protruding into the femoral vein is thought to be benign, evidence of a protruding thrombus from the saphenous vein into the femoral vein should be looked for in every postprocedural examination. Evidence of a noncompressible GSV with thickened walls and absence of flow on color ultrasound analysis are signs of successful obliteration. However, partial closure may be accompanied by skin discoloration.

Discussion

Compression therapy and surgery have been the cornerstone of chronic venous insufficiency treatment for years but are of diminishing importance. New minimally invasive techniques including radiofrequency ablation of saphenous veins, endovenous laser therapy and venous ablation with sclerofoam have been demonstrated to be safe, effective and more acceptable to the patient. The contribution of ultrasound in general, and duplex technology in particular, has given reliability to the diagnosis of chronic venous insufficiency and has enhanced the development of minimally invasive treatments. Intraprocedural and postprocedural duplex ultrasound monitoring provides the best control of the entire procedure. This ensures early prevention of complications and minimizes the chance of failure.

Conclusion

Duplex ultrasound sonography is essential in every phase of patient care for chronic venous insufficiency, and has played a pivotal role in the recent revolution in venous therapy. Experience, critical thinking, uniform testing and insight into the pathologic process are necessary to achieve satisfactory results.

References

1. Labropoulos N, Leon LR Jr. Duplex evaluation of venous insufficiency. Semin Vasc Surg 2005; 18: 5–9.
2. Ballard J, Bergan J, DeLange M. Venous imaging for reflux using duplex ultrasonography. In: AbuRahma A, Bergan J, eds. Noninvasive Vascular Diagnosis. London: Springer-Verlag, 2000: 329–34.
3. Depalma RG, Kowallek DL, Barcia TC, Cafferata HT. Target selection for surgical intervention in severe chronic venous insufficiency: comparison of duplex scanning and phlebography. J Vasc Surg 2000; 32: 913–20.

4. Yamaki T, Sasaki K, Nozaki M. Preoperative duplex-derived parameters and angioscopic evidence of valvular incompetence associated with superficial venous insufficiency. J Endovasc Ther 2002; 9: 229–33.
5. Flückiger P. Nicht-operative retrograde Varicenverödung mit Varsylschaum. Schweiz Med Wochenschr 1956; 48: 1368–70.
6. Cabrera J, Redondo P, Becerra A, et al. Ultrasound-guided injection of polidocanol microfoam in the management of leg ulcers. Arch Dermatol 2004; 148: 667–73.
7. Cabrera, J. Dr J Cabrera is the creator of the patented polidocanol microfoam. Dermatol Surg 2004; 30: 1605; author reply 1606.
8. Kistner RL, Eklof B, Masuda EM. Diagnosis of chronic venous disease of the lower extremities: the "CEAP" classification. Mayo Clin Proc 1996; 71: 338–45.
9. Eklof B, Rutherford RB, Bergan JJ, et al. Revision of the CEAP classification for chronic venous disorders: consensus statement. J Vasc Surg 2004; 40: 1248–52.
10. Mekenas L, Bergan J. Venous reflux examination: technique using miniaturized ultrasound scanning. J Vasc Tech 2002; 2: 139–46.
11. Lynch TG, Dalsing MC, Ouriel K, et al. Developments in diagnosis and classification of venous disorders: non-invasive diagnosis. Cardiovasc Surg 1999; 7: 160–78.
12. Labropoulos N, Tiongson J, Pryor L, et al. Definition of venous reflux in lower-extremity veins. J Vasc Surg 2003; 38: 793–8.
13. Masuda EM, Kistner RL, Eklof B. Prospective study of duplex scanning for venous reflux: comparison of Valsalva and pneumatic cuff techniques in the reverse Trendelenburg and standing positions. J Vasc Surg 1994; 20: 711–20.
14. Markel A, Meissner MH, Manzo RA, et al. A comparison of the cuff deflation method with Valsalva's maneuver and limb compression in detecting venous valvular reflux. Arch Surg 1994; 129: 701–5.
15. Vasdekis SN, Clarke GH, Nicolaides AN. Quantification of venous reflux by means of duplex scanning. J Vasc Surg 1989; 10: 670–7.
16. Sadick NS. Advances in the treatment of varicose veins: ambulatory phlebectomy, foam sclerotherapy, endovascular laser, and radiofrequency closure. Dermatol Clin 2005; 23: 443–55.
17. Bergan JJ, Pascarella L. Severe chronic venous insufficiency: primary treatment with sclerofoam. Semin Vasc Surg 2005; 18: 49–56.
18. Caggiati A, Bergan JJ, Gloviczki P, et al. Nomenclature of the veins of the lower limbs: an international interdisciplinary consensus statement. J Vasc Surg 2002; 36: 416–22.
19. Delis KT, Husmann M, Kalodiki E, et al. In situ hemodynamics of perforating veins in chronic venous insufficiency. J Vasc Surg 2001; 33: 773–82.
20. Caggiati A, Bergan JJ, Gloviczki P, et al. Nomenclature of the veins of the lower limb: extensions, refinements, and clinical application. J Vasc Surg 2005; 41: 719–24.
21. Goldman M. Mechanisms of action of sclerotherapy. In: Goldman MP, ed. Sclerotherapy: Treatment of Varicose and Telangiectatic Leg Veins, 2nd edn. St Louis, MO: Mosby, 1995: 244–79.
22. Bergan J, Pascarella L. Severe chronic venous insufficiency: primary treatment with sclerofoam. Semin Vasc Surg 2005; 18: 49–56.
23. Tessari L, Cavezzi A, Frullini A. Preliminary experience with a new sclerosing foam in the treatment of varicose veins. Dermatol Surg 2001; 27: 58–60.
24. Coleridge Smith P. Saphenous ablation: sclerosant or sclerofoam? Semin Vasc Surg 2005; 18: 19–24.
25. Guex JJ, Allaert FA, Gillet JL, Chleir F. Immediate and midterm complications of sclerotherapy: report of a prospective multicenter registry of 12 173 sclerotherapy sessions. Dermatol Surg 2005; 31: 123–8; discussion 128.
26. Bergan JJ, Weiss RA, Goldman MP. Extensive tissue necrosis following high-concentration sclerotherapy for varicose veins. Dermatol Surg 2000; 26: 535–41; discussion 541–2.

7 A personal method for foam sclerotherapy: technique and results

Philip D Coleridge Smith

Introduction

Sclerotherapy has been used to treat varicose veins for 150 years. A detailed review of the history of this subject has been published[1] and is covered in Chapter 1 of this book. In the 1980s, ultrasound was introduced for the diagnosis of venous disease of the lower limb. In France, where enthusiasm for the use of sclerotherapy was well established, Schadeck and Vin improved the efficacy of their treatment by using ultrasound imaging to guide injections into incompetent saphenous trunks.[2,3] This method of treatment was found to achieve obliteration of the saphenous trunks in a substantial proportion of patients, resulting in long-term relief from varices. As with conventional sclerotherapy, the problem of recanalization of veins was encountered in up to one quarter of patients at 1 year.[4] Proponents of sclerotherapy argue that even if recurrence occurs, the resulting varices and incompetent saphenous trunk are easily managed by further sessions of sclerotherapy.

In 1944, Orbach described the "air block" technique. A small volume of air is included in the syringe with the sclerosant. The air is injected ahead of the sclerosant in order to prevent blood diluting the sclerosant and reducing its efficacy. In 1950, Orbach published a further paper describing the use of a foam that he created by vigorously shaking a syringe containing air and sclerosant to produce a froth.[5]

The next significant advance came in 1993, when Cabrera suggested that foam could be created using carbon dioxide mixed with polidocanol, a detergent sclerosant.[6] Cabrera published a further article in 1997 describing his experience in 261 limbs with long saphenous varices and 8 patients with vascular malformations.[7] He had used sclerotherapy with foam, guiding his injections by ultrasound imaging. Some of the varicose veins reached 20 mm in diameter. He considered that foam greatly extended the range of vein sizes that could be managed by sclerotherapy. He felt that the increased efficacy of foam was attributable to it displacing blood from the treated vein and increasing the contact time between the sclerosant and the vein. He used a "microfoam," that is, a foam made of very small bubbles that was created by the use of a small rapidly rotating brush. This distinguished his foam from the "froth" made by Orbach.

I have used the method of sclerotherapy described below with improvements developed over the last 7 years. The aim is to treat patients over the fewest possible sessions and fits the expectations of patients from the United Kingdom as well as the medical insurance companies.

Patient selection–indications and contraindications

Suitability of a patient for foam sclerotherapy depends on the aims of treatment as well as the venous anatomy demonstrated by duplex ultrasonography. Foam sclerotherapy can be carried out successfully in almost any patient with clinically significant venous disease, no matter how elderly, frail, obese or ill that patient is. In patients with leg ulcers, more aggressive treatment may be indicated or more ambitious treatment (very large varices) than in those seeking cosmetic improvement. The adverse factors shown in Table 7.1 are not (in the author's experience) absolute contraindications to treatment, but should be taken into consideration when deciding on whether or not to treat a patient. Only the absolute

Table 7.1 Relative and absolute contraindications to treatment

Adverse patient factors
Morbid obesity (body mass index >30)
Extreme age or frailty
Severe concomitant disease (malignancy, cardiovascular, respiratory)
Known thrombophilia or history of previous deep vein thrombosis
"Needle-phobic" patients or those preferring treatment under general anaesthesia
Very thin patients may be left with lumps where the veins were obliterated following sclerotherapy, and are less suitable for treatment
Adverse venous anatomy
Severe post-thrombotic damage in the deep veins (little advantage of treating varicose veins)
Very large varices (more complications of skin pigmentation and lumps following treatment)
The lesion is an arteriovenous malformation (more difficult to treat)
Absolute contraindications to treatment
Severe allergy to sclerosants.
Obliteration of deep vein system (e.g., following extensive previous deep vein thrombosis with no recanalization of deep veins)

contraindications of severe allergy and obliterated deep veins prevent any treatment being performed.

Patient consent

Patients should be fully informed of the method of treatment as well as the complications that may arise. In general, it is best to provide written information (or reference to a website) during an initial consultation and perform the treatment on a separate occasion. Return for treatment on a separate occasion is good evidence of consent. Some surgeons like to ask patients to sign a consent form, but it is more important to record that the patient has received standard written advice, covering methods of treatment, management after treatment and common problems during follow-up. My patient information warns of the lumps and skin pigmentation, but since I have never seen extensive skin ulceration, this is not mentioned. Visual disturbance, chest tightness and coughing occur occasionally and are included. Deep vein thrombosis is also mentioned, as is severe allergy, although these are very uncommon. I support this information with a website reference to more extensive information.

Patients on whom to begin a sclerotherapy practice

When I am teaching others how to use ultrasound-guided foam sclerotherapy, I suggest that the easiest varices to manage are those in patients with moderate-size great or small saphenous trunks (5–8 mm in diameter) who have never been treated previously. In general, the saphenous trunks are straight and easy to canulate and the varices are not very extensive. Patients with recurrent varices following previous surgery are more difficult, especially if several operations have been performed in the past. Residual nontortuous saphenous trunks are relatively easy to canulate, but very tortuous recurrent vessels near the saphenofemoral junction (SFJ) and saphenopopliteal junction (SPJ) need significant previous experience.

Ultrasound-guided canulation

I treat saphenous trunks and major tributaries through an intravenous canula or butterfly needle. There are two groups of reasons for this: the first is safety. It is easy to check that a vein is being injected (not an artery), that there is no extravasation when injecting some saline prior to sclerotherapy and that the saline emerges in the correct vessel following injection. Second, I try to treat most veins in a limb in one session, which patients and healthcare providers in the United Kingdom find desirable. Once sclerosant foam is injected into a limb, it reaches many veins, making further canulation difficult because the needle cannot be identified in the vein lumen. Placing needles or a canula in most veins before putting in any foam makes treatment much easier. Superficial varices do not need ultrasound guidance and can be treated by direct needle injection without prejudicing safety or efficacy. Once all trunks and major tributaries have been canulated, the limb can be elevated to empty the veins and maximize efficacy. Foam can then be injected into all veins requiring treatment without any further difficulty.

Ultrasound venous canulation is difficult for beginners but with practice becomes much easier. I prefer to scan the vein in transverse section, but it is essential to track the tip of the needle (only) when using this method. I regularly inject veins of 1 mm diameter and less using this strategy, and find that it is the most effective. Canulation of a straight section of vein is the easiest, but this can be difficult to find in cases of recurrent varices. In primary great saphenous vein (GSV) incompetence, the best place is just above the knee (for the thigh section) and in the mid-calf when treating calf varices. In primary small saphenous vein (SSV) reflux, the best place is 10–15 cm below the SPJ. I inject local anesthetic for insertion of an 18 g canula but use no anesthetic for 23–30-gauge needles.

Foam preparation

At present there is no commercial foam, and the majority of phlebologists prepare foam from either polidocanol (Sclerovein, Resinag, Zurich; Aethoxysclerol, Kreussler, Germany) or sodium tetradecyl sulphate (STS) (Fibrovein, STD Pharmaceuticals, Hereford, United Kingdom; Sotradecol). The most widely used method is the Tessari technique, in which 1 part of sclerosant and 4 parts of air are mixed by passing the components between two syringes connected together (Figure 7.1).

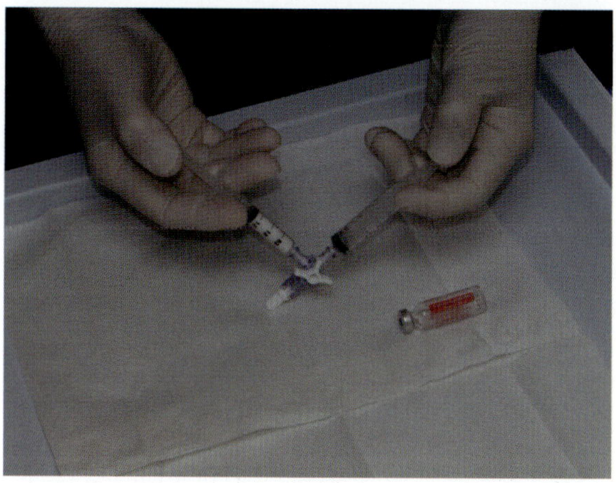

Figure 7.1 Preparation of sclerosant foam using the Tessari technique

Carbon dioxide-based foams

Since the case of "stroke" reported by Forlee et al from Professor Greg Shanik's department in Dublin,[8] there has been an increase in the anxiety level of sclerotherapists about using air to inject veins. There is accumulating scientific evidence that the use of carbon dioxide (CO_2) foams reduces the number of post-treatment episodes of visual disturbance and coughing. CO_2 is much more soluble in blood and water than nitrogen (in air) and is less likely to travel to more distant organs. However, pure CO_2 makes poor foam, and my current practice is to use a mixture of 70% CO_2 and 30% O_2.

Position of the patient

I position the patient supine before placing any needle or canula, to minimize the risk of syncope. The SSVs are most easily accessed with the patient lying on his or her left side, facing away from the surgeon. The leg to be treated is moved toward the operator as shown in Figure 7.2. For the left GSV, the same position works well. The left lower limb is drawn toward the operator, giving easy access to the medial aspect of the thigh and calf. For the right GSV, the patient lies on his or her right side (Figure 7.3).

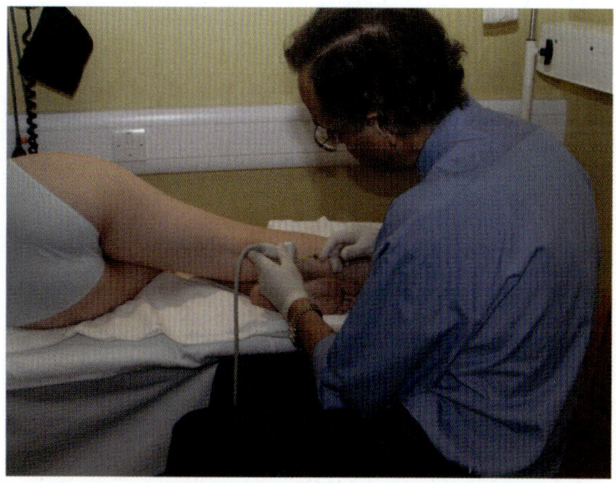

Figure 7.2 The patient lies in the left lateral position, which is comfortable for canulation of the small saphenous veins and left great saphenous vein

Strategy for primary great saphenous vein varices

In those cases where the GSV lies in the saphenous compartment throughout the thigh, I place an 18-gauge canula in the GSV in the lower third of the thigh. This will treat the vein proximal to this level as far as the SFJ.

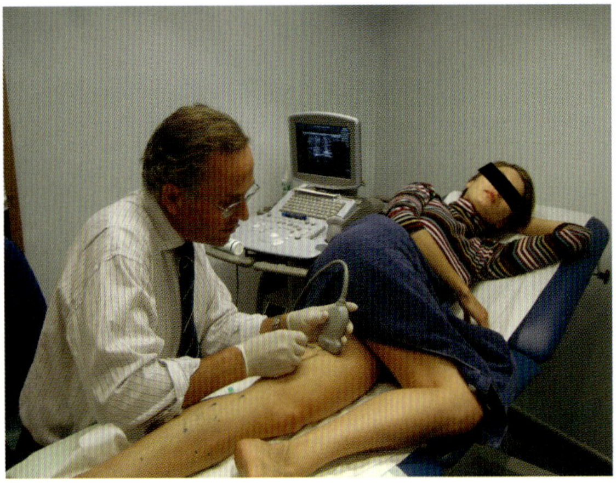

Figure 7.3 The right great saphenous vein can be canulated with the patient lying in the right lateral position

If the GSV lies more superficially in part of its track, this is strictly speaking an accessory vein and *not* the main saphenous trunk. It is better to inject less strong sclerosants here. In these cases I place an 18-gauge canula in the saphenous trunk where it lies within the saphenous fascia. I then place a butterfly in the superficial accessory vein, usually in the distal third of the thigh. I treat any further accessory veins in the region of the GSV by placing further butterflies in these. These may be the source of recurrence if left untreated.

I then identify any major tributary of the GSV in the thigh, especially those above the level of canulation of the GSV. Larger tributaries (3 mm diameter and above) may supply enough venous flow to the GSV to keep it open above the level of the junction of the GSV with its tributaries. I usually manage these by direct needle injection with foam.

In the calf I use a 23-gauge butterfly needles to canulate the saphenous trunk and any varices, again inserting all canulae and butterflies before any treatment is commenced. In patients with primary varicose veins, between 2 and 6 canulations are required to treat GSV reflux and associated varices.

Strategy for primary small saphenous vein varices

SSV varices are usually much less complex to treat than GSV varices, since they have fewer tributaries and accessory veins. With the patient lying in the left lateral position, I canulate the SSV in the mid-calf region using an 18-gauge canula. This avoids making an injection in the "tiger country" of the popliteal fossa and then injecting foam close to the popliteal vein. I use a 23-gauge butterfly to treat the distal SSV. Varices can be managed using a further butterfly or by direct needle injection. I usually employ two or three canulations for the management of SSV varices.

Combined great and small saphenous vein reflux

For patients in whom both the GSV and SSV are incompetent, I canulate both veins in order to treat the two saphenous trunks in one session. More limited treatment of superficial varices may be required to minimize the number of canulations and volume of foam injected during the first treatment session.

Incompetent perforating veins

In the calf, most incompetent perforating veins can be managed by canulation of a superficial vein immediately fed from the perforator. This works for ankle (Cockett's) perforators as well as more proximal paratibial perforating veins. I prefer to use 3% STS in liquid form for medial calf perforators to avoid producing thrombosis in the posterior tibial veins. I use foam for proximal calf perforating veins, popliteal fossa perforators and perforating veins in the thigh. In the popliteal fossa, I place a canula within the perforator so that the tip of the canula lies at or near the fascial opening. For medial thigh perforating veins, I canulate with an 18-gauge canula to ensure reliable injection of the source of varices.

Treatment–injecting the foam

I start by injecting any superficial varices with 1% sclerosant foam using a syringe and a 30- or 25-gauge needle. I use 1 mL per injection and distribute the foam to varices near the point of injection by massaging the leg with the ultrasound probe or by hand. Next I treat all the previously placed butterflies and canulae. I elevate the leg well above the heart to minimize the diameter of the veins – this achieves Fegan's "empty vein" requirement, although it is not universally used by sclerotherapists (Figure 7.4). I inject no more than 2 mL of foam at a time, even into the largest veins. In small veins in the calf, I usually inject 1 mL at a time.

After each injection of foam, I ask the patient to perform a series of ankle dorsiflexions to clear any foam that has reached the deep veins. Foam always reaches the deep veins within a few moments of injection. There is significant difference of opinion amongst phlebologists over this point, some recommending that the patient lies very still after injection of foam. My own experience is that occasional calf vein thrombosis, seen in the earlier part of my clinical experience, is now a rare occurrence following frequent dorsiflexions by the patient during treatment.

I make further injections of 1–2 mL of foam into each needle and canula to reinforce the treatment already given. This strategy results in the veins being treated and then re-treated. Re-treatment has been suggested by French and Italian phlebologists as a method of achieving more effective sclerosis of veins than a single injection. The first injection produces spasm of the treated vein and facilitates the passage of foam to more proximal veins with the subsequent injections.

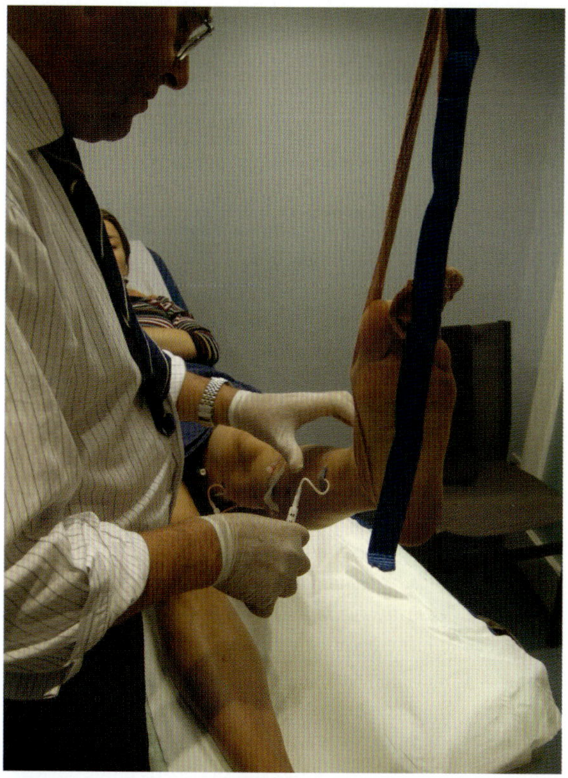

Figure 7.4 Once all butterflies and canulae have been inserted, the limb is elevated and foam injected

Then I move to the next more proximal injection site and inject some foam, asking the patient to dorsiflex at the ankle after each injection. The last vein to be treated is the GSV in the thigh, for which I use 2 mL of 3% STS foam, repeating this twice more making sure the patient dorsiflexes between each one. I monitor the extent of spread of the foam using duplex ultrasonography and discontinue injection at any site where extravasation of foam is seen. Butterflies work well but sometimes cut through the side of the vein The development of spasm in treated veins is widely regarded as a measure of success following sclerotherapy of a vein.

The total amount of foam required to treat the GSV in the thigh is usually 6 mL, or 8 mL if it is a large vein. In the calf section of the GSV, 2–4 mL of 1% STS foam is sufficient. In the SSV, 4–6 mL of 3% STS foam is required, depending on the size of the vein. Additional foam is required for accessory veins and varices. In perforating veins other than the medial ankle (Cockett's) perforators, I use 2–4 mL of 3% foam. Robust treatment of perforators is required to achieve a permanent result. For medial calf perforators connecting directly to the posterior tibial vein, I use 1 mL of 3% liquid STS.

Compression following sclerotherapy

I bandage the treated limb for 7–14 days using a short-stretch cohesive bandage (PehaHaft, Hartmann, Germany). I employ eccentric compression by placing a roll of "bubble-wrap" covered in Tubigauze between the layers of the bandage to increase compression over the treated veins. I apply a complete 20 m roll full-leg bandage after treating the GSV. I start proximally at the thigh and apply a very loose layer, leaving a small gap at the knee. The direction is reversed once the ankle is reached, and the "bubble-wrap" roll is incorporated in the next layer, using the marks over the saphenous trunks and varices as guidance. Foam rubber pads have traditionally been used for this purpose. A final, third layer is applied from the thigh to the ankle, finishing at the ankle. This strategy allows the stocking, which will be applied next, to slide more easily over the layers of the bandage. The bandage is secured with Medipore (3M Company, United States) 100 mm wide adhesive tape and covered with a class 2 compression stocking over all of this. The compression regime should be repeated after each treatment session.

Follow-up sessions

I usually review patients 2 weeks after their first treatment, which is about optimum for managing the consequences of treatment (Figure 7.5). Patients usually return having removed bandages themselves. I inspect the limb with the patient standing and to identify any obvious residual varices and those with excess retained thrombus. I check the treated trunks, accessory veins and varices using duplex ultrasonography I check for extension of thrombus into the femoral and popliteal veins, although only rarely have I seen this. In the calf, I assess the gastrocnemius veins for thrombus.

Veins have two common appearances at this stage on ultrasonography. The more echogenic (speckly) ones are also the more solid and are firmly obliterated, with resolution well advanced. Some are echolucent, containing liquid thrombus with no evidence of early resolution. This is commonly seen in saphenous trunks and some varices, especially those presenting with residual "lumps."

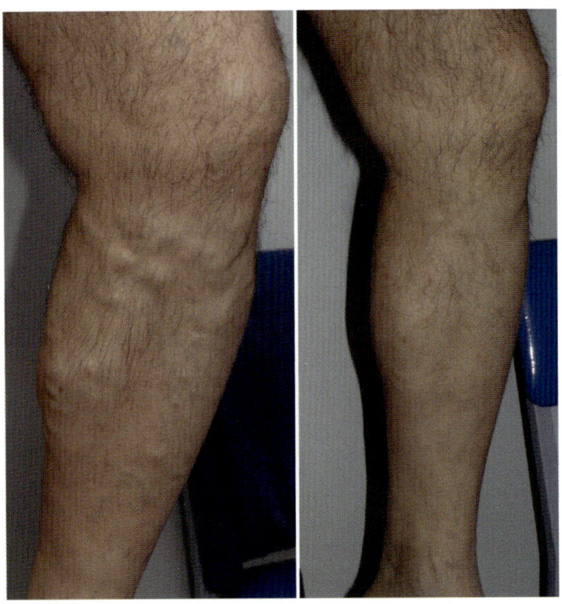

Figure 7.5 Before and 2 weeks after treatment of the left great saphenous vein with ultrasound-guided foam sclerotherapy

I position the patient supine and manage any veins with excessive retained echolucent thrombus. I use a 5 mL syringe and a 21-gauge or 19-gauge needle, which can be guided into saphenous trunks or varices under ultrasound guidance or by palpation. As much thrombus as possible is aspirated to abolish lumps and distended saphenous trunks. This rapidly resolves painful veins and lumps. Thrombophlebitis can be managed in an identical fashion.

If I find any residual segment of vein that should have been closed, then I treat this by direct needle injection, although occasionally I use a canula or butterfly if a major saphenous trunk has remained open. I use the same strategy as before and inject further sclerosant foam in 2 mL aliquots. Re-bandaging the leg in the region of further sclerotherapy is usually appropriate.

Problems

The most frequent problem is thrombophlebitis. This can be managed with compression and analgesia. Affected veins can be drained using a large needle (19-gauge) under ultrasound control and some local anesthesia. If a vein or varix contains a large amount of thrombus, this can be aspirated via a large needle within 1–2 weeks of treatment, and has the advantage that the palpable lump is rapidly removed. After this, the thrombus becomes more solid and incompressible, with increased echogenicity on ultrasound imaging. It is impossible to aspirate this. After 4–8 weeks, echolucency returns to some veins. These appear to be the ones that cause the thrombophlebitis. The thrombus can usually be retrieved with the large needle at this stage, with removal of lumps and any associated discomfort.

I have occasionally injected STS foam outside a vein due to a technical problem with a canula. This resulted in an inflammatory lump at the injection site, which resolved completely over 2 weeks. I have not seen a classical injection ulcer, and these are rarely reported in published work, since ultrasound monitoring of treatment allows discontinuation of injection where extravasation has occurred. Polidocanol is much safer in this respect. It causes no significant problem if injected at low concentrations and amounts outside the vein. Extravascular injection of sclerosant foam usually causes pain. I always check with the patient that my injection is causing no discomfort as a further measure to avoid this problem.

Deep vein thrombosis has been seen occasionally after this treatment, most frequently affecting the calf veins. This should be managed conventionally with compression and exercise or heparin/warfarin anticoagulation if it extends to major veins.

Systemic complications

Visual disturbance occurs in about 2% of patients and is probably dose-related. This occurs following both liquid and foam sclerotherapy, but is more frequent after foam treatments. It occurs most frequently in patients who have a previous history of migraine, but may occur in anyone. A scotoma develops, associated with other visual phenomena such as a ground glass appearance in part of the visual field and irregular coloured patterns. This resolves within 30 minutes in most patients. It is highly likely to return in subsequent sessions of treatment, and we recommend that affected patients lie supine for up to 30 minutes following injection of foam to prevent this problem.

Some patients may develop tightness in the chest or coughing afterwards. I believe that this is a direct effect of the foam on the lungs and can also occur following injections of liquid sclerosant. This also resolves in about 30 minutes. Again lying supine for some time after treatment may be useful. The incidence of visual disturbance and chest symptoms has been reported to be reduced by the use of CO_2 foams.

Allergic reactions may follow injection of either of the sclerosants mentioned here. Appropriate drugs and equipment must be available to manage this problem.

More difficult cases

Patients with recurrent varicose veins following surgery are much easier to manage using foam sclerotherapy than by further surgery. However, they often have few straight veins, and canulation may be more difficult than with primary varicose veins. Patients with recurrence at the SFJ and SPJ can be readily managed by foam sclerotherapy. I place a canula or butterfly fairly close to the junction and inject 4–6 mL of 3% STS foam. Residual varices and segments of saphenous trunk may require the placing of more needles prior to the start of injection in order to ensure that all varices are filled with foam during the treatment. Recanalization of SFJ and SPJ recurrences managed by foam sclerotherapy is no more frequent than following treatment of primary incompetent junctions. This is therefore a very useful strategy in patients who have had many previous operations for varicose veins.

Later follow-up

In reviewing the outcome of foam sclerotherapy in initial series of patients, I found that recanalization was most likely in the first 6–12 months after treatment. My current practice is to review all patients at 6 months after treatment to identify any vein in which recanalization has begun. This is usually on a minor scale, with recanalized channels 2–3 mm in diameter being the norm. These are readily treated by further foam injections, following which permanent obliteration of veins is usually achieved. The most frequently treated veins in my experience are the proximal SSV and GSV in the thigh.

Outcomes of treatment

My own experience of the use of ultrasound-guided foam sclerotherapy is based on an analysis of all patients treated for varicose veins during the period January 2002 to August 2005.[9] A total of 808 patients (666 women, 142 men) were managed by ultrasound-guided foam sclerotherapy for truncal saphenous incompetence. In all, 1411 limbs were affected by varices (CEAP C_1 $n = 212$, 15%; CEAP C_2 $n = 1154$, 82%). Treatments were selected according to the preference of the patients and upon the advice of the author. This was not a randomized study. Patients often requested foam sclerotherapy, since they considered that surgery was excessively invasive, and many of them had previous experience of surgical treatment. Nearly one-third of patients treated for GSV reflux had had previous surgical treatment.

I investigated patients by clinical examination and duplex ultrasonography. Those with isolated saphenous varices and reticular varices are not included in this analysis. All treatments were carried out in a consulting room without sedation or general anesthesia. The methods of treatment were based on those published by Cabrera in which ultrasound-guided canulation of the GSV or SSV is used to deliver foam to the saphenous trunk. Direct needle injection of foam was used to manage superficial varices.

The sclerosants used to prepare the foam were either polidocanol or STS. Polidocanol was used as a 1% solution to create the foam to treat saphenous trunks and STS was used as either a 1% or 3% solution for saphenous trunks. Foam was prepared in a ratio of 0.5 mL of sclerosant to 1.5 mL of air, in keeping with the practice reported in previous publications.

Compression bandaging was applied to limbs where saphenous trunks and varices had been injected. Pehahaft cohesive bandage (Pehahaft®, Hartmann, Germany) was used most often with Velband (Velband®, Johnson & Johnson Medical, Ascot, Berkshire, United Kingdom); cotton wool padding was applied over the saphenous trunks to increase compression. This results in a thin bandage that fits beneath most clothes and shoes. A class 2 medical compression stocking was measured and applied over the bandage to secure the bandage (Credelast®, Credenhill, Ilkeston, Derbyshire, United Kingdom). In the early part of the series, bandaging was applied for 3–5 days, but later in the series this was increased to 10–14 days to minimize the incidence of thrombophlebitis.

Treatment sessions were carried out at intervals of 2 weeks. Duplex ultrasonography was used to check the treated veins for completeness of occlusion and additional segments of saphenous trunk and associated varices were treated as required.

All patients were invited to return for review after 6 months following completion of treatment. Those who did not attend were sent further appointments. Despite this, not all patients attended for follow-up.

Not all venous disease detected on clinical and ultrasound examination underwent ultrasound-guided foam sclerotherapy, since in some limbs clinically insignificant varices were present. Some patients considered that only one limb required treatment. In all, 1109 limbs were managed by foam sclerotherapy. In these limbs, duplex ultrasonography showed that the main cause was GSV or SSV reflux. GSV reflux alone was present in 766 limbs (69%), SSV reflux alone in 223 limbs (20%) and combined GSV and SSV reflux in 120 (11%). A surprisingly high proportion of patients had undergone previous surgery for varicose veins in the vessel being treated ($n = 267$, 30% of GSVs and $n = 60$, 17% of SSVs). The median diameter of the GSVs treated was 5 mm (interquartile range [IQR] 4–6 mm) and for the SSVs 5 mm (IQR 4–6 mm). In this series, 4 limbs were treated in which post-thrombotic damage was found leading to deep vein incompetence in association with GSV or SSV reflux.

Thrombophlebitis occurred in a small number of patients (5%), and was managed by analgesia, compression and aspiration of thrombus. Calf vein thrombosis was confined to isolated gastrocnemius veins or to part of the posterior tibial vein (10 cases). All resolved with compression by stocking or bandage and exercise without use of anticoagulants.

In one case, a short occlusive thrombus arose in the common femoral vein 2 weeks following treatment of the GSV. The mechanism appeared to be due to direct extension of thrombus from the GSV into the femoral vein. This case was managed by anticoagulation using low-molecular-weight heparin and warfarin continued for 6 months. The occluded femoral vein recanalized within 4 weeks, and at 6 months of follow-up no residual scarring or valve damage could be demonstrated on duplex ultrasonography. In two further cases, thrombus extended from the SFJ and SPJ (one case each) into the femoral and popliteal vein. The extent of the thrombus was limited and firmly adherent to the vein wall. This was managed by compression stockings and exercise whilst monitoring the extent of the thrombus by duplex ultrasonography. In these cases, the thrombus resolved without further intervention. No major systemic complication such as anaphylaxis, stroke or transient ischemic attack occurred in this series. A number of patients (14 of them, 2% of all patients treated) reported visual disturbance following treatment. Patients with a previous history of migraine were especially at risk of this problem. In all but one case, the only effect was to produce a scotoma with flashing lights or ground glass appearance in part of the visual field. This resolved in most cases within 30 minutes and in all but one case within an hour.

In all, 457 limbs have been reviewed at 6 months or more following treatment (average 11 months, range 6–46 months). This includes 367 of 886 GSVs and 145 of 263 SSVs that had been treated. A substantial improvement in clinical venous disease was obtained. Duplex examination of the GSVs showed that occlusion was obtained in 322 of 364 (88%). In the SSVs, occlusion was present in 118 of 143 (83%). The median diameter of the GSVs and SSVs fell from 5 mm before treatment to 2 mm and 1 mm, respectively, at follow-up of 6 months or more.

The only residual adverse events still present at 6 months or more of follow-up were skin pigmentation and palpable lumps. Skin pigmentation was seen in 115 of 457 limbs and palpable lumps were present in 21 limbs. The skin pigmentation was almost always of a minor extent and continued to fade with the passage of time. In those patients reviewed 1 year or more following treatment, skin pigmentation was present in 11 of 115 limbs. Small palpable lumps were sometimes detectable in the calf, and comprised residual elements of treated veins. These could be identified by ultrasound imaging, but were not otherwise visible. In contrast to surgery, no scars, neurologic damage or lymphatic injuries were encountered.

Conclusions

Foam sclerotherapy can be used to manage primary and recurrent varicose veins arising from truncal saphenous incompetence, perforating veins and saphenous tributaries. It requires a minimum of equipment, but a skilled operator is needed with good competence at ultrasound-guided canulation of vessels. The long-term obliteration of saphenous trunks is 85–90%, although this can be improved by adding a further review and treatment session after 6 months. This method is especially useful in patients with recurrent varicose veins in whom further surgery carries a substantial risk of complications and further recurrence of varices. Recurrent varices managed by ultrasound-guided foam sclerotherapy have the same long-term recurrence rate as primary varices.

References

1. Wollmann JC. The history of sclerosing foams. Dermatol Surg 2004; 30: 694–703.
2. Schadeck M, Allaert F. Echotomographie de la sclérose. Phlébologie 1991; 44: 111–30.
3. Vin F. Echo-sclérothérapie de la veine saphène externe. Phlébologie 1991; 44: 79–84.
4. Kanter A, Thibault P. Saphenofemoral incompetence treated by ultrasound-guided sclerotherapy. Dermatol Surg 1996; 22: 648–52.
5. Orbach EJ. The thrombogenic activity of foam of a synthetic anionic detergent (sodium tetradecyl sulfate NNR). Angiology 1950; 1: 237–43.
6. Cabrera Garido JR, Cabrera Garcia-Olmedo JR, Garcia Olmedo Dominguez. Nuevo metodo de esclerosis en las varices tronculares. Pathologia Vasculares 1993; 1: 55–72.
7. Cabrera Garrido JR, Cabrera Garcia-Olmedo JR, Garcia-Olmedo Dominguez MA. Elargissement des limites de la schlérothérapie:nouveaux produits sclérosants. Phlebologie 1997; 50: 181–8.
8. Forlee MV, Grouden M, Moore DJ, Shanik G. Stroke after varicose vein foam injection sclerotherapy. J Vasc Surg 2006; 43: 162–4.
9. P. Coleridge Smith. Chronic venous disease treated by ultrasound guided foam sclerotherapy. Eur J Vasc Endovasc Surg 2006; 32: 577–83.

8 Foam sclerotherapy with and without duplex ultrasound guidance

Jean-Jérôme Guex and Jean-Luc Gillet

Rationale for the use of foamed sclerosing agents (sclerofoam)

The sclerosing reaction is due to the effect of molecules of sclerosing agent on venous endothelium and whole venous wall.[1] In veins smaller than 3 mm diameter, an injection of liquid produces laminar flow, ensuring complete contact without dilution only if the vein is filled entirely with sclerosing solution. The effect is almost uniform throughout the injected length of the vein (Figure 8.1). However, in larger veins, dilution occurs and the concentration of the sclerosing agent diminishes progressively from the point of injection distally (Figure 8.2). When foam does not mix with blood, the concentration of sclerosing molecules in contact with the venous wall is constant throughout the length of the foam contact (Figure 8.3). Unfortunately, in very large veins, foam floats and, to some extent, contact is optimal only at the superior surface of the treated vein (Figure 8.4). This fact could explain, at least partly, the benefit of venous spasm after the injection of foam. Such spasm may be provoked by intermittent compression by the ultrasound transducer.

These theoretical considerations are only a small part of actual phenomena of foam sclerotherapy. We can also observe the following:

- Microfoam is made up of microbubbles and surrounding liquid. The total volume of each phase is determined at the time of preparation by the Tessari method.

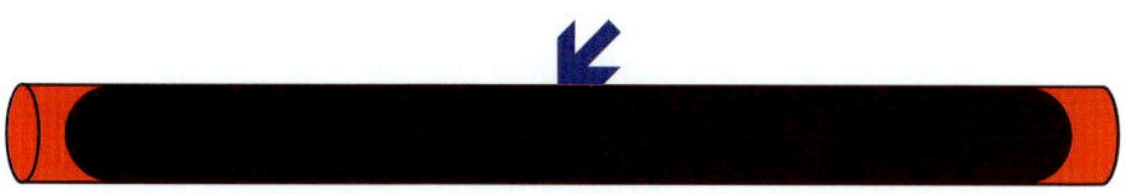

Figure 8.1 Injection of liquid in veins of diameter <3 mm: dilution does not happen

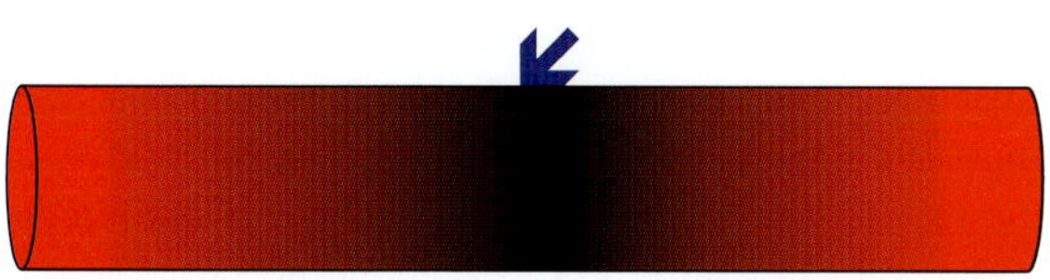

Figure 8.2 In bigger veins, liquid sclerosants are quickly diluted

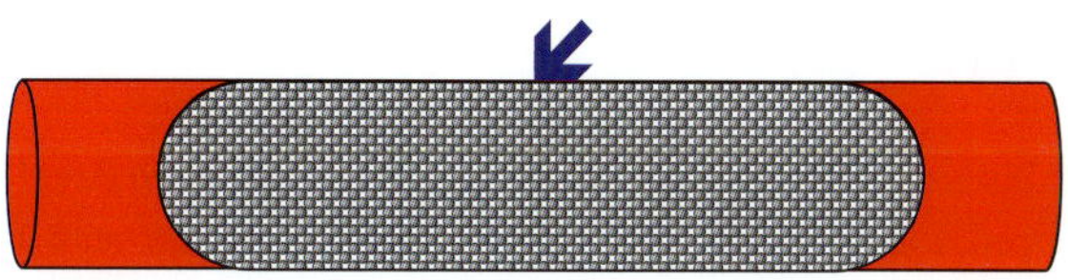

Figure 8.3 Foam does not mix with blood, and the concentration of sclerosing molecules in contact with endothelium is even

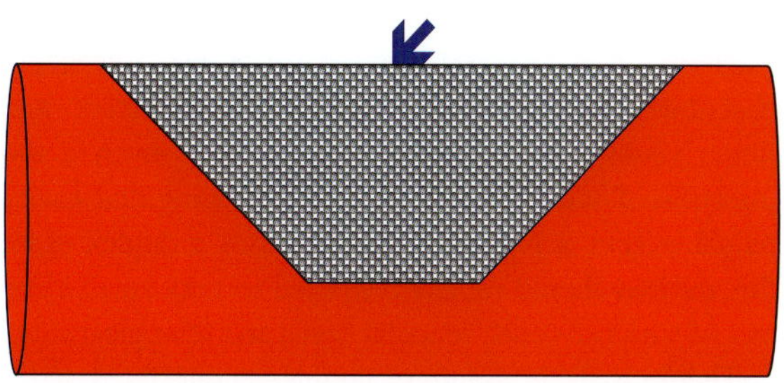

Figure 8.4 In very big veins, foam floats and is in better contact with the upper venous wall

- Microfoam microbubbles coalesce into larger bubbles, thus reducing the amount of bubble-bound sclerosing solution.
- The liquid film present between bubbles is diluted by the liquid blood, thus diminishing the sclerosing action as time passes.
- The sclerosing molecules that are present on the microbubble surface are used up by their action on the endothelium, thus decreasing their concentration.

There are many unanswered questions regarding the use of sclerofoam:

- Nobody knows the actual composition of the residual bubbles that are observed in the general circulation. Do they carry sclerosing molecules? Does their size matter? Is it better to have them circulate as soon as possible, or is it better to trap them in the limb first (leg elevation, saphenofemoral junction compression, etc.)?
- Are other gases better than air? Do these gases change the quality of foam, its efficacy, its side-effects? Would a cerebral gas embolus be of lesser importance if the gas were oxyen or carbon dioxide?

Despite these unanswered questions, the global observation of results of sclerotherapy treatment reveals great efficacy and a very limited rate of complications.[2]

Duplex guidance

Duplex guidance of sclerosing injections has been developed and has contributed to the rebirth of sclerofoam. It represents an improvement over classical sclerotherapy, since it provides more accuracy and better safety.

In classical (duplex guided) sclerotherapy, the injected liquid was not very visible in the lumen of the treated vein. The revolution occurred when phlebologists observed that ultrasound guidance and foam could be used together. Several techniques were ultimately described both with ultrasound-guided puncture and direct visible vein access. We believe that even if the injection of sclerofoam in a visible, bulging and easily palpable vein is feasible without use of a duplex scan, this method should remain restricted to very small clusters of varicose veins, reticular veins and telangiectasias.

Thanks to its thousands of liquid–gas interfaces, foam is an excellent contrast medium for ultrasonography, and this facilitates monitoring. Ultrasonography also identifies venous spasm, and that is the main criterion of efficacy. Newest technologies use high-frequency probes allowing imaging of small vessels down to 1–2 mm in diameter.

The permanent presence of an ultrasound scanner in the office must be now considered an absolute requirement. Similarly, the physician's skills in duplex ultrasound practice must be excellent. Detection of immediate complications such as extravasation, and of delayed adverse events such as deep venous thrombosis, is only possible with ultrasonography.

Another important element is who is actually doing the duplex scan, following the tip of the needle, following the diffusion of the foam, massaging the vein with the probe, etc. Or, to simplify this aspect, we should ask, "who's holding the probe?"

The current position in this respect is variable, reflecting with each country's habits and previous regulations. Some countries, such as France, have no vascular technicians and rely on physicians to carry out the examination and follow the treatment. In other countries such as the United States and the United Kingdom, registered vascular technologists are available to carry out a duplex scan. We believe that the physician injecting the vein must also hold the probe, since the movement of both hands must be continuously coordinated. Since many things need to be done at the same time, with only two hands, we prefer placing a fixed venous access such as a butterfly needle or a short catheter in order to have plenty of time to prepare the sclerofoam and allow injection of additional volumes of foam.

Practical techniques

Basic principles of the closed needle technique

Treatment with foam sclerotherapy can only be planned after precise duplex mapping of the normal and the varicose veins.

(a) Injection site

Since the major complication of sclerotherapy is the injection of sclerosing agent into an artery, the operator must avoid injecting the great saphenous vein (GSV) at the junction and the small saphenous vein (SSV) in the popliteal fossa. For the GSV, except in special cases, it is preferable to inject the trunk or a superficial accessory branch of the GSV.

For the small saphenous vein, it is compulsory to look closely for the presence of the small saphenous artery. It is preferable to use a micro-catheter or a butterfly needle to insure safety, rather than to perform needle puncture directly.

For a perforating vein, the injection is given at some distance, never into the perforator itself, because of the constant presence of an arteriole, with the perforator. This is true even if the arteriole is not identified with duplex scanning.

(b) Four successive phases can be described:

1. Ultrasound localization of the vein with B-mode ultrasonography (transverse and longitudinal views);
2. Puncture of the vein under ultrasound control, with transverse or longitudinal views, according to each physician's individual preference. The needle tip in the lumen of the vein must be identified; and obtaining a reflux of blood is essential before going on to the next step.
3. Injection of the sclerosing agent under continuous ultrasound guidance ensures the absence of sclerosant extravasation. With the direct puncture method, continuous ultrasound observation is essential for two reasons:
   - Getting an initial reflux is important but is not sufficient, since the bevel of the needle can penetrate the wall of the vein;
   - Making sure that the needle bevel did not escape the vein during the injection.
4. Postinjection ultrasound control: since microscopic bubbles can be easily identified with B-mode utrasonography, diffusion of the agent is visualized. Using the ultrasonographic probe, it can be ascertained that the foam is distributed into the whole target varicose vein cluster. Finally, obtaining venous spasm is an important event that is predictive of efficacy.

(c) Operator's position

1. The operator's hand used for injecting the sclerosant foam should be resting on the patient's limb to avoid any movement during the injection;
2. The other hand should not leave the probe during the injection, and the operator should be positioned in a manner that enables both hands and the ultrasonography screen to be in his or her field of vision simultaneously.

(d) Choice of syringes

We prefer to use syringes without silicone to allow better preservation of the foam quality, but the injection is slightly more difficult, with jerky movements. It requires training, experience, proper positioning of the operator and a correct choice of needle.

(e) Choice of needles

1. The needle diameter should be from 21 to 25 gauge.
2. It is important to choose a needle whose *length* allows the syringe to rest on the skin, limiting the risk of dislodging the needle from the vein during the injection.

Basic principles of open vein access

This approach is similar to all medical venous accesses, for example, in the emergency room and in intensive care units. This approach provides both safety and time for sclerofoam preparation and injection. Once the vein is cannulized, the physician has plenty of time to check reflux and to prepare fresh foam. It also allows controlled diffusion of foam remote from the puncture site during the infusion, which is not possible during a direct puncture injection.

Different materials can be used. Butterfly needles are the simplest, and can be used for all veins that are not deeper than 10 mm. We recommend keeping the bevel down for both puncture and injection and attaching the needle wings to the skin with tape. The short length of the needles requires a transverse placement of the ultrasonic probe, but after adequate placement a very safe injection is achieved, since blood reflux through the attached tubing demonstrates accurate placement. In addition, butterfly needles are very cheap.

In the case of deeper veins, an injection kit can be prepared with a longer needle and a short, narrow connector. Except for the absence of wings, the longer needle is used exactly in the same way as the butterfly.

The microcatheter and Seldinger techniques are a little more complicated. However, they allow injection into deeper veins with maximal safety. The access must be attached to a small connector and fixed to the skin.

Indications

Varicose veins are a sign of a chronic venous disorder, but are not the cause. However, hemodynamic abnormalities associated with reflux in the varicose network are likely to worsen the condition and increase the risk of complications. Varicose veins are responsible for troublesome symptoms such as plebalgia, pruritus, external hemorrhage, superficial thrombosis, and skin changes, including hyperpigmentation, atrophie blanche and even ulceration. For these reasons, elimination of varicose veins is necessary. It is not, however, a goal in itself and partial preservation of a varicose network should always be taken into consideration.

The aims of the treatment of varicose veins are:

- to answer the patient's demands and needs, whether clearly formulated or not
- to restore satisfactory hemodynamics
- to avoid worsening of the disease, recurrence and/or complications.

The patient's point of view is of utmost importance, and understanding his or her reasons to seek treatment is a priority.

1. The patient's point of view

It is important to understand what are the reasons that push the patient to request treatment. Reasons for consultation are variable: symptoms, aesthetics, fear of aggravation or of complications (especially with a family history), restriction of activities, and emotional problems.[83] For patients referred by their physician, the analysis of needs must be as precise as for patients who consult spontaneously. Satisfaction with the main reason for consultation is the major objective of treatment. If the patient is not satisfied, it will represent a failure of the treatment, even though the reflux has been abolished.

Popularization of medicine and word of mouth information can cause some patients to have a preference for one method of treatment. Similarly, some patients reject surgery or sclerotherapy for personal reasons. Respecting their preferences is necessary. Therapeutic indications among patients referred by their physician are especially delicate and justify clear and detailed preliminary explanation. In all cases, the consent of the patient must be obtained; it must be based on the benefits, alternatives and risks (BAR).

2. The practitioner's point of view

The treatment must be based on sound and validated pathophysiologic concepts. It must be the least dangerous, least painful, least immobilizing and cosmetically satisfactory, with no or few scars, no discoloration and no matting, at an acceptable price. The treatment must also be efficient: disappearance of the varicose veins, disappearance of the reflux, global improvement of hemodynamics with an absence of recurrence, and validated. It must respect the patient's wishes as much as possible. For the practitioner, suppression of symptoms and prevention of complications remain mandatory objectives.

Because of the polymorphous presentation of chronic venous disorders, it is easier to decide treatment according to the principal lesions, which constitute each individual case. The final treatment will then be a mixture of the various methods that are most adapted to each of the abnormalities.

In GSV insufficiency, detailed hemodynamic mapping is a compulsory prerequisite. This is true for all varicosities – even those that are clinically minimal.

Measurement of diameters of veins at various levels and determination of the topography of reflux are fundamentally important. Competence of the most proximal valves (terminal and preterminal), location of tributaries, amount of reflux in incomplete truncal insufficiency, and presence of incompetent perforators of the femoral tract re-entry perforators in the lower leg predominant extrafascial tributaries, etc., are the elements that permit a specific approach to each case.

Until recently, the prevailing principle in surgery of varicose veins was the superiority of the performance of stripping the GSV in combination with its division and resection of tributaries.

In the meantime, endovenous methods demonstrated that the junction could be preserved. Other work has demonstrated the importance of the removal of the varicose reservoir in order to restore or to improve the function of truncal valves. This is described elsewhere in this volume.

Nowadays, it is necessary to think very carefully about the usefulness of eliminating a GSV, especially when its incompetence is not complete, or when its diameter is only moderately increased, and when the varicose reservoir is dominant. Ablation of a small dystrophic saphenous vein in a young patient is a procedure that might be regretted later, in case material is needed for bypass surgery. For example, cases where the medial thigh tributary is larger than the GVS trunk and joins it just distal to the saphenofemoral junction lead one to respect both the trunk and the junction.

Given that some recent work has questioned the

dogma of conventional saphenous stripping, which was previously validated by several studies, it is likely that such questioning arises from better duplex scan analysis, and from better selection of patients.

Classical surgery remains a valid technique for many severe varicosities. It is now true that classical surgery can be performed under local anesthesia and in an ambulatory setting.

Since the birth of echo-guided sclerofoam sclerotherapy, indications for conventional sclerotherapy of saphenous veins with liquid, with or without echo guidance, have been reduced to almost nothing.

Therefore, in the case of valvular incompetence of the GSV, it is necessary to choose amongst conservation of the saphenous vein, traditional surgery (in its less invasive form), thermal endovenous methods (laser, radiofrequency Closure®, ClosureFAST®) and echo-guided sclerofoam.

The French Health Authority[4] recognizes several methods: surgery (crossectomy + stripping), endovenous laser, radiofrequency Closure® and echo-guided sclerofoam.

Results at short- and mid-term follow-up demonstrate that echo-guided sclerofoam treatment is not inferior to other methods, but long-term results are not yet available. To choose to treat saphenous veins by echo-guided sclerofoam is more and more frequently chosen, but it has prerequisites and fundamental corollaries:

- the practitioner's knowledge of the technique
- good understanding, and the patient–practitioner agreement of a program of treatment requiring several sessions, repeat injections and repeat duplex examinations
- important benefits such as a short and completely ambulatory procedure, without even local anesthesia, excellent aesthetic results, and excellent cost-effectiveness.

3. Is the assessment of results possible, and will it influence the choice of treatment?

By what criteria can we judge the efficacy of a treatment of varicose veins? For most patients with severe chronic venous insufficiency, an easy outcome to appreciate is ulcer healing: one can know the time necessary for its healing, the delay before recurrence (or onset), the rate of recurrence, and the speed of healing (measuring surface area).

C_5 and C_6 patients are infrequent and are far from being the only ones to make themselves treated. For other patients, we lack criteria of assessment; the VDS and the VCSS scales associated with the CEAP classification are hardly sensitive in C_1 to C_3 patients, and these are evaluated by the practitioner. To avoid bias, evaluation by an external audit is recommended.

It is usual to judge the results of varicose vein treatment on the disappearance of the reflux in one or several target veins; but this is only a hemodynamic criterion, imperfectly correlated with clinical improvement, and the risks of error are not negligible. The total venous reflux measured with plethysmography is not used very often, but it would be an interesting global measurement. We do not have a specific biological criterion, or a simple means to measure the importance of varicose veins. Measurement of edema is possible, but not all patients have swollen legs.

Finally, the evolution of varicose disease is extremely variable from one patient to another. This aspect of the problem is often misunderstood and only observed in hindsight. Yet, the progression of varicosis not only affects the follow-up, but should also determine the choice of the initial treatment. Predisposing factors such as heredity, number of future pregnancies and professional status need to be taken into account.

One should recognize that the problem becomes complicated because the methods of treatment are very different. Moreover, the secondary effects and expected inconveniences are likely to modify the choice of treatment. Inevitably, one concludes that we need new tools of assessment. For example, injections of foam are simple, cheap, repeatable and do not cause any incapacity. Assessment of results and comparison with other methods cannot be done with the same tools or the same objectives. The treatment of varicose veins is not the same as the treatment of cancer, and recurrence does not have the same consequences. Patients readily accept re-injection of a recanalized varicose vein.

This problematic issue is not resolved yet. It is necessary to evaluate results not only on suppression of reflux but also by composite, sensitive and specific patient reported outcomes such as the SQOR-V.[3]

A unique, ideal and indisputable treatment of varicose veins does not exist. Two contradictory choices can be perfectly applicable.

Table 8.1 indicates all possible indications. Decisions will be made according to the physician's experience and knowledge, patient's preferences, inconveniences of techniques, and so on.

Table 8.1 Summary of all *possible* therapeutic options in GSV incompetence

Diameter of GSV 15 cm below SFJ	Upper level of	GSV trunkal valve	Incompetence
	TERMINAL	PRETERMINAL	TRUNCAL
Diameter <5 mm	Abstention, sclerofoam	Abstention, sclerofoam	Abstention, sclerofoam
5mm<Diameter < 8mm	Sclerofoam laser EV, Closure®, crossectomy–stripping	Sclerofoam, laser EV, Closure®, ambulatory phlebectomy	Sclerofoam, ambulatory phlebectomy
8mm<Diameter <12 mm	Crossectomy–stripping, laser, Closure®, sclerofoam	Laser EV, Closure®, sclerofoam	Sclerofoam, ambulatory phlebectomy
Diameter > 12 mm	Crossectomy–stripping, laser EV	Laser EV, sclerofoam	Sclerofoam, laser EV

SFJ, saphenofemoral junction; EV, endovenous.

Small saphenous vein (SSV)

Sclerofoam is suitable for almost all cases of SSV insufficiency. Other methods are either more aggressive (crossectomy–stripping) and/or the local anatomic situation leads to fear of neurologic complications (Closure® and endovenous laser). The question of recurrence by recanalization deserves to be better assessed, but recurrence is easily taken care of by a simple "re-do" injection. Only several varicose veins of exceptional diameter are still an indication for ligation and stripping. When a surgical treatment is indicated, general anesthesia must be avoided.

Tributaries react very well to sclerofoam. Varicose veins may develop progressively upward, beginning at lower leg level and not from junctional or truncal reflux. The varicose reservoir is a fundamental hemodynamic element, as important as truncal reflux. It is therefore necessary to insist on the complete treatment of the varicose network. So far, nothing demands that it is necessary to treat everything at once and/or all by the same method.

Perforating veins

Perforating veins connected to the saphenous network must be classified in two main theoretical categories (it is not always simple): first as sources of reflux, and second as re-entries (meaning that they drain the varicose network situated proximal to them).

The majority of lower medial leg perforators are re-entries. Most of the time, they regress spontaneously after suppression of the pathologic medial varicose network (superficial axial reflux). We suggest not treating them initially, but rather waiting for 3–6 weeks and re-assessing them at that time. On the other hand, more proximal perforators (of the femoral canal, for example) participate in the reflux and may feed the varicose reservoir. These are pathogenic and must be treated at the outset. Sclerofoam is the treatment of choice for this, since it will avoid large incisions to find veins whose pathways are very often complicated.

Efficacy of ultrasound-guided sclerofoam

We present in this chapter only the main results of major studies. Elsewhere in this book, Chapter 7 by Coleridge-Smith is devoted to the assessment of the results of foam sclerotherapy.

Barrett, Goldman and colleagues[5] analyzed foam sclerotherapy results in legs with GSV (n = 89) or SSV (n = 23) insufficiency, or both (n = 12). The average follow-up was 22.5 months (range 20–26 months). Overall satisfaction was high in terms of treated varices (complete success in 85% and partial success in 15% of patients). Symptoms were assessed by quality of life questionnaire and visual assessment.

Hamel-Desnos'[6] and Yamaki's[7] studies demonstrated that the efficacy of sclerotherapy was greater using foam than liquid. Even injecting low volumes of foam (2–3 mL), the rate of success at 1 year was 73.3% and 75.7%, respectively, in these two studies.

Bergan[8] reported his experience of treatment using foam sclerotherapy in patients with various venous disorders: uncomplicated varicose veins; chronic venous insufficiency, including 50 limbs with active ulcer; and venous angiomas, including Klippel–Trenaunay syndrome. Ulcer healing was achieved in all patients treated with foam sclerotherapy. The result of the treatment was satisfactory in the other groups of patients.

Cabrera[9] reported a series of 116 patients with active ulcer. At 6 months follow-up, treatment with foam achieved complete healing in 83% of the patients.

Cavezzi[10] published two series including 194 patients with varicose veins treated with foam sclerotherapy. At 1 month follow-up, 91% (161/177) of patients included in the first series and all (17/17) in the second series presented obliteration of the vein or an antegrade flow, without reflux.

Coleridge Smith[11] treated 808 patients (1109 limbs) with foam sclerotherapy for chronic venous disease due to truncal saphenous incompetence. The total amount of foam injected in one treatment session was limited to 20 mL. A total of 459 limbs were available for assessment at a follow-up interval of 6 months (mean, 11 months) or greater. The GSV was obliterated in 88% of limbs and the SSV in 82% of limbs.

In the Varisolve® study,[12] success defined as occlusion of the trunk vein (GVS or SSV) and elimination of reflux was achieved at 3 months and 12 months in 83.4% and 78.9% of patients, respectively.

Although foam sclerotherapy is widely used and most often the treatment of first choice in recurrent varicose veins after surgery, few data have been published on this issue. Recently, Kakkos[13] showed that the immediate results at 3 weeks follow-up were satisfactory, with 87% of patients showing complete elimination of varicose veins and reflux.

Adverse events: prevention

Description, explanation, and most of all the evaluation of benefit/risk ratio of adverse events after sclerofoam injection remain controversial. Frequency of complications and side-effects vary according to method of study, and according to the authors' background and personal practice. The incidence of adverse events remains low and severe complications are exceptional. They are not greater than for other techniques.[2] However, several elements appear to be common. Even if there is some difference in interpretation, management and consequences, a certain consensus has begun to form.

Types of reported complications are neurologic/sensory (visual troubles, migraine, resembling or actual transient ischemic attack, or strokes), cardiac (heart constriction/chest compression), thrombotic (superficial thrombophlebitis, muscular thrombosis, deep venous thrombosis or pulmonary emboli), necrotic (intra-arterial injection), and various nonspecific side-effects varying from vaso-vagal fainting to septicemia.

Most specialists concentrate on neurologic and thrombotic complications, since they are clearly directly related to the treatment and must be addressed with much care.

The explanation for neurologic adverse events is unclear, but associations with previous episodes of migraine with aura and presence of a patent foramen ovale have been implicated. The importance of the nature of the gas used to prepare the foam has been emphasized by some, but disputed by others, without much evidence so far. Some advocate the need for a search for a patent foramen ovale before using sclerofoam. Considering the very small number of reported complications, this remains unproven so far. Limiting the volume of injections as proposed by the Second European Consensus of Tegernesee[14] seems a logical option, even if the preventive effects are unknown. Any supposed ischemic lesion would be less severe with a lower volume of foam. Leg elevation after foam injection, as proposed by Bergan, can trap the bubbles for some time, but since air is not resorbed it will return to the circulation at some point. We do not know much about the fate of the bubbles when they circulate in the body: are they bound to a significant amount of sclerosing molecules? Or have they been washed out? Are these bubbles potentially responsible for neurologic ischemia? Does the nature of the gas change something? All these questions deserve serious attention and further research. For the time being, patients should be informed of both the potential risks and the extremely rare manifestations of foam sclerotherapy.

Regarding thrombotic complications, most are benign. They can be interpreted as excessive reactions of either too strong local reactions or too remote extensions (perforator, muscular, junctions), thus emphasizing the need for appropriate dosage. However, several cases of true deep venous thrombosis (DVT) and pulmonary embolism have been described, and prevention must be undertaken. Excessive amounts of foam have been seen to increase the incidence of DVT. Patients with known thrombophilia, personal or even family history of DVT and pulmonary embolism must be approached with additional care. Prevention with low-molecular-weight heparin or oral anticoagulation is an interesting option. Most authors use compression and ambulation after injection.

Finally, sclerofoam is a very powerful tool for the treatment of varicose veins, but as such it has potential drawbacks. In our opinion, sclerofoam should be used for the treatment of varicose veins only. Telangiectasias and reticular veins react without side-effects very well to liquid sclerosing agents such as polidocanol 0.5%.[2]

Summary

The use of foam instead of sclerosant liquid has revolutionized sclerotherapy. With its power and reliability, an injection of sclerofoam equals a surgical procedure. Safety and accuracy have been increased by duplex guidance as the monitoring of results and prevention of some adverse events has been aided by ultrasound surveillance. However, the technique is demanding in terms not only of theoretical knowledge but also of practical experience. It should not be used without a preliminary extensive learning and training experience. At present, several complications remain that should become better understood and prevented. The future development of sclerofoam will require more theoretical studies and mid/long-term clinical trials to improve both clinical results and safety of the procedure.

References

1. Goldman MP, Bergan JJ, Guex JJ. Sclerotherapy: Treatment of Varicose and Telangiectatic Leg Veins, 4th edn. St Louis, MO: Mosby-Elsevier; 2007: 163–88.
2. Guex J-J MD, Allaert F-A, Gillet J-L, Chleir F. Immediate and mid-term complications of sclerotherapy. Report of a prospective multi-center registry of 12 173 sclerotherapy sessions. Dermatol Surg 2005; 31: 123–8.
3. Guex JJ, Zimmet SE, Boussetta S, et al. Construction and validation of a patient-reported outcome dedicated to chronic venous disorders: SQOR-V (specific quality of life and outcome response – venous). J Mal Vasc 2007 Jul; 32(3): 135–47.
4. Haute Autorité de Santé (HAS). Recommandations pour le Traitement des Varices; 2004 Available at www.has-sante.fr/portail/upload/docs/application/pdf/Varices_synth.pdf.
5. Barrett JM, Allen B, Ockelford A, Goldman MP. Microfoam ultrasound-guided sclerotherapy of varicose veins in 100 legs. Dermatol Surg 2004; 30: 6–12.
6. Hamel-Desnos C, Desnos P, Wollmann JC, et al. Evaluation of the efficacy of polidocanol in the form of foam compared with liquid form in sclerotherapy of the greater saphenous vein: initial results. Dermatol Surg 2003; 29: 1170–5.
7. Yamaki T, Nozaki M, Iwasaka S. Comparative study of duplex-guided foam sclerotherapy and duplex-guided liquid sclerotherapy for the treatment of superficial venous insufficiency. Dermatol Surg 2004; 30: 718–22.
8. Bergan J, Pascarella L, Mekenas L. Venous disorders: treatment with sclerosant foam. J Cardiovasc Surg 2006; 47: 9–18.
9. Cabrera J, Cabrera JJR, Garcia-Olmedo MA, Redondo P. Treatment of venous malformations with sclerosant in microfoam form. Arch Dermatol 2003; 139: 1409–16.
10. Cavezzi A, Frullini A, Ricci S, Tessari L. Treatment of varicose veins by foam sclerotherapy: two clinical series. Phlebology 2002; 17: 13–18.
11. Coleridge-Smith P. Chronic venous disease treated by ultrasound guided foam sclerotherapy. Eur J Vasc Endovasc Surg 2006; 32: 577–83.
12. Wright D, Gobin JP, Bradbury AW, et al. Varisolve® polidocanol microfoam compared with surgery or sclerotherapy in management of varicose veins in the presence of trunk vein incompetence: European randomized controlled trial. Phlebology 2006; 21: 180–90.
13. Kakkos SK, Bountouroglou DG, Azzam M, et al. Effectiveness and safety of ultrasound-guided foam sclerotherapy for recurrent varicose veins: immediate results. J Endovasc Ther 2006; 13: 357–64.
14. Breu FX, Guggenbichler S, Wollmann JC. 2nd European Consensus Meeting on Foam Sclerotherapy 2006, Tegernsee, Germany. Vasa 2008; 37(Suppl 71): 3–29.

9 Foam sclerotherapy for varicose veins: medium-term results as assessed by ultrasound

Kenneth Myers and Damien Jolley

Ultrasound-guided sclerotherapy (UGS) has become increasingly popular for treating superficial venous disease. The larger proportion of patients with or without complications have underlying superficial reflux rather than deep venous disease. Younger patients are attracted by the minimal disruption of activities and absence of surgical scarring. Older patients are well suited to UGS rather than surgery to avoid morbidity from anesthesia and immobility.

Sclerotherapy has been practiced for more than 100 years. Hobbs showed that blind treatment injecting tributaries with a fluid sclerosant in limbs with saphenous reflux was inferior to surgery.[1] Clearly, "pruning the branches" is inadequate, as long-term control relies on eliminating the saphenous trunk. Subsequently, UGS was introduced to direct treatment to the saphenous veins so that they could be permanently obliterated.[2,3] Early results with fluid sclerosant were acceptable, but it was considered that results improved after methods were developed to convert sclerosants to foam.[4–10] The technique for foam UGS uses ultrasound to guide the needle to the vein and to follow the passage of foam.

Various techniques have been described and studies have presented results for liquid and foam UGS,[11–16] but there is no objective evidence that any one technique has an advantage over others in clinical practice. For most studies, outcome was not assessed by long-term objective surveillance and results were not determined by appropriate statistical techniques. This chapter presents a prospective observational study describing a technique for UGS and outcome assessed by surveillance with serial ultrasound scans using survival analysis. Medium-term success rates are determined by life-table analysis, and the influence of covariates that might affect outcome are assessed by Cox regression analysis. This chapter updates a previous publication.[16] The findings have led to changes in patient selection and technique for UGS that we consider should improve results in the future.

Selection of patients for foam ultrasound-guided sclerotherapy

Any patient with superficial venous disease can be treated by UGS. However, we avoid UGS during pregnancy and lactation as the effects of sclerosants on a fetus or infant are not known. UGS may be used in patients with a past deep vein thrombosis or thrombophilia, but usually only if there are venous complications and always under full anticoagulation with low-molecular-weight heparin. Associated lower limb arterial disease is not necessarily a contraindication to UGS. Venous stasis from chronic venous disease may contribute to ischemia from arterial disease to cause trophic changes or ulceration. However, severe arterial disease is always treated first. We have little concern about losing the vein as a result of UGS, since diseased veins have been shown to have poor patency rates when used as arterial bypass grafts.[17]

Most limbs treated in this study were in patients presenting with uncomplicated varicose veins, either with symptoms or for cosmetic reasons. However, the presence of complications from venous disease was often an indication to perform UGS. Unlike surgery, where our previous attitude was always to insist that a venous ulcer be healed before operation for fear of infection, we consider it safe to perform UGS in the presence of an active ulcer, thus potentially shortening the healing time.

Patients may have presented for treatment for the first time, but many had recurrences after previous surgery and we consider these ideally suited to UGS. Most patients with recurrent varicose veins after past surgery have little enthusiasm for another operation.

Any superficial vein can be treated by UGS. However, we have confined treatment to saphenous veins and tributaries and have avoided deliberate injection of incompetent perforators. Endovenous treatment is now preferred for most patients. Operation is now rarely recommended for great saphenous reflux and never recommended for small saphenous reflux. Surgery is offered to a small group of patients with saphenofemoral incompetence leading to large thigh varices but without great saphenous reflux. These are treated by proximal great saphenous ligation and excision of tributaries without saphenous stripping. With experience, it became apparent that larger-diameter veins were more difficult to control with UGS than small-diameter veins. This was noted at about the time that endovenous laser therapy (EVLT) became available, and EVLT has now replaced UGS in our practice for most patients with reflux in saphenous veins of diameter >5 mm. The relative numbers of the two procedures since the introduction of EVLT in our practice are shown in Figure 9.1.

Preoperative clinical assessment

At the first consultation, a full medical history is taken and clinical examination of the venous system performed to establish the severity and general nature of the venous disorder. A history is also taken for general medical diseases, risk factors for arterial disease, potential bleeding or clotting disorders, allergies or asthma, migraine headaches, an obstetric history, and medications. A past severe allergic disorder or asthma may influence the choice of polidocanol rather than sodium tetradecyl sulfate as the sclerosant. Patients with migraine are warned that treatment may precipitate a transient visual aura. If a woman is taking the oral contraceptive pill, then there is discussion as to whether or not it should be discontinued, although the final decision is left to the patient. Discussion relates to a theoretical increased risk of thrombosis if the pill is continued against a theoretical risk to a fetus from injecting sclerosant in the presence of an unrecognized pregnancy if it is discontinued. The decision as to whether or not to continue hormone replacement therapy is also left to the patient. We do not consider that warfarin or aspirin therapy should be stopped before UGS. The clinical examination shows the extent of disease, and this will influence the likely total

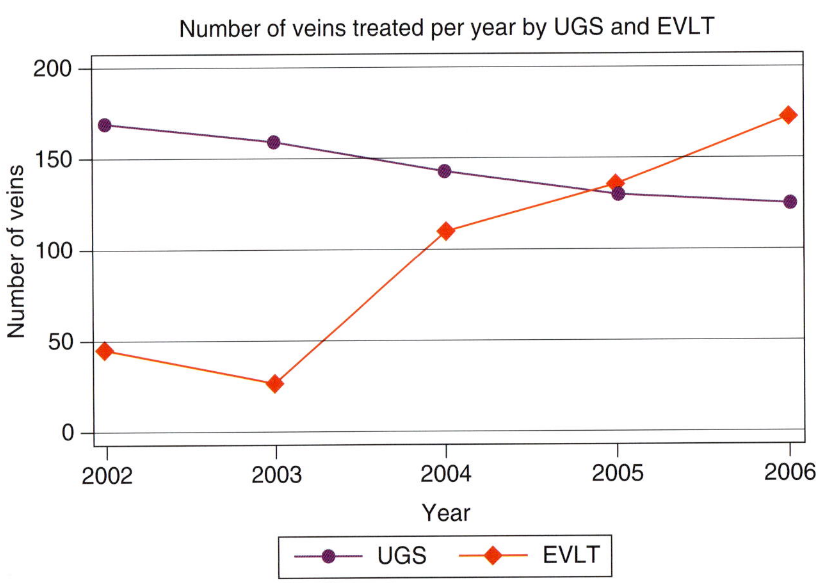

Figure 9.1 The relative numbers of veins treated by ultrasound-guided sclerotherapy and by endovenous laser therapy from 2002 to 2006

volume of foam to be given and the possible number of treatment sessions. Examination attempts to determine which saphenous system or perforator veins are connected to varices, although this is largely deferred until preoperative duplex ultrasound scanning. Examination identifies complications of lipodermatosclerosis and past or present ulceration.

We consider that clinical assessment alone is insufficient to plan treatment, and all patients are sent for a venous duplex ultrasound scan performed by a specialist vascular sonographer.[18] We no longer use the hand-held continuous-wave Doppler unit to evaluate pathology. A decision not to rely on clinical judgment alone has been supported by studies that found that it misses 25–30% of communications between deep and superficial veins when compared with duplex ultrasound.[19,20]

The second consultation after the duplex scan allows discussion of recommended treatment based on the ultrasound findings as well as an appreciation of the clinical assessment. If UGS is advised, then the limbs are measured to be fitted for class 2 thigh high-compression stockings. The patient is advised not to apply moisturizer to the legs on the day of treatment and to wear loose trousers and shoes to allow for the thickness of the bandages and stockings.

As well as discussion, each patient is given printed material that details the anatomy, physiology, pathology, results and potential complications for the proposed treatment in lay terms. For medico-legal reasons, patients are required to sign a consent form for treatment that states that they have read the pamphlet and understand the nature of UGS and current knowledge of using foam sclerosants. Whether this is sufficient in law has not yet been tested by the authors.

Preoperative venous duplex ultrasound examination

The scan is of value only if performed by a specialist vascular sonographer who thoroughly understands venous anatomy and physiology after experience of working with the phlebologist. Scanning is performed with the patient standing or on a tilt table supported with weight taken on the opposite limb. Reflux is defined as retrograde flow lasting for greater than 0.5 s, but it is usual for reflux to persist for at least 2–3 s, the duration depending on the capacitance of the varicose veins. Reflux is easily assessed by color flow, and it is rare for an experienced sonographer to need to record a spectral tracing. Incompetence at the saphenofemoral junction is elicited by the Valsalva maneuver, and reflux from low abdominal or pelvic tributaries into the great saphenous vein is elicited by a calf or thigh squeeze. Incompetence at the saphenopopliteal junction is elicited by augmentation with a calf squeeze. The scan routinely assesses incompetence at either saphenous junction, alternative sources of reflux, and presence or absence of reflux in each saphenous vein, major tributaries, perforators and deep veins. Whether or not the saphenopopliteal junction is present is noted and the level of the junction in relation to the knee crease is measured. The level of perforators in relation to the knee or ankle is measured. In addition, the examination records the extent of involvement and measurements of diameters at the junctions and representative diameters of the saphenous veins and major tributaries for veins that show reflux.

Techniques for treatment

Preparation of sclerosant

The sclerosant agents used and their preparation in this study varied from patient to patient according to the size and extent of the varicose veins and the attitude of the treating surgeon (KM) at different times throughout the study. This provides an opportunity to compare success rates for different treatment techniques. The agent used was either sodium tetradecyl sulfate or polidocanol, and these were not used in combination in any patient. No more than 4 mL of 3% sodium tetradecyl sulfate or 2 mg/kg of 3% polidocanol was used at any one treatment session, as recommended by the Australian Therapeutic Goods Administration (TGA).

For the first year of the series, injection was with liquid sclerosant at the 3% concentration, and this was used for 98 treatment sessions in the primary group. From early 2000, treatment changed, with foamed sclerosant used for all subsequent procedures. The sclerosant to be foamed was either undiluted at 3% or commonly diluted with normal saline to provide concentrations ranging from 2% down to 0.6%. Diluted solutions were used to provide greater volumes of foam for more extensive varicose disease. Foam was made by a modification of the Tessari method,[7,8] with two parts of sclerosant combined with three parts of gas mixed between two syringes. A 5 μm filter in the system was added into the mixing system about two years ago, and it has been shown to produce a finer foam. Initially, the gas was air, but this has been changed to a mixture of 70% oxygen and 30% carbon dioxide over the past two years in an attempt to eliminate nitrogen passing into the general circulation. The gas is contained in a plastic bag connected to the gas cylinder. Three-way taps allow a volume to be drawn up into a 20 mL syringe for each session. The 3% sclerosant solution, now always diluted with 0.9% saline to 1.5%, is drawn up into a 10 mL syringe. Each is then connected in turn to a 5 mL syringe through a three-way tap to draw up the mixture of 2 mL of fluid and 3 mL of gas. Foaming is performed to another 5 mL syringe through the three-way tap and filter. It takes at least 10 exchanges between the syringes to produce a consistent, fine foam. In the early years, no limit was placed on the maximum volume of foam given at one session, although it is now arbitrarily restricted to no more than 20 mL of foam. The volume ranged from 3 to 40 mL foam (median 5 mL) throughout the study.

Selection of veins to be treated

The policy throughout has been to inject as far distally and away from connections between superficial and deep veins as possible. The aim is to find a "strategic vein" that appears from the preoperative scan to provide the best avenue for foam to fill the full length of the venous system to be treated. With distal injection, it is surprising how far up the limb foam will travel, thus avoiding the need for a second injection. Patients are in the supine position or tilted slightly, feet down, to fill the veins. Foam sclerosant causes immediate intense venospasm, so that the feet-down position does not increase "trapped blood."

It is usual practice to inject only one leg at each session in most patients with bilateral disease. We consider it better to inject the full amount of sclerosant that can be used to comprehensively treat one side, in the hope that this will limit the number of treatment sessions per leg. Injecting both legs with a volume limit could result in too little sclerosant on each side to be effective for either. In addition, bandaging both legs is more inhibiting for the patient. A common strategy is to alternate treatment for the two legs at 7–10-day intervals until both are controlled, as this is the usual period that we leave the patients in compression. However, some patients prefer to concentrate on the worse limb to ensure that they are satisfied with the outcome before accepting the further discomfort and expense of treating the less affected side.

Needling the vein using ultrasound guidance

This technique uses ultrasound to guide the needle into a saphenous vein or prominent tributary and to confirm that there is no extravasation during injection. The entire procedure is performed using B-mode, but we consider it essential to use a modern duplex ultrasound scanner with a high-frequency linear array probe. All procedures in this series were performed with the assistance of a sonographer. We prefer to hold the probe in the longitudinal view to guide the needle into the vein, since this shows a length of foam in the vein as it is injected and also shows the first signs of extravasation. It is easier to aim for a deeper vein. The sonographer must hold the probe perpendicular to the skin, and the phlebologist must place the needle in the midline of the probe axis to guide the needle; otherwise parallax will make it more difficult to find the vein (Figure 9.2). Injection is made with a 5 mL syringe and 3.3 cm length 25-gauge needle. This allows the needle to be seen well into the middle of the ultrasound screen. A longer, 23-gauge needle is available for injecting a deep vein in an obese thigh. Blood is aspirated to confirm that the needle tip is in the lumen, sclerosant is injected slowly, and ultrasound confirms that foam is flowing within the vein. Extravasation is uncom-

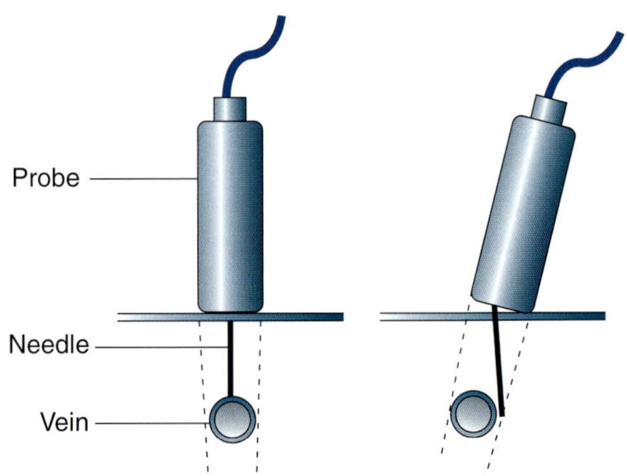

Figure 9.2 Position of the ultrasound probe. Left: the correct position – held vertically so as to line up the needle in the axis to pass directly to the vein lumen. Right: incorrect angling of the probe causes parallax so that the needle passes to one side of the vein

mon and avoided, as it results in pain that persists for approximately one hour, but extravasated foam appears to be inert and we have never encountered persisting damage to fat or skin from this event.

Blind needling of a tributary

Injection into a tributary can be performed blind using a 23-gauge butterfly needle. This allows the 5 mL syringe to be changed for greater volumes to be injected. The sonographer looks at a proximal vein to ensure that foam is appearing within the lumen. For a right-handed phlebologist, the left hand steadies the needle, with the thumb and index finger holding the hub and syringe, the middle finger steadies the wings, and the ring and little fingers placed lightly on the skin beyond the needle confirm that there is no extravasation. If this occurs, then the needle is removed and a fresh puncture made at a different site with a new needle.

Following the passage of foam

If scanning shows that sclerosant has not filled the veins, then it is gently massaged along their length until it appears at the appropriate saphenous junction. The sonographer follows the foam and applies pressure by the probe or finger to saphenous junctions or large perforators as foam approaches, whether they are incompetent or not. The sonographer can direct flow of sclerosant along one vein by compressing other veins. Once the saphenous vein is filled to the junction, the distal vein and tributaries are inspected, and foam can be milked down to fill them if they do not contain foam, although this may not be possible if valves are competent. Usually, only one injection is required to fill the vein, but further injections at the proximal limit are performed if necessary, although this is usually more difficult due to venous spasm.

It is common to see foam pass from one saphenous system to the other through communicating veins. If foam is seen to enter muscular or deep axial veins, then injection is stopped, the needle is removed and the patient is asked to exercise the calf muscles for a few minutes.

Management after injection

After completing the injections, compression is immediately applied with the limb horizontal. A soft strip is placed around the knee to prevent rubbing. Combine pads are placed along the treated superficial veins to aid compression. Crepe bandages are then applied firmly from the ankle along the full length of the limb. A self-adhering outer elastic bandage is then applied firmly along the full length. A class 2 above-knee stocking is placed over the bandages to provide maximum compression using an applicating frame. Patients are then immediately mobilized and asked to walk for 15 minutes. It is recommended that they be driven home with the leg elevated.

Initial compression is maintained constantly for 48 hours and then changed to compression with the class 2 stocking worn just through the day and removed at night and for the morning shower. Compression is maintained for 1–3 weeks depending on the degree of reaction in superficial veins. Patients are instructed to walk regularly each day. It is recommended that they avoid more strenuous exercise throughout this period. All of these instructions are empirical, since we know of little evidence to provide guidance for best postsclerotherapy management.

Postoperative reviews

All patients are assessed by clinical examination and an ultrasound scan at 3–5 days after every treatment session. The patients are informed verbally and in printed postoperative instructions that it is common for there to be mild pain, tender lumps and some discoloration and that these do not need to be reported prior to the review. They are reassured that all should gradually fade over a few weeks. Any trapped blood is released by puncture with a 19-gauge needle, best performed at about 10–14 days after injection. Evacuation can be aided by aspiration with a 1 mL syringe. The ultrasound is performed to determine whether the treatment had been effective, to detect residual patent veins that might require further treatment, and to detect or exclude deep vein occlusion. The postoperative scan frequently showed residual foam in veins up to several days after treatment (Figure 9.3). Clinical review and an ultrasound scan are then repeated at 6 weeks, 6-monthly for 2 years and then annually to determine whether treated veins are absent, occluded, patent or refluxing. Reflux in non-treated veins is also recorded.

There can be a dilemma as to what to do if recurrence is noted on ultrasound but without clinical evidence of recurrent disease. Patients are advised that further

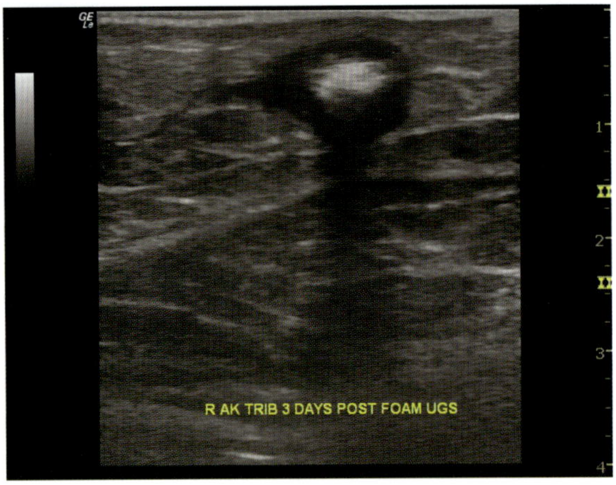

Figure 9.3 Ultrasound performed three days after foam ultrasound-guided sclerotherapy, showing residual foam in a large tributary

varicose veins will become apparent with time. Some patients elect to have further UGS while veins are still small to avoid future problems, while others prefer to defer further treatment until veins appear or at least until the next scheduled review. Patients appreciate our aggressive approach to surveillance; most are well aware of accounts of large, neglected recurrent varices after surgery.

Characteristics of treated patients

There have been 852 patients treated from early 1999 to April 2007. UGS was the primary treatment in 578 patients (the primary group), and these will be examined by survival analysis. A further 274 patients were treated with UGS for tributaries or distal segments of saphenous veins after EVLT for proximal saphenous veins, and these will not be analyzed separately though included for assessment of complications. The numbers of patients, limbs, veins treated and treatment sessions in each group and the particular venous systems treated are shown in Table 9.1. For the primary group, the 578 patients had treatment in 836 limbs involving 989 vein segments. Treatment was for one vein in 283 patients, two veins in 215, three veins in 55 and four or more in 25 patients.

For the primary group, the patients' ages ranged from 19 to 92 (median 53) years, with 473 females (83%) and 105 males. There were 763 limbs with clinical CEAP category $C_{2/3}$ (91%) and 73 limbs with clinical CEAP category $C_{4–6}$ (45 C_4, 21 C_5 and 7 C_6). Treatment was for primary varicose veins without previous surgery in 678 limbs (81%) and for recurrent varicose veins after previous surgery in 159 limbs.

For the first treatment in the primary group, reflux affected the great saphenous territory in 530 limbs (53%), including 5 where reflux was into the anterior accessory saphenous vein; the small saphenous territory in 198 limbs (20%), including 9 with involvement of the thigh extension or vein of Giacomini; or tributaries alone without reflux in either saphenous system in 261 limbs (27%).

No attempt was made to ensure that treatment was finalized in one session, although this often proved to be the case. For the primary group, there were 1457 treatment sessions to treat the 989 vein systems, so that an

Table 9.1 Number of treatment sessions, veins treated, limbs and patients for ultrasound-guided sclerotherapy (UGS) alone or after endovenous laser therapy (EVLT)

	All veins	Great saphenous	Small saphenous	Tributaries only
UGS alone				
Sessions	1457	823 (56%)	275 (19%)	359 (25%)
Veins	989	530 (53%)	198 (20%)	261 (27%)
Limbs	836	–	–	–
Patients	578	–	–	–
UGS after EVLT				
Sessions	472	157 (33%)	19 (4%)	296 (63%)
Veins	451	149 (33%)	18 (4%)	284 (63%)
Limbs	389	–	–	–
Patients	274	–	–	–

average of 1.47 sessions was required to accomplish adequate occlusion of each vein system. A second session was required in 251, a third in 43 and more than 3 in 12 limbs. Of the 989 veins initially successfully treated, subsequent failure due to development of reflux in the treated veins as shown by ultrasound resulted in the patient returning for a second series of treatments in 109, a third series in 17 and a fourth in 5 patients.

Statistical analysis of results

Results have been analyzed in those patients presenting for limbs with saphenous reflux, usually with associated tributaries, and for treatment of tributaries alone without saphenous reflux. Analysis for those with saphenous reflux will combine the great saphenous vein and anterior accessory saphenous vein as one group, and the small saphenous vein, thigh extension and vein of Giacomini as another group.

Data were entered prospectively into an Excel spreadsheet and statistical analysis was performed with Stata software. Primary success was defined as persistent occlusion or absence of reflux in the treated venous segment. Secondary success was defined as persistent occlusion or absence of reflux in the treated venous segment after further UGS for primary failure. The time for commencement of surveillance was the date at which the last treatment session was performed that achieved occlusion of the treated venous system. The time to failure was the interval at which reflux was noted on the follow-up scan at the next scheduled appointment. If the patient had missed a scheduled appointment, then the time to failure was dated back to that missed appointment.

Univariate life-table analysis using Kaplan–Meier curves was performed for primary and secondary success for all veins and for primary and secondary success for great saphenous reflux, small saphenous reflux and tributaries alone without saphenous reflux. Multivariate Cox regression analysis was used to estimate hazard ratios for covariates that might affect outcome for all veins and for all saphenous veins. The covariates studied were age and sex, right or left side, date of procedure (which indicated the experience of the operator), primary or recurrent varicose veins, vein treated, representative diameter of the vein, technique of injection into tributaries or the saphenous trunk, use of foam or liquid, sodium tetradecyl sulfate or polidocanol, concentration of sclerosant, and volume of liquid or foam infused.

For covariates with continuous rather than categorical data, an arbitrary point was taken to separate approximately equal subgroups. To avoid linearity assumptions, we categorized continuous covariates. We selected categories based on quartiles of the variable's distribution, independent of its association with the outcome variable. We used a likelihood-ratio χ^2 test to assess the contribution of each predictor variable in a final model. The unit of analysis for Cox proportional hazard regression was the vein. We used the Huber/White sandwich estimator of variance to accommodate clustering of veins within the same patient. Each vein inherited the higher-level characteristics of its "parent" limb and patient within the regression model.

Results of treatment with ultrasound-guided sclerotherapy

Primary and secondary success rates

Primary success rates at 3 years for all veins were 53.6% (95% confidence interval [CI] 48–59%) (Figure 9.4). Secondary success rates at 3 years for all veins were 77.4% (95% CI 72–82%) (Figure 9.5). Primary success rates at 3 years for great saphenous veins, small saphenous veins and tributaries alone were 55.5%, 36.8% and 78.9%, respectively (Figure 9.6). Secondary success rates at 3 years for great saphenous veins, small saphenous veins and tributaries alone were 81.4%, 64.4% and 86.7%, respectively (Figure 9.7).

Covariates affecting primary success rates

Cox regression analysis for all veins treated showed significantly worse primary success rates compared with tributaries alone (hazard ratio [HR] 2.67; 95% CI 1.6–4.5). Cox regression analysis for all saphenous veins and related tributaries is shown in Table 9.2. It showed worse primary success rates for small compared with great saphenous veins (HR 1.60; 95% CI 1.2–2.2), and for veins >5 mm diameter compared with veins ≤5 mm diameter (HR 1.78; 95% CI 1.3–2.3) (Figure 9.8) and for liquid compared with foam sclerotherapy (HR 1.75; 95% CI 1.2–2.5) (Figure 9.9). Subdivision of success rates for each of the sclerosant concentrations used showed best results for a 1.5% solution compared with either stronger or weaker concentrations (Figure 9.10). In addition, hazard ratios suggested better results for patients older

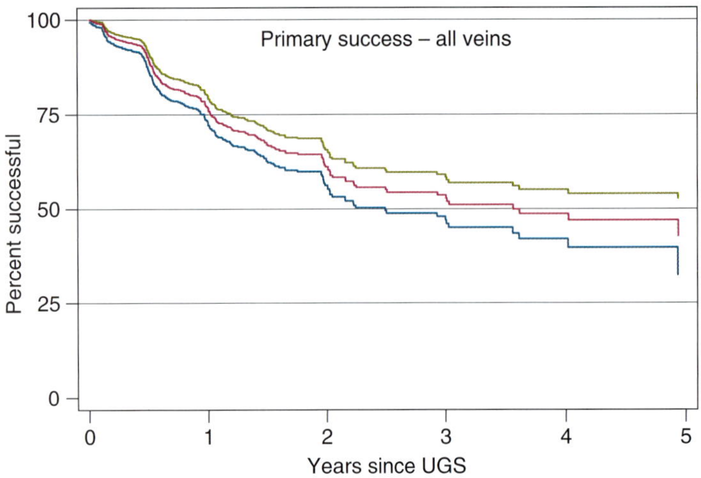

Figure 9.4 Kaplan–Meier curves showing primary success rates with 95% confidence intervals for all veins treated by ultrasound-guided sclerotherapy

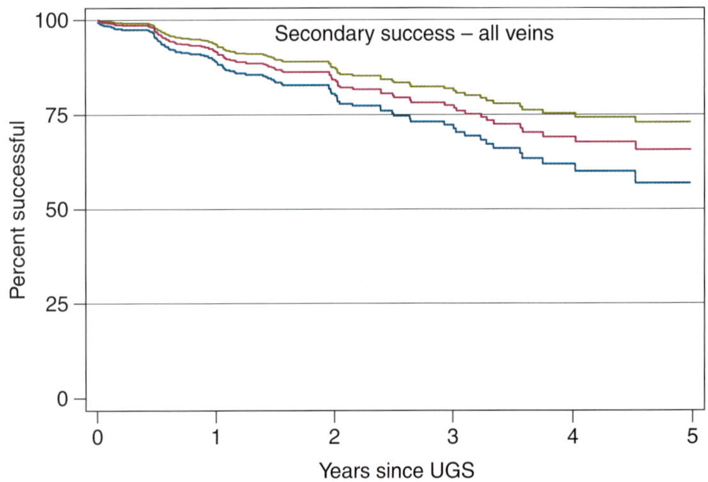

Figure 9.5 Kaplan–Meier curves showing secondary success rates with 95% confidence intervals for all veins treated by ultrasound-guided sclerotherapy

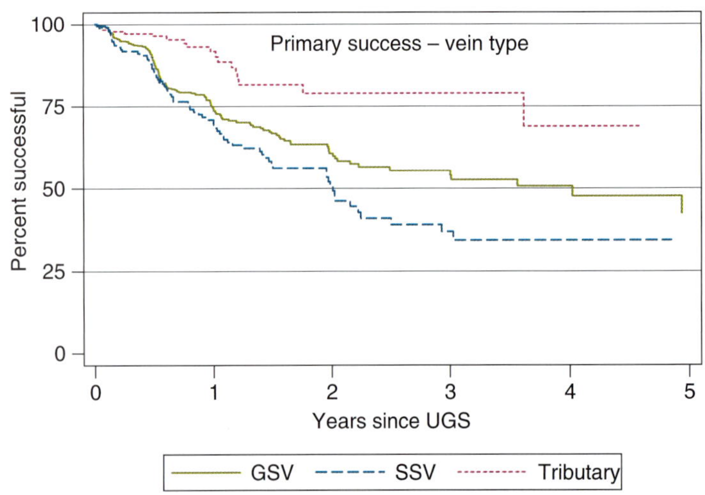

Figure 9.6 Kaplan–Meier curves showing primary success rates after ultrasound-guided sclerotherapy for great saphenous veins, small saphenous veins and tributaries alone

Table 9.2 Cox regression analysis of covariates studied for outcome of ultrasound-guided sclerotherapy for saphenous veins (n = 727)

Covariate	Hazard ratio	Standard error	$P > \|z\|$	95% confidence interval
Type of saphenous vein				
Great[a]	1			
Small	1.635	0.273	0.003	(1.179 to 2.267)
Vein diameter				
≤5 mm[a]	1			
>5 mm	1.694	0.246	<0.001	(1.275 to 2.253)
Type of sclerosant				
Foam[a]	1			
Liquid	1.854	0.519	0.027	(1.071 to 3.209)
Concentration of sclerosant				
0.6%	1.981	0.575	0.018	(1.122 to 3.499)
0.75–1.2%	1.738	0.559	0.085	(0.926 to 3.264)
1.5%[a]	1			
2–3%	1.608	0.527	0.148	(0.846 to 3.058)
Patient age group (years)				
<40	1.606	0.391	0.052	(0.996 to 2.588)
40–49	1.172	0.260	0.474	(0.759 to 1.810)
50–59[a]	1			
60–69	1.063	0.223	0.772	(0.705 to 1.603)
70+	0.646	0.182	0.121	(0.372 to 1.122)
CEAP grading				
C2/3[a]	1			
C4–6	1.378	0.350	0.207	(0.838 to 2.268)

[a]Baseline category.

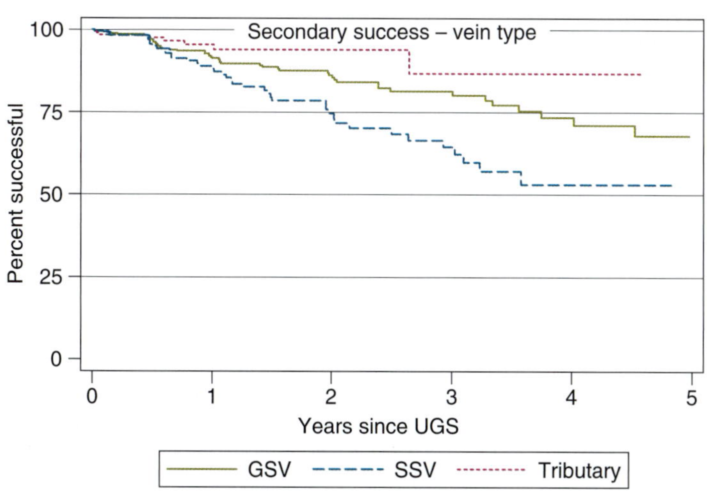

Figure 9.7 Kaplan–Meier curves showing secondary success rates after ultrasound-guided sclerotherapy for great saphenous veins, small saphenous veins and tributaries alone

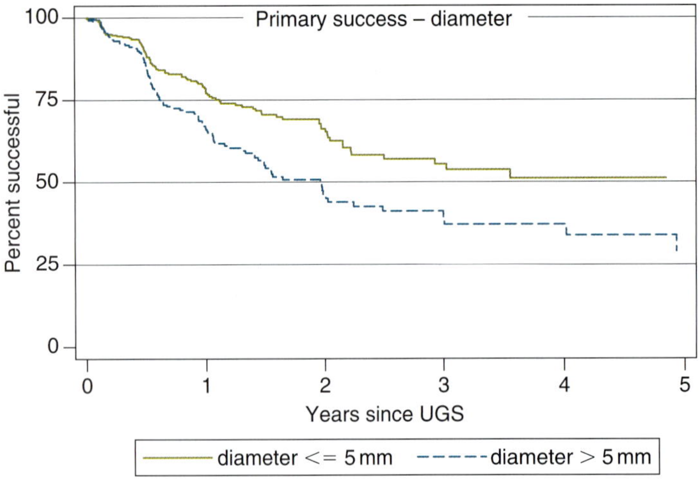

Figure 9.8 Kaplan–Meier curves showing primary success rates for all saphenous veins after ultrasound-guided sclerotherapy according to the vein diameter

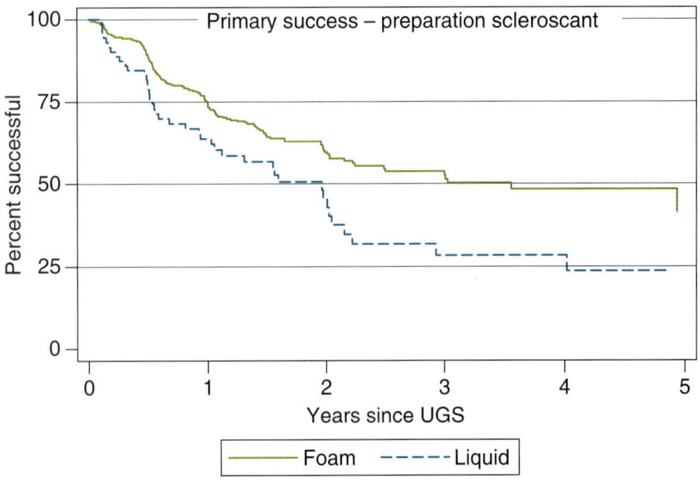

Figure 9.9 Kaplan–Meier curves showing primary success rates for all saphenous veins after ultrasound-guided sclerotherapy comparing liquid and foam

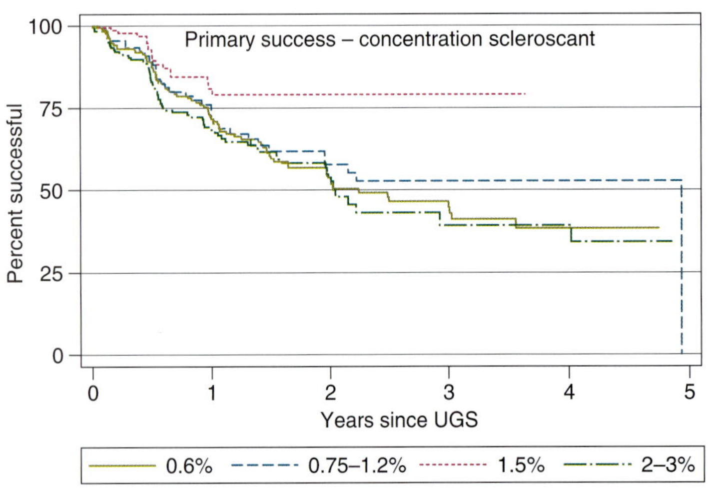

Figure 9.10 Kaplan–Meier curves showing primary success rates for all saphenous veins after ultrasound-guided sclerotherapy according to the concentration of sclerosant

than 70 years compared with patients aged 50–59 years (HR 0.65; 95% CI 0.4–1.1) and worse for CEAP category C_{4-6} compared with $C_{2/3}$ (HR 1.50; 95% CI 0.9–2.4). Other covariates studied showed little or no association with primary success outcome.

Postoperative complications

The routine early postoperative scan after all 1822 treatment sessions for foam UGS in both groups detected deep vein occlusion after 25 sessions. There were 13 fully occlusive posterior tibial vein occlusions and 12 partially occlusive femoropopliteal occlusions (3 femoral and 9 popliteal). All were asymptomatic, and the axial vein occlusions all resolved within a short period. Follow-up scans showed persisting reflux after recanalization in the posterior tibial segment in 5 limbs and persisting occlusion of the rest. All deep vein occlusions followed use of foam, and the volume infused ranged from 5 to 35 mL (median 13 mL). The risk of deep venous occlusion in relation to the number of veins treated increased from 0% in veins in which less than 5 mL of foam was infused up to 3.3% in veins in which more than 20 mL of foam was infused (Table 9.3).

The treatment policy for above-knee axial vein occlusions was to give therapeutic levels of subcutaneous low-molecular-weight heparin for 1–2 weeks until ultrasound showed that the occlusion was well incorporated into the vein wall. Tibial vein occlusions were simply observed with a further scan at 1 week to confirm that there had been no extension. We did not observe any instance of damage to overlying skin, cutaneous sensory nerves, deeper nerves or other structures in the limbs.

No clinical episodes of pulmonary embolism or other cardiovascular complications were observed after UGS. Three patients with a prior history of migraine headaches developed visual aura during mobilization after injection, all typical of previous symptoms, and all settled within 20 minutes without headache or residual neurologic deficit. No other neurologic symptoms were observed. No other complications were noted.

Table 9.3 Relation of deep venous occlusion to volume of foam infused for each vein treated

	Deep vein occlusion		
Volume of foam (mL)	No	Yes	Total
1–4	166 100.00%	0 0.00%	166
5–9	953 99.48%	5 0.52%	958
10–19	472 97.32%	13 2.68%	485
20+	206 96.71%	7 3.29%	213
Total	1,797 98.63%	25 1.37%	1822

Discussion

Action of sclerosants

Sclerosants denude vein endothelium, and this leads to some degree of thrombosis. The amount of thrombus is reduced by immediate vein spasm and subsequent compression. It is anticipated that there will be rapid fibrosis across the lumen, although the greater the residual thrombus in the lumen then the more likely it is that the vein will recanalize with recurrent reflux. There is inadequate knowledge of the rate of vein shrinkage and fibrosis after UGS, and this requires further study by serial ultrasound examinations to measure diameter changes and objectively measure ultrasound echogenicity within the vein lumen.

The present study showed no significant difference for results comparing sodium tetradecyl sulfate and polidocanol as the sclerosant in terms of medium-term technical success. However, some phlebologists advocate one or the other for reasons of reducing pain, phlebitis, pigmentation and other effects. This needs to be studied in more detail by randomized trials comparing the two sclerosants.

Preparation of sclerosants

Initially, sclerosants for UGS were injected as a liquid, but this has several constraints. Only a limited volume can be administered to stay within dosage limits and this volume is frequently inadequate to occlude the vein. Liquid sclerosant stays in contact with the endothelium for only a short time before flowing away, so that endothelial damage may be inadequate. The fluid mixes with blood, leading to the possibility of excess "trapped blood" in the veins. These problems are greatly reduced by converting the sclerosant into foam. The sclerosants used readily make foam as they are detergents. Foam stays in the lumen acting on the endothelium for far longer – it can frequently be seen on a review scan up to several days later. A diluted solution can be given, since the effect is so much more prolonged. Foam largely displaces blood, reducing the amount of "trapped blood." Finally, foam is easily seen and followed with ultrasound as it is highly echogenic.

In the present study, there were significantly better long-term results for foamed sclerosant rather than liquid sclerosant, independent of experience. The use of foam rather than liquid is strongly supported in the contemporary literature.[4,9,10] French phlebologists performed a randomized prospective multicenter trial of injection for great saphenous reflux in 88 patients using polidocanol.[9] They found that a single injection controlled 84% in the foam group and only 40% in the liquid sclerosant group. Of those that were occluded, ultrasound at 6 months showed recanalization in two veins in the foam group and six in the liquid sclerosant group. Japanese workers performed a similar study of UGS with polidocanol for 77 great saphenous veins.[10] They showed occlusion in 68% of the foam group and only 18% for the liquid group, and recanalization in three veins in the foam group compared with ten veins in the liquid group. It is unlikely that these types of trials will be repeated.

Initially, we could find no compelling clinical evidence to favor any technique for preparation of foam sclerosant or its administration. Accordingly, we chose to use various techniques in an attempt to intuitively select the best method in different patients. This differs from some arbitrary recommendations made by other phlebologists. The most commonly used technique in Australia is to administer a 3% solution of either sclerosant, but we elected to dilute this to increase the volume of foam in many patients. The present study showed significantly better medium-term results for 1.5% sclerosant rather than more diluted or undiluted 3% sclerosant. This is not intuitive, and needs to be explained by further research. It is starting to become apparent that the two sclerosant agents have either procoagulant or anticoagulant effects according to their dilution, but much needs to be done to unravel why this should influence clinical outcome.

The total maximum dose of sclerosant used for each treatment session was that allowed by the Australian regulatory TGA. The use of sclerosant as foam is allowed by the TGA as an "off the label" product provided that patient consent is obtained. The total volumes of foam used in the present study were frequently considerably more than used by many phlebologists, although no more than recommended by Cabrera.[4] Concerns have been expressed regarding the maximum volume of foam that should be used at one session, and a European consensus group and a German national group have established guidelines,[21,22] but these have not yet been subjected to scientific analysis. No conclusive evidence is available that larger volumes are associated with any increased risk to the patient other than the increased likelihood of deep vein occlusion observed in the present study.

The technique that we used to prepare foam is different to that initially recommended by Cabrera[4] or Tessari.[6] It is considered that inclusion of a 5 μm filter in the system increased foam stability. We could find little published information describing objective techniques to determine which preparation provided the finest and most stable microfoam. There is a need for further research to determine the best gas to use, the optimal proportion of gas to liquid, the most effective concentration of the sclerosant and the best way to mix the fluid and gas.

Commercial preparations are being developed, but these are still not available for general use. They use gases that do not contain nitrogen, as this is much less soluble than alternatives such as oxygen or carbon dioxide. Commercial preparations contain agents that stabilize foam. The optimal mixture for the gas is a balance between those that dissolve before they pass into the general circulation, yet remain as foam for long enough to be effective in the treated superficial veins. The various combinations have yet to be tested widely in clinical practice. It is not yet certain whether these mixtures reduce the incidence of systemic side-effects or complications. The stability and efficacy of foam sclerosant is believed to be inversely proportional to the bubble size in the foam, but the texture of foam in most studies (including our own) is usually not known. Whether microfoam is indeed more effective than foam with larger bubble size has yet to be widely tested.

Techniques for injection

There are many techniques advocated by phlebologists, ranging from injecting as far proximal to as far distal as possible. We elect to inject as far away from connections to deep veins as possible, but whether this reduces systemic spillage is not known. Some phlebologists prefer to inject with the limb elevated or at least horizontal. Some prefer to wait for some time after injection before applying the bandages or stocking or mobilizing the patient. The various techniques appear to result from perceptions as to how best to avoid displacing foam from the leg into the general circulation. Further research is required using ultrasound to study passage of foam bubbles into the right heart or through a patent foramen ovale or pulmonary circulation into the arterial circulation in an attempt to show which technique results in the least volume and duration of systemic bubbles.

Selection of patients

When saphenous veins were considered in this study, no significant independent influence on outcome was demonstrated for date of procedure, sex, side, or primary or recurrent varicose veins. However, primary success rates were independently significantly better for several covariates relating to the veins and treatment techniques. Treatment was more likely to be effective for great saphenous compared with small saphenous veins, and smaller compared with larger diameter veins. There were other covariates where hazard ratios suggested better outcome in older patients and for clinical C_2 rather than C_{4-6}. Others have shown better outcome for small-diameter compared with large-diameter veins,[6] although satisfactory results for large veins have also been reported.[4] The findings relating to the difference between the great and small saphenous veins are not intuitive, which suggests the need for further research.

Any size vein can be treated, particularly if the patient has been warned that repeat treatment may be required in the future. However, we now increasingly advise EVLT for larger diameter saphenous veins and consider phlebectomy for large tributaries of the thigh.

In the present study, adequate control of the veins was frequently achieved with one treatment session, in agreement with the experience of Cabrera and colleagues.[4,5] Success was far more likely for tributaries alone compared with saphenous veins. Primary success rates at 3 years determined by ultrasound for great saphenous veins were approximately 55%, so that patients should be warned that repeat treatment may be required at some time in the future, preferably when the veins are still relatively small. However, the secondary success rate at 3 years for great saphenous veins was more than 80%, indicating that UGS provides a satisfactory outcome. The improved secondary success rate presumably would have been even higher if all patients had agreed to repeat treatment, but many did not as they had not developed clinical recurrence. The excellent primary and secondary success rates for tributaries indicates that UGS is an appropriate option for treatment in all patients. However, the success rates were not as good for the small saphenous vein as for the great saphenous, prompting us to prefer EVLT if possible.

Statistical analysis of results

Ultrasound surveillance provides the most stringent test for success after any treatment for varicose veins. It is also important to determine factors such as clinical recurrence rates, patient satisfaction, quality of life and cost-effectiveness, but these were not assessed in this study. It is unfortunate that guidelines for presentation of results have not yet been adequately developed in phlebology. Many articles present interval success rates at some time after treatment representing the number who remain successful in the small group who have persisted with follow-up. This is meaningless and misleading as it represents the persisting successes and ignores the earlier failures. Life-table analysis to present a cumulative success rate is essential for honest assessment of outcome allowing different series to be compared. Multivariate Cox regression analysis allows independent comparison of outcome in subgroups over a period of time.

Comparison with other forms of treatment

Ultrasound surveillance has been used by van Rij and colleagues to determine outcome after surgery, with success at 3 years in 79% of limbs after great saphenous surgery and 49% of limbs after small saphenous surgery.[23] Ultrasound surveillance has also been used to determine success after radiofrequency closure for great saphenous reflux[24] and after EVLT for great and small saphenous reflux.[25] However, there are few studies after UGS. Kanter and Thibault reported cumulative success of 76% at 2 years from an early experience with liquid sclerosant,[9] while Belcaro and colleagues showed 56% success at 10 years with foam sclerotherapy.[11] Cabrera and colleagues have pioneered foam sclerotherapy and report good results for large-diameter great saphenous veins,[4,5] although the statistical techniques used to calculate outcome are not clear. Randomized studies with ultrasound follow-up are needed to compare different treatment techniques and to determine whether alternative methods provide superior results to those described in this chapter.

Complications

The only complication observed in this study was deep vein occlusion, which occurred in 3.2% of patients. This is somewhat higher than reported in other studies,[26] but this may reflect an aggressive policy to scan the deep veins within a few days after treatment for every session, since this unearthed asymptomatic thromboses that otherwise probably would not have become apparent. This rate is similar to that described with ultrasound evaluation after surgery for varicose veins.[27] We consider that the deep vein occlusions seen differ from spontaneous deep vein thrombosis as the appearances on ultrasound are different. After UGS, an occluded segment of deep vein has a far more echogenic appearance than fresh clot and the "sclerus" appears to be quite adherent to the wall. The partial occlusions in above-knee axial deep veins all quickly resolved to become incorporated into the vein wall.

Neurologic complications have been reported in the literature[28,29] but were not observed in this series, other than occasional visual aura in patients with a known history of migraine headaches with aura. Further analysis of series looking carefully with objective techniques are required to see if there are high-risk patients for arterial embolism, such as those with patent foramen ovale, in whom UGS may be contraindicated.

Future directions

The findings from this study support the use of UGS for varicose disease with or without saphenous reflux, provided that patients are warned of the possible need for repeat treatment to achieve secondary success. Results are not as good for large-diameter veins or the small saphenous vein, and a personal preference now is to treat these by EVLT or radiofrequency closure. The study encourages us now to dilute the sclerosant to a 1.5% concentration before preparing the foam and to use as much foam as is necessary to fill the diseased venous segments. Patients should be warned that there is a risk of postoperative deep vein occlusion, and we will continue the practice of early postoperative ultrasound scanning to detect asymptomatic thromboses. There is a great need for further objective research to find ways to improve outcome and minimize complications.

References

1. Hobbs JT. Surgery and sclerotherapy in the treatment of varicose veins. A random trial. Arch Surg 1974; 109: 793–96.
2. Knight RM. Treatment of superficial venous disease with accurate sclerotherapy. Proceedings of the Canadian Society of Phlebology. Whistler, British Columbia, Canada. 1991.
3. Grondin L, Soriano J. UGS, a Canadian study. In: Raymond Martimbeau P, Prescott R, Zummo M, eds. Phlebologie 1992, Paris: John Libbey Eurotext, 1992: 828–31.
4. Cabrera J, Cabrera J Jr, Garcia-Olmedo MA. Treatment of varicose long saphenous veins with sclerosant in microfoam form: long-term outcomes. Phlebology 2000; 15: 19–23.
5. Cabrera J, Cabrera J Jr, Garcia Olmedo MA. Sclerosants in microfoam. A new approach in angiology. Int Angiol 2001; 20: 322–9.
6. Tessari L, Cavezzi A, Frullini. A preliminary experience with a new sclerosing foam in the treatment of varicose veins. Dermatol Surg 2001; 27: 58–60.
7. Frullini A, Cavezzi A. Sclerosing foam in the treatment of varicose veins and telangiectases: history and analysis of safety and complications. Dermatol Surg 2002; 28: 11–15.
8. Cavezzi A, Frullini A, Ricci S, Tessari L. Treatment of varicose veins by foam sclerotherapy: two clinical series. Phlebology 2002: 17; 13–18.
9. Hamel-Desnos C, Desnos P, Wollmann JC, et al. Evaluation of the efficacy of polidocanol in the form of foam compared with liquid form in sclerotherapy of the greater saphenous vein: initial results. Dermatol Surg 2003; 29: 1170–5.
10. Yamaki T, Nozaki M, Iwasaka S. Comparative study of duplex-guided foam sclerotherapy and duplex-guided liquid sclerotherapy for the treatment of superficial venous insufficiency. Dermatol Surg 2004; 30: 718–22.
11. Kanter A, Thubault P. Saphenofemoral incompetence treated by ultrasound-guided sclerotherapy. Dermatol Surg 1996; 22: 648–52.
12. Belcaro G, Cesarone MR, Di Renzo A, et al. Foam-sclerotherapy, surgery, sclerotherapy, and combined treatment for varicose veins: a 10-year, prospective, randomized, controlled, trial (VEDICO trial). Angiology 2003; 54: 307–15.

13. Barrett JM, Allen B, Ockelford A, Goldman MP. Microfoam ultrasound-guided sclerotherapy treatment for varicose veins in a subgroup with diameters at the junction of 10 mm or greater compared with a subgroup of less than 10 mm. Dermatol Surg 2004; 30: 1386–90.
14. Smith PC. Chronic venous disease treated by ultrasound guided foam sclerotherapy. Eur J Vasc Endovasc Surg 2006; 32: 577–83.
15. Darke SG, Baker SJ. Ultrasound-guided foam sclerotherapy for the treatment of varicose veins. Br J Surg 2006; 93: 969–74.
16. Myers KA, Jolley D, Clough A, Kirwan J. Outcome of ultrasound-guided sclerotherapy for varicose veins: medium-term results assessed by ultrasound surveillance. Eur J Vasc Endovasc Surg 2007; 33: 116–21.
17. Davies AH. Vein factors that affect the outcome of femorodital bypass. Ann R Coll Surg Engl 1995; 77: 63–6.
18. Myers KA, Ziegenbein RW, Zeng GH, Matthews PG. Duplex ultrasonography scanning for chronic venous disease: patterns of venous reflux. J Vasc Surg 1995; 21: 605–12.
19. Wills V, Moylan D, Chambers J. The use of routine duplex scanning in the assessment of varicose veins. Aust NZ J Surg 1998; 68: 41–4.
20. Mercer KG, Scott DJ, Berridge DC. Preoperative duplex imaging is required before all operations for primary varicose veins. Br J Surg 1998; 85: 1495–7.
21. Breu FX, Guggenbichler S. European Consensus Meeting on Foam Sclerotherapy, April 4–6, 2003, Tegernsee, Germany. Dermatol Surg 2004; 30: 709–17.
22. Rabe E, Pannier-Fischer F, Gerlach H, et al. German Society of Phlebology. Guidelines for sclerotherapy of varicose veins (ICD 10: I83.0, I83.1, I83.2, and I83.9). Dermatol Surg 2004; 30: 687–93.
23. Van Rij AM, Jiang P, Solomon C, et al. Recurrence after varicose vein surgery: a prospective long-term clinical study with duplex ultrasound scanning and air plethysmography. J Vasc Surg 2003; 38: 935–43.
24. Almeida JI, Raines JK. Radiofrequency ablation and laser ablation in the treatment of varicose veins. Ann Vasc Surg 2006; 20: 547–52.
25. Myers K, Fris R, Jolley D. Treatment of varicose veins by endovenous laser therapy: assessment of results by ultrasound surveillance. Med J Aust 2006; 185: 199–202.
26. Guex JJ, Allaert FA, Gillet JL, Chleir F. Immediate and midterm complications of sclerotherapy: report of a prospective multicenter registry of 12 173 sclerotherapy sessions. Dermatol Surg 2005; 31: 123–8.
27. van Rij AM, Chai J, Hill GB, Christie RA. Incidence of deep vein thrombosis after varicose vein surgery. Br J Surg 2004; 91: 1582–85.
28. Hanisch F, Muller T, Krivokuca M, Winterholler M. Stroke following variceal sclerotherapy. Eur J Med Res 2004; 9: 282–4.
29. Forlee MV, Grouden M, Moore DJ, Shanik G. Stroke after varicose vein foam injection sclerotherapy. J Vasc Surg 2006; 43: 162–4.

SPECIAL CONSIDERATIONS

10 Varisolve® polidocanol microfoam compared with surgery or sclerotherapy in the management of varicose veins in the presence of trunk vein incompetence: European randomized controlled trial

David DI Wright, Jean Pierre Gobin, Andrew W Bradbury, Philip D Coleridge Smith, Harry Spoelstra, David Berridge, Cees HA Wittens, Anja Sommer, Olle Nelzen, Dennis Chanter, on behalf of the Varisolve® European Phase III Investigators Group

Introduction

Varicose veins are a common problem, present in approximately 25% of the Western adult population.[1] Early varicose veins are relatively benign, but some patients will progress to develop severe and irreversible problems of chronic venous insufficiency, including venous ulcers.[2,3]

Surgery, by high ligation and stripping of trunk veins, is still considered the "gold standard" for treatment of varicose veins in association with trunk vein incompetence. Surgery has been demonstrated to be more efficacious and durable than sclerotherapy, but its position as the standard of care has been challenged more recently by heat ablation therapy: radiofrequency ablation (RFA) or endovenous laser therapy (EVLT).[4,5] Recurrence following surgery remains a problem, and the occurrence of surgical complications, although infrequent, highlights the need for an effective, safe and patient-friendly treatment.[6,7] Heat ablation treatments have met this need in part, but are linked to pain and bruising, skin burns, paresthesias, phlebitis, deep vein thrombosis (DVT) and pulmonary embolism (PE).[8–13] Sclerotherapy using liquid sclerosant is effective for the treatment of telangiectasias and small varicose veins; however, controlling the dose and its distribution are problematic.[14]

There is no consensus about which treatment is most effective for varicose veins. A review comparing surgery and sclerotherapy concluded that there was insufficient evidence to recommend either treatment preferentially.[15] However, the application of ultrasound guidance to sclerotherapy has led to improvements in this technique.[16,17]

The invention of sclerosant microfoam that displaces blood from the vessel has resulted in succesful treatment of larger veins, including the great saphenous vein (GSV).[14,18] In comparative studies, polidocanol microfoam was more efficacious than liquid in the treatment of saphenous veins.[19–21] It is also effective in the treatment of some vascular malformations and chronic venous insufficiency causing leg ulcers.[14,18,21]

Varisolve® polidocanol microfoam was developed to provide several advantages over investigator-generated foams, including consistent microfoam quality, bubble size and sterility.

The aim of this study was to compare the safety and efficacy of the defined technique using polidocanol 1% microfoam formulation against that of alternative treatments (surgery or sclerotherapy) for varicose veins and trunk vein incompetence.

Methods

Patients

Patients, aged from 18 to 75 years, with varicose veins and great and/or small saphenous incompetence were recruited from the clinical practice of investigating physicians. Eligible patients were assessed and assigned to receive either surgery or sclerotherapy based on the extent of their disease and physician preference. Once the alternative treatment had been selected, they were randomized to either the Varisolve® technique or the chosen alternative treatment. Thus, two separate cohorts were created: Varisolve®/surgery and Varisolve®/sclerotherapy. The key inclusion and exclusion criteria for the study are shown in Table 10.1.

Regulatory and local ethics committee approval was obtained for each center and all patients gave written informed consent.

Study design

This study was an open-label, international, multicenter, randomized Phase 3 trial to evaluate the safety and efficacy of the Varisolve® technique using polidocanol 1% microfoam in comparison with alternative treatments in the management of patients with moderate to severe varicose veins. The investigators were selected on the basis of their expertise in venous disease management and ability to recruit adequate patient numbers. These were either experienced vascular surgeons, some with limited experience of sclerotherapy prior to the study, or experienced phlebologists, primarily from France. Investigators were provided with the Varisolve® Training Manual and accompanying video and were supervised during the first five treatments or until basic proficiency was demonstrated.

Screening assessments included physical examination, medical history, hematology and biochemistry laboratory tests. Clinical examination and duplex scanning of the leg determined the patients' CEAP classification[22] and allowed the investigator to select a suitable treatment for each patient.

Patients underwent central randomization to either the Varisolve® technique or alternative treatment at a ratio of 2 : 1 in favor of the Varisolve® technique (Figure 10.1). The surgical or sclerotherapy approach used as an alternative to Varisolve® was not specified. Any marketed sclerosant at any marketed concentrationas was permitted either as liquid or as investigator-generated foam. Efficacy and safety were assessed by duplex scanning on days 7 and 28 and at months 3 and 12. If additional treatment was necessary, this was performed on days 7 and 14

Table 10.1 Key inclusion and exclusion criteria

Inclusion	Exclusion
• Male or female • Aged 18–75 years • SFJ or SPJ incompetence or both with retrograde blood flow for >1 s and <7 s demonstrated by duplex scanning • Great saphenous incompetence and/or short saphenous incompetence • Minimum of 10 cm of proximal trunk vein incompetence • Normal arterial circulation; ankle:brachial pressure ratio >0.9 • Hematology and blood chemistry profiles within normal/acceptable limits, i.e., abnormalities not clinically significant • Normal deep venous system on duplex scanning, no evidence of occlusion or incompetence. Evidence of reflux acceptable, however, if confined to a limited segment caused by filling of the superficial system	• History of major superficial thrombophlebitis • Venographic or ultrasonographic evidence of current or previous DVT • Immobility—unable to walk a minimum of 5 min/h per day • Body mass index >32 kg/m² • Contraindications for polidocanol: severe hypertension, glomerulonephritis and nephroses, hepatopathy, active phlebitis, general febrile disease, diabetes, asthma, advanced arteriosclerosis • Serious coexisting illness, including carcinoma, cardiac or respiratory disease, past or present venous ulcers, pregnancy, or lactation • Concomitant treatment with disulfiram, systemic corticosteroids, estrogen, or anticoagulants • Known allergic response to polidocanol or severe allergic diathesis • Abnormal, clinically significant hematology or biochemistry profiles

for patients treated with Varisolve® and between days 7 and 21 for surgery or sclerotherapy patients.

Varisolve® treatment

Varisolve® polidocanol microfoam is a uniform foam of physiological gases, principally oxygen and carbon dioxide, combined with a 1% aqueous solution of polidocanol. It is generated at the point of use from an aerosol canister. The maximum total dose of microfoam was initially set at 60 mL, which was subsequently reduced to 30 mL. The aims of the Varisolve® technique are to eliminate all deep to superficial vein reflux and occlude associated trunk veins and superficial varicosities.

The Varisolve® technique was carried out under ultrasound guidance in five stages in accordance with the Training Manual.

1. Cannulation of the trunk vein and proof of venous access to avoid intra-arterial injection.
2. Injection of microfoam into the trunk vein, filling the vein from the cannulation site to its termination with the deep vein, while carefully monitoring either the saphenofemoral junction (SFJ) or saphenopopliteal junction (SPJ) for the arrival of microfoam. After foam was seen at the junction, the trunk vein was compressed to stop microfoam from freely passing into the deep veins.
3. Spasm of the injected vein segment was confirmed by ultrasound before further injection of the distal trunk vein through the same cannulation site with digital compression of the GSV proximal to the cannula tip.
4. Any residual varicosities were injected with Varisolve® using a butterfly needle.
5. Once treatment was complete, compression was applied consisting of an under bandage from ankle to groin, foam pads along the treated veins, a second layer of bandage, a thin overstocking, and finally 30–40 mmHg and thigh length compression stocking (Sigvaris). Compression was worn for 14 days post-treatment, day and night for the first 7 days; patients were advised to walk for 5 minutes in each waking hour for the first 7 days post-treatment.

Varisolve® technique changes. During the study, modifications to the treatment procedure were implemented, intended to reduce the risk of DVT. The amendments reduced the maximum total dose of microfoam per treatment session to 30 mL and required the injection to be stopped and compression applied to the terminal GSV or small saphenous vein (SSV) when microfoam was seen 5 cm from the SFJ or SPJ. In addition, the maximum volume of the initial injection of the trunk vein was calculated based on the distance (in centimeters) from the point of cannulation to the junction. Retrograde filling of the SSV trunk was prohibited.

Duplex scanning

Duplex scans were carried out by experienced technologists or physicians. They were trained to follow a detailed protocol that required the imaging of all major veins. The deep calf veins were repeatedly checked throughout their length for the presence of thrombus, and their competence was monitored by compression and color flow filling during and following calf compression. The status of each vein was scored at screening and at each follow-up visit after treatment.

Efficacy assessment

The primary end-point was the response to treatment at month 3, defined as the occlusion of incompetent trunk vein(s) from the source of deep to superficial flow, and the elimination of reflux greater than 0.5 s in the treated vein(s) 2–5 cm from its point of termination, as determined by duplex scanning. In order to be considered a responder, both occlusion (or, for surgery, absence) of the treated vein and elimination of junctional reflux were required. If the GSV and SSV had been treated, both veins had to meet both criteria in order for the patient to be classified as a responder.

The secondary end-points included severity of post-procedure pain (day 1–6 measured using a visual analog scale [VAS]), time taken to return to normal activities, the number of treatment sessions required and the month-12 response rate.

Statistical analysis

The statistical analysis was based on comparison of the whole population by meta-analysis to test a noninferiority hypothesis. The intended sample size of 650 patients was chosen to demonstrate noninferiority of Varisolve®, assuming an 85% response rate with alternative treatment. Noninferiority was to be deemed established if the lower bound of the 95% confidence interval (CI) for the treatment difference (Varisolve® – alternative treatment)

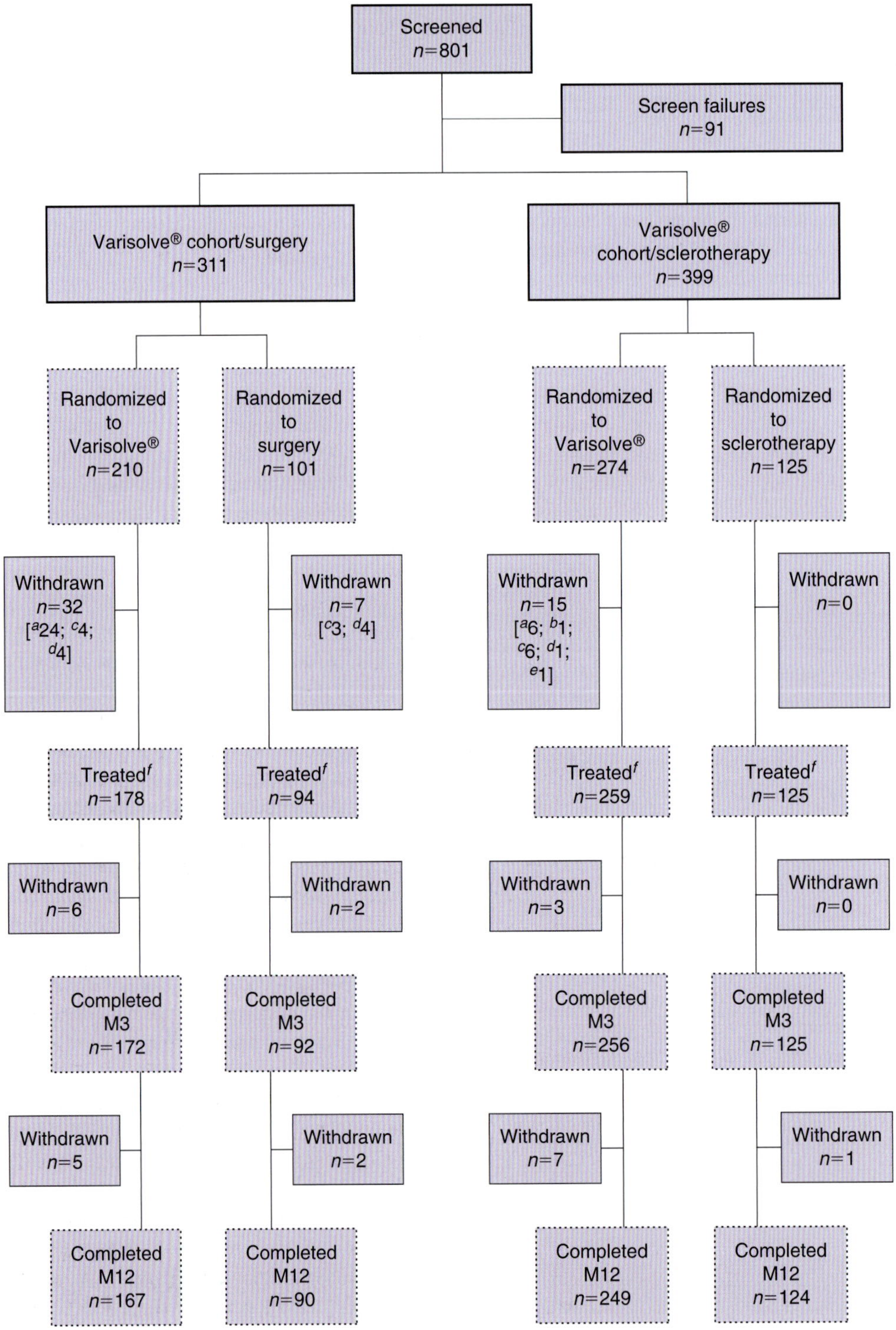

Figure 10.1 Patient disposition. M3, month 3; M12, month 12. [a]Study interupted by sponsor. [b]Adverse event. [c]Patient decision. [d]Other reasons. [e]Missing. [f]First treatment (Leg 1)

did not lie below −15 percentage points. The two independently randomized cohorts (Varisolve®/surgery and Varisolve®/sclerotherapy) were analyzed separately. The proportions of patients responding at month 3 were compared between the treatment groups using a logistic regression analysis, with covariate adjustment for a number of prespecified factors, including gender, disease status, and study center. Missing data were imputed using the last observation carried forward technique, provided that data were available for at least one post-treatment visit.

Results

Patient demography

Seven hundred and ten patients were randomized, of whom 54 were withdrawn before treatment, which was delayed to permit a review of potential causes of DVT. Six hundred and fifty-six patients were treated, of whom 26 withdrew from the study after treatment (Figure 10.1). In the Varisolve®/surgery cohort, 178 patients were treated with Varisolve® and 94 with surgery, while 259 were treated with Varisolve® and 125 with sclerotherapy in the Varisolve®/sclerotherapy cohort. Of the treated patients, all but 2, who provided no post-treatment data (both were treated with Varisolve® in the Varisolve®/surgery cohort), were included in the statistical analysis.

Patient demographics were typical of varicose-vein treatment populations (Table 10.2), with the majority being female, of mean age of 50 years, and few patients with recurrent disease following previous treatment.

The two cohorts were similar in most respects. However, the Varisolve®/sclerotherapy cohort had more female patients (71.9% vs 63.2%; $P = 0.022$, Fisher's exact test), more recurrent varicosities (16.9% vs 8.9%; $P = 0.003$, Fisher's exact test), a smaller baseline GSV diameter (7.1 mm vs 7.9 mm; $P < 0.001$, Student's t-test), and a higher proportion of patients with SSV disease (23.4% vs 13.0%; $P < 0.001$, Fisher's exact test) than the Varisolve®/surgery cohort.

The CEAP classification was recorded at entry and was dominated by C_2, E_p, A_s, and P_r patients. All patients had to have varicose veins (C_2) to be included, and

Table 10.2 Patients' baseline demographic data

	Varisolve®/surgery cohort		Varisolve®/sclerotherapy cohort		All Varisolve®
	Varisolve® (*n* = 178)	Surgery (*n* = 94)	Varisolve® (*n* = 259)	Sclerotherapy (*n* = 125)	(*n* = 437)
Gender					
Male, *n* (%)	66 (37.1%)	34 (36.2%)	76 (29.3%)	32 (25.6%)	142 (32.5%)
Female, *n* (%)	112 (62.9%)	60 (63.8%)	183 (70.7%)	93 (74.4%)	295 (67.5%)
Mean age ± SD, y	49.9 ± 12.6	49.0 ± 11.2	50.7 ± 12.3	49.6 ± 12.2	50.4 ± 12.4
Vein disease, *n* (%)					
Primary					
GSV	141 (79.2%)	77 (81.9%)	169 (65.3%)	76 (60.8%)	310 (70.9%)
SSV	12 (6.7%)	8 (8.5%)	47 (18.1%)	23 (18.4%)	59 (13.5%)
GSV + SSV	8 (4.5%)	0	3 (1.2%)	1 (0.8%)	11 (2.5%)
Recurrent					
GSV	11 (6.2%)	6 (6.4%)	29 (11.2%)	20 (16.0%)	40 (9.2%)
SSV	1 (0.6%)	2 (2.1%)	11 (4.2%)	5 (4.0%)	12 (2.7%)
GSV + SSV	3 (1.7%)	1 (1.1%)	0	0	3 (0.7%)
CEAP classification[a]					
C_3	14 (7.9%)	11 (11.7%)[b]	58 (22.4%)	35 (28%)[b]	72 (16.5%)
C_4	20 (11.2%)	10 (10.6%)[c]	18 (6.9%)	11 (8.8%)[c]	38 (8.7%)

DVT, deep vein thrombosis; GSV, great saphenous vein; SFJ, saphenofemoral junction; SSV, small saphenous vein; SPJ, saphenopopliteal junction; SD, standard deviation.

[a] All patients were C_2 and above: C_5 and C_6 were exclusion criteria.

[b] C_3 more frequent in Varisolve®/sclerotherapy cohort, $P < 0.001$.

[c] C_4 more frequent Varisolve®/surgery cohort, $P < 0.075$ not significant.

edema or skin changes (C_3, C_4) were permitted. Patients with healed and open ulcers (C_5, C_6) and evidence of post-thrombotic deep vein disease were excluded. Etiology was primary in 98.2% and all patients had incompetent superficial veins. Incompetent perforator veins were present in only 12.1% of patients and deep vein incompetence was present in only 2.5% (only permitted if isolated and draining into superficial veins; all but 3 of 19 incompetent deep vein segments became competent after treatment). There were differences in the proportions of patients classified as C_3 and C_4 between the two groups of Varisolve®-treated patients: significantly more patients in the Varisolve®/sclerotherapy cohort were (C_3) 22% vs 7.9% in the Varisolve®/surgery group; $P < 0.001$); conversely, more patients had C_4 recorded in the Varisolve®/surgery cohorts but this difference was not statistically significant (11.2% vs 6.9%; $P =$ 0.075, Fisher's exact test).

Alternative treatments

Surgery. High ligation was performed in 91.5% of patients randomized to this approach, stripping in 88.3%, and avulsion phlebectomy in 53.2%. General anesthesia was used in 57.4% of surgical procedures and local anesthesia (including regional) in 42.6%; median operating time was 49 minutes (range: 15–200 minutes). Prophylactic perioperative anticoagulation was used in 22% of patients.

Sclerotherapy. Polidocanol and sodium tetradecyl sulfate were used with approximately equal frequency (61 and 64 patients, respectively). Investigators used their own, home-made foam rather than liquid in 92% of treatments. Sclerosants were used in concentrations ranging from 0.5% to 3%; the mean volume was 9.8 mL for foam and 3.5 mL for liquid.

Efficacy

Response rates at month 3 and month 12 are shown in Table 10.3. The overall response rate was 83.4% for Varisolve® and 88.1% for alternative therapy at month 3 and 78.9% and 80.4%, respectively, at month 12. At month 3, the lower limit of the 95% CI for the difference in response rate between Varisolve® and alternative treatment was –13%. This confirmed the noninferiority of the Varisolve® technique relative to the combined alternative treatments.

Analyzing the cohorts separately at month 3, the response rates were 68.2% for Varisolve® and 87.2% for surgery (Varisolve®/surgery), and 93.8% for Varisolve® and 88.8% for sclerotherapy (Varisolve®/sclerotherapy). Noninferiority of the Varisolve® technique to surgery was not demonstrated, while conversely there was a small but nonsignificant trend ($P = 0.06$) in favor of the Varisolve® technique relative to sclerotherapy in the Varisolve®/sclerotherapy cohort.

At month 12, overall noninferiority was again demonstrated: efficacy was 78.9% for Varisolve® and 80.4% for alternative therapies (lower limit of 95% CI for difference of –10%). The superiority of surgery over Varisolve® was maintained (86.2% vs 63.1%). In the Varisolve®/sclerotherapy group, when comparing month 3 and month 12 response rates, there was greater loss of efficacy with sclerotherapy than with Varisolve® (12.8% for sclerotherapy vs 4.2 % for Varisolve®) such that the Varisolve® response rate at month 12 (89.6%) was statistically superior to the response rate for sclerotherapy (76.0%; $P < 0.001$).

Secondary end-points

Surgery was associated with more pain than the Varisolve® treatment, and this difference extended throughout the first week (day 6: surgery median VAS score 9, Varisolve® VAS score 2, full scale 0–100; $P < 0.001$, Mann–Whitney test).

In the Varisolve®/surgery cohort, the median time to resumption of normal activities following treatment was considerably shorter in the Varisolve® group (2 days) than in the surgery group (13 days; $P < 0.001$, Mann–Whitney test). No difference was observed between the treatment groups in the Varisolve®/sclerotherapy cohort for time to resumption of normal activities (1 day each).

More patients completed treatment in one treatment session in the Varisolve® group than in the sclerotherapy group (92.2% vs 74.4%, respectively) (Table 10.4). When vascular surgeons performed the Varisolve® technique, only 82.0% completed the treatment in a single session, 16.9% required two sessions and 1.2% required three sessions.

Vascular surgeons used a mean of 24.9 mL (range: 5.0–55.0 mL) of Varisolve® microfoam during the initial treatment in the Varisolve®/surgery cohort compared with 14.9 mL of Varisolve® (range: 2.0–60.0 mL; $P < 0.001$, Student's t-test) for patients treated by phlebologists in the Varisolve®/sclerotherapy cohort.

Table 10.3 Response rates at month 3 and month 12

Response defined as occlusion of trunk vein and elimination of reflux at months 3 and 12

	Varisolve®		Alternative treatment		Statistical analysis	
	Response rate, *n/N*	%	Response rate, *n/N*	%	Difference[a] (%)	95% CI (%)
Month 3						
Varisolve®/surgery cohort	120/176	68.2	82/94	87.2	–27	–33 to –17
Varisolve®/sclerotherapy cohort	243/259	93.8	111/125	88.8	7	–0 to 15
Overall[b]	363/435	83.4	193/219	88.1	–8	–13 to 0
Month 12						
Varisolve®/surgery cohort	111/176	63.1	81/94	86.2	–25	–33 to –17
Varisolve®/sclerotherapy cohort	232/259	89.6	95/125	76.0	17	7 to 26
Overall[b]	343/435	78.9	176/219	80.4	–2	–10 to 6

Response defined as elimination of reflux at months 3 and 12

	Varisolve®		Alternative treatment		Statistical analysis	
	Response rate, *n/N*	%	Response rate, *n/N*	%	Difference[a] (%)	95% CI (%)
Month 3						
Varisolve®/surgery cohort	143/176	81.3	84/94	89.4	–18	–22 to –8
Varisolve®/sclerotherapy cohort	248/259	95.8	120/125	96.0	–1	–4 to 4
Overall[b]	391/435	89.9	204/219	93.2	–7	–10 to –2
Month 12						
Varisolve®/surgery cohort	130/176	73.9	83/94	88.3	–21	–27 to –10
Varisolve®/sclerotherapy cohort	235/259	90.7	104/125	83.2	8	0 to 17
Overall[b]	365/435	83.9	187/219	85.4	–3	–9 to 5

[a] Adjusted difference, backtransformed from the odds ratio obtained from logistic analysis.
[b] Overall adjusted results are based on a meta-analysis of the combined individual cohort results.

Table 10.4 Number of sessions required to complete the course of treatment at month 3

No. of treatment sessions	Varisolve®/surgery cohort		Varisolve®/sclerotherapy cohort			
	Varisolve® (*n* = 172)[a]		Varisolve® (*n* = 256)[a]		Sclerotherapy (*n* = 125)[a]	
	n	%	*n*	%	*n*	%
1	141	82.0	236	92.2	93	74.4
2	29	16.9	19	7.4	20	16.0
3	2	1.2	1	0.4	9	7.2
≥4	0		0		3	2.4

[a]Only patients who completed the study are included.

Adverse events

The most common adverse events related to the use of Varisolve® were mild contusion, skin discoloration, and limb pain; there were no cardiac or pulmonary adverse events suggestive of gas embolism related to the administration of microfoam (Table 10.5). There were six reports of nonspecific transient neurologic symptoms occurring within 24 hours of treatment, including paresthesias and visual and speech disorders; these were short-lived and there were no clinical findings during follow-up examinations.

Deep vein thrombosis. By protocol, all DVTs, including asymptomatic cases, were classified as serious adverse events (SAEs). DVT was the most frequent SAE, occurring in 11 Varisolve®-treated patients (9 [4.5%] in the Varisolve®/surgery cohort and 2 [0.8%] in the Varisolve®/sclerotherapy cohort) and in 1 sclerotherapy patient (0.8%). Of these, all but 2 were detected post-treatment at the safety duplex scan on day 7. Four DVTs were symptomatic, but only two involved symptoms directly attributable to DVT. Two patients were hospitalized for intravenous anticoagulant therapy. One patient developed a DVT at 9 months after treatment, which was considered unrelated to treatment and caused by a Baker's cyst. (Table 10.6). There were no clinically apparent cases of PE, and no diagnostic tests for PE were required. Most cases of DVT were treated with anticoagulants, and all but one resolved without sequelae. The incidence of DVT prompted technique changes (see Methods) and, following their implementation, no further DVTs were reported in the 95 patients treated subsequently.

There were no other SAEs related to Varisolve® treatment. There were two treatment-related SAEs reported in patients treated with surgery, both associated with anesthesia (one episode of nausea requiring hospital admission and one failure of regional anesthesia), which resolved without sequelae. There were no clinically significant changes in clinical chemistry, hematology, or coagulation test results.

Discussion

This randomized, multicenter study is the first to compare the Varisolve® technique with alternative treatments for varicose veins and is one of the largest and most rigorous studies performed to date for this condition. In other studies, either occlusion of the vein or, more commonly, elimination of reflux has been used to determine the efficacy of treatment.[15] In this study, patients were required to demonstrate both elimination of reflux and occlusion of the treated vein in order to be considered a responder. Furthermore, if both the GSV and SSV were treated, only patients with elimination of reflux and occlusion in both of the treated veins were classified as responders, highlighting the rigorous efficacy end-point employed in this trial.

Varisolve® proved to be inferior to surgery when delivered by vascular surgeons (68% Varisolve®, 87% surgery).

Where treatment was delivered by phlebologists (mostly in France), a remarkable 93.8% response rate was achieved at month 3. Possible explanations for the reduced efficacy when Varisolve® was delivered by the

Table 10.5 The five most common treatment-related[a] adverse events

	Varisolve®/surgery cohort				Varisolve®/sclerotherapy cohort				All Varisolve®	
	Varisolve® (*n* = 178)		Surgery (*n* = 94)		Varisolve® (*n* = 259)		Sclerotherapy (*n* = 125)		(*n* = 437)	
	n	%	*n*	%	*n*	%	*n*	%	*n*	%
Contusion	122	68.5	80	85.1	153	59.1	57	45.6	275	62.9
Skin discoloration	98	55.1	39	41.5	119	45.9	57	45.6	217	49.7
Pain in limb	73	41.0	39	41.5	77	29.7	31	24.8	150	34.3
Headache	41	23.0	20	21.3	14	5.4	7	5.6	55	12.6
Hematoma	11	6.2	1	1.1	29	11.2	9	7.2	40	9.2

[a] Related was defined as related, possibly related, or probably related to study treatment.

Table 10.6 Deep vein thrombosis (DVT) distribution and outcome

Patient No.	Gender/ age (y)	Specialist delivering treatment	Diagnosis, days following treatment	Microfoam volume (mL)	Treated vein	DVT location	DVT type	DVT symptoms	DVT treatment	Outcome
1	M/55	VS	7	50	GSV	GSV > CFV	1	No	Heparin IV + warfarin	Resolved
2	M/66	VS	7	12	SSV	Popliteal vein	2	No	LMWH + warfarin	Resolved
3	F/56	Ph	7	17	GSV	GSV > CFV	1	No	LMWH	Resolved
4	F/35	Ph, Derm	7	9	SSV	Popliteal vein	2	Yes	LMWH + coumarin	Resolved
5	M/74	VS	7	30	GSV	GSV > CFV	1	?Yes	Heparin IV + warfarin	Resolved
6	M/62	VS	3	20	SSV	Popliteal and soleal veins	2	Yes	LMWH	Resolving, with mild symptoms
7	F/33	VS	7	21	GSV	CFV	4	No	LMWH	Resolved
8	F/48	VS	7	25	SSV + GSV	Medial gastrocnemius vein	3	No	None	Resolved
9	F/37	VS	30	20	GSV	Soleal vein	3	No	Compression stocking	Unchanged
10	F/43	VS	7	12.3	SSV	Gastrocnemius vein	3	No	None	Resolved
11	M/59	VS	9mo	20	GSV	Peroneal vein	3	Yes	LMWH + warfarin	Resolved with sequelae

CFV, common femoral vein; LMWH, low-molecular-weight heparin; VS, vascular surgeon; Ph, phlebologist; Derm= dermatologist. For other abbreviations, see Table 10.2.

DVT type

1 = Thrombus extending from superficial vein into a deep vein (GSV into CFV); 2 = thrombus arising small deep veins, extending proximally; 3 = isolated muscular calf vein thrombi; 4 = Extension of sclerosis with thrombus formation at SFJ.

vascular surgeons include the fact that most vascular surgeons had limited experience of sclerotherapy for large veins and that they tended to use ultrasound technologists to carry out and report the duplex scans. To deliver the Varisolve® technique, surgeons either had to learn to coordinate the ultrasound probe and their hand movements or needed to develop an interdependent working practice with the ultrasound technologist. By contrast, phlebologists use ultrasound-guided sclerotherapy as their routine management of varicose veins of truncal origin. Some of the differences might also be accounted for by less severe disease in the Varisolve®/sclerotherapy cohort in which vein diameters were smaller and fewer C_4 patients were recorded, although this was offset by the higher frequency of recurrent vein disease and C_3 patients reported in this group. The differences in skill base and outcome between the cohorts suggest that additional training and experience may improve Varisolve® technique outcomes, even though analyses did not demonstrate a training effect or learning curve.

Between month 3 and month 12 in the Varisolve®/sclerotherapy cohort, the response rate with Varisolve® fell by 4%, whereas with sclerotherapy the response fell by 12%; those who underwent surgery had the smallest reduction in response (1%). Further studies will be required to determine the durability of microfoam sclerotherapy treatment beyond 1 year; however, since most believe varicose disease to be progressive and retreatment is straightforward, the importance of long-term efficacy is diminished. It is also anticipated that once the Varisolve® technique is fully evolved and executed by experienced practitioners – whether surgeon, phlebologist or interventional radiologist – the response rate will be similar to that seen in the Varisolve®/sclerotherapy cohort (around 90%), and therefore equivalent to the surgical outcome response rate.

It is surprising to find that at month 3, 15% of patients treated surgically still had residual venous reflux in the saphenous trunk. However, this emphasizes that surgical treatment is imperfect when treating varicose veins.

The Varisolve® technique was generally well tolerated; local adverse events, such as contusion, skin discoloration and limb pain, were generally mild in intensity and resolved without sequelae. The only SAE associated with the Varisolve® treatment was DVT. Here again there was a striking difference between Varisolve® delivered by vascular surgeons and by phlebologists: an incidence rate of 4.5% compared with 0.8%, respectively, the latter being equal to the rate with sclerotherapy. No patients treated surgically developed DVT, which may reflect the use of pharmacologic DVT prophylaxis in 22% of patients in conjunction with nonpharmacologic prophylaxis. The high rate reported for DVT also reflects the detailed and systematic duplex scanning required by the study protocol, which may have revealed the true rate of thrombotic events, but not their clinical significance. No cases of PE were clinically apparent and most of the DVTs were detected by routine duplex scanning at 1 week after treatment.

DVT is a recognized complication of all varicose vein treatments, including surgery, sclerotherapy, radiofrequency and laser ablation.[23–27] The incidence of DVT following varicose vein surgery has generally been reported as low, but two studies with routine prospective duplex scanning reported incidences of 4% and 5.3%,[28,29] comparable with this study. PE has been reported as rare following vein surgery, but in systematic reviews of over 4000 and 1000 patients, the incidence of clinically suspect PE was found to be 0.39% and 0.73%, respectively.[30,31]

There were no DVTs after changes were made to the Varisolve® technique used in the study. It is thus reasonable to conclude that DVT may be minimized by administration of Varisolve® by experienced practitioners using smaller volumes of microfoam and stopping the microfoam 5 cm distal to the termination of the trunk vein. It is advisable to continue using the follow-up scan after 1 week, so that any minor thrombotic events can be treated before they become clinically evident, thus avoiding serious sequelae.

Foam sclerotherapy deliberately introduces gas into the venous system, which was previously considered dangerous unless in very small quantities, but complications that could be attributed to pulmonary gas embolism were absent in both Varisolve®- and sclerotherapy-treated patients (92% air foam). Minor neurologic and ocular events, including migraine that could be attributed to cerebral gas embolism, following the presumed passage of bubbles across a right to left circulatory shunt, were infrequent and transient. Similar findings have been reported by others, including Guex et al.[32] The passage of gas bubbles through the microvasculature has been studied experimentally by Eckmann et al, whose results suggest that method of foam manufacture and gas composition have a highly significant influence over the potential for gas bubbles to occlude the microvasculature and by inference cause cerebral symptoms.[33] In the current study, there were few neurologic or visual events reported; there was no difference between physician generated air-based foam and Varisolve®, predominantly made with oxygen and carbon dioxide.

In conclusion, the Varisolve® technique is capable of sclerosing major incompetent trunk veins and tributaries in a single outpatient session. This study showed the Varisolve® technique to be effective in over 80% of patients and a well-tolerated treatment for varicose veins and trunk vein incompetence. In experienced hands, the Varisolve® technique caused only mild discomfort, permitting rapid return to normal activities. Long-term efficacy has yet to be established and the relative merits in comparison with RFA and EVLT need to be studied. These benefits make the Varisolve® technique an appropriate future treatment for patients with varicose veins and trunk vein incompetence.

Acknowledgements

We would like to gratefully acknowledge the other members of the Varisolve® investigator group who participated in this trial: Jean-Patrick Benigni; Roeland Ceulen; Alun Davies; Gilles Gachet; Pierre Ouvry; Patrick Patural; Paolo Ruscelli; Peter Rutter; Symon Sadoun; Uli Taucher; Stephen Tristram; Joep Veraart. We would also like to thank Janet Rush for her assistance and careful review and Sigvaris Ltd for the provision of compression stockings.

References

1. Callam MJ. Epidemiology of varicose veins. Br J Surg 1994; 81: 167–73.
2. Evans CJ, Fowkes FG, Ruckley CV, Lee AJ. Prevalence of varicose veins and chronic venous insufficiency in men and women in the general population: Edinburgh Vein Study. J Epidemiol Community Health 1999; 53: 149–53.
3. Callam MJ, Harper DR, Dale JJ, Ruckley CV. Chronic ulcer of the leg: clinical history. BMJ 1987; 294: 1389–91.
4. Lurie F, Creton D, Eklöf B, et al. Prospective randomized study of endovenous radiofrequency obliteration (closure procedure) versus ligation and stripping in a selected patient population (EVOLVeS Study). J Vasc Surg 2003; 38: 207–14.
5. Min RJ, Khilnani N, Zimmet SE. Endovenous laser treatment of saphenous vein reflux: long-term results. J Vasc Interv Radiol 2003; 14: 991–6.
6. Neglen P, Einarsson E, Eklöf B. The functional long-term value of different types of treatment for saphenous vein incompetence. J Cardiovasc Surg (Torino) 1993; 34: 295–301.
7. Fischer R, Chandler JG, De Maeseneer MG, et al. The unresolved problem of recurrent saphenofemoral reflux. J Am Coll Surg 2002; 195: 80–94.
8. Rautio T, Ohinmaa A, Perala J, et al. Endovenous obliteration versus conventional stripping operation in the treatment of primary varicose veins: a randomized controlled trial with comparison of the costs. J Vasc Surg 2002; 35: 958–65.
9. Dauplaise TL, Weiss RA. Duplex guided endovascular occlusion of refluxing saphenous vein. J Vasc Technol 2001; 25: 79–82.
10. Weiss RA, Weiss MA. Controlled radiofrequency endovenous occlusion using a unique radiofrequency catheter under duplex guidance to eliminate saphenous varicose vein reflux: a 2-year follow-up. Dermatol Surg 2002; 28: 38–42.
11. Goldman MP, Amiry S. Closure of the greater saphenous vein with endoluminal radiofrequency thermal heating of the vein wall in combination with ambulatory phlebectomy: 50 patients with more than 6-month follow-up. Dermatol Surg 2002; 28: 29–31.
12. Merchant RF, DePalma RG, Kabnick LS. Endovascular obliteration of saphenous reflux: a multicenter study. J Vasc Surg 2002; 35: 1190–6.
13. Proebstle TM, Gul D, Kargl A, Knop J. Endovenous laser treatment of the lesser saphenous vein with a 940-nm diode laser: early results. Dermatol Surg 2003; 29: 357–61.
14. Cabrera J, Cabrera J Jr, Garcia-Olmedo MA, Redondo P. Treatment of venous malformations with sclerosant in microfoam form. Arch Dermatol 2003; 139: 1409–16.
15. Rigby KA, Palfreyman SJ, Beverley C, Michaels JA. Surgery versus sclerotherapy for the treatment of varicose veins. Cochrane Database Syst Rev 2004: CD004980.
16. Knight RM, Vin F, Zygmunt JA. Ultrasonic guidance of injections into the superficial venous system. In: Davy A, Stemmer R, eds. Phlebologie 89. Paris: John Libbey Eurotext Ltd, 1989: 339–41.
17. Schadeck M, Allaert F. [Ultrasonography during sclerotherapy.] Phlebologie 1991; 44: 111–30 [in French].
18. Cabrera J, Cabrera J Jr, Garcia-Olmedo MA. Sclerosants in microfoam. A new approach in angiology. Int Angiol 2001; 20: 322–9.
19. Hamel-Desnos C, Desnos P, Wollmann JC, et al. Evaluation of the efficacy of polidocanol in the form of foam compared with liquid form in sclerotherapy of the greater saphenous vein: initial results. Dermatol Surg 2003; 29: 1170–5.

20. Yamaki T, Nozaki M, Iwasaka S. Comparative study of duplex-guided foam sclerotherapy and duplex-guided liquid sclerotherapy for the treatment of superficial venous insufficiency. Dermatol Surg 2004; 30: 718–22.
21. Cabrera J, Redondo P, Becerra A, et al. Ultrasound-guided injection of polidocanol microfoam in the management of venous leg ulcers. Arch Dermatol 2004; 140: 667–73.
22. Eklöf B, Rutherford RB, Bergan JJ, et al, for the American Venous Forum International Ad Hoc Committee for Revision of the CEAP Classification. Revision of the CEAP classification for chronic venous disorders: consensus statement. J Vasc Surg 2004; 40: 1248–52.
23. Guex JJ. Thrombotic complications of varicose veins. A literature review of the role of superficial venous thrombosis. Dermatol Surg 1996; 22: 378–82.
24. Manfrini S, Gasbarro V, Danielsson G, et al. Endovenous management of saphenous vein reflux. Endovenous Reflux Management Study Group. J Vasc Surg 2000; 32: 330–42.
25. USA Food and Drug Administration. Manufacturer and User Facility Device Experience Database (MAUDE). Available at www.fda.gov.
26. Bhogal R, Hickey NC, Nyamekye IK. Selective venous duplex imaging detects all clinically relevant DVT after varicose veins surgery [Abstract]. Phlebology 2005; 20: 97.
27. Critchley G, Handa A, Maw A, et al. Complications of varicose vein surgery. Ann R Coll Surg Engl 1997; 79: 105–10.
28. Puttaswamy V, Fisher C, Neale M, Appleberg M. Venous thromboembolism following varicose vein surgery: a prospective analysis [Abstract]. Presented at the Australian and New Zealand Society of Phlebology 18th Scientific Meeting, 2001.
29. Van Rij AM, Chai J, Hill GB, Christie RA. Incidence of deep vein thrombosis after varicose vein surgery. Br J Surg 2004; 91: 1582–5.
30. Lofgren EP, Coates HLC, O'Brien PC. Clinically suspect pulmonary embolism after vein stripping. Mayo Clin Proc 1976; 51: 77–80.
31. Huber O, Bounameaux H, Borst F, Rohner A. Postoperative pulmonary embolism after hospital discharge. An underestimated risk. Arch Surg 1992; 127: 310–3.
32. Guex J-J, Allaert F-A, Gillet J-L, Chleir F. Immediate and midterm complicatios of sclerotherapy: a report of a prospective multicenter registry of 12 173 sclerotherapy sessions. Dermatol Surg 2005; 31: 123–8.
33. Eckmann DM, Kobayashi S, Li M. Microvascular embolization following polidocanol microfoam sclerosant administration. Dermatol Surg 2005; 31: 636–43.

11 Ultrasound-guided foam sclerotherapy of large varicose veins

John M Barrett

Introduction

Ultrasound-guided sclerotherapy (UGS) with foam sclerosants has become an integral part of modern phlebology for the treatment of varicose veins since Cabrera first published his medium-term results in 2000.[1] But is foam UGS appropriate for large varicose veins?

Large varicose veins are those with a diameter of >10 mm at the saphenofemoral junction (SFJ) and/or mid-thigh, or saphenopopliteal junction (SPJ) and/or mid-calf, which are measured while the patient is standing. Such veins present special issues for patients and phlebologists by virtue of their common association with significant symptoms and associated pathology such as varicose eczema, edema, lipodermatosclerosis and varicose ulcers. Large veins often involve several sources of reflux, including reflux from the SFJ and SPJ, pelvic and abdominal veins, and multiple perforators. The large diameters of the saphenous trunks, which define "large" varicose veins, present particular issues for treatment with foam UGS (Figure 11.1). Large volumes of foam are required to displace the blood, but once the vein is in spasm, there is potential for large volumes of foam to traverse perforators or pass directly into the deep vein system via the common femoral or popliteal veins, and thus potentially pass into the cardiac, pulmonary and cerebral circulation. Higher volumes of foam can be associated with other adverse effects, such as phlebitis or deep vein thrombosis (DVT). The thrombosclerotic process formed in large veins is potentially more prone to recanalization than smaller veins. Blood trapping in large varicose tributaries is also an issue, often requiring aspiration.

Despite these potential issues, foam UGS remains a remarkably safe and effective procedure for large varicose veins. Given that chronic venous insufficiency is a condition that is controlled rather than cured, it behooves phlebologists to use a technique with a high efficacy and safety profile. Surgery alone has not historically eliminated the possibility of recurrence and in fact has relatively high long-term recurrence rates.[2,3] Surgery also has significant potential for adverse effects of its own, such as wound infection, venous thromboembolism,[4] nerve damage,[5–7] lymphatic damage and arterial injury.[8] Endovenous ablative techniques such as endovenous laser ablation and radiofrequency ablation look very promising, but are relatively new techniques and their efficacy is yet to be confirmed in studies beyond five

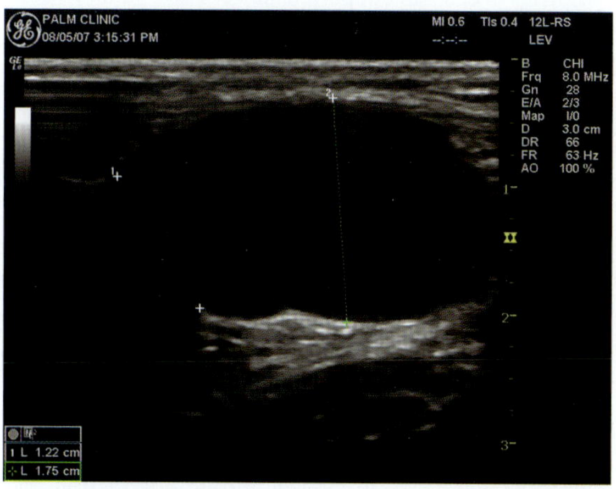

Figure 11.1 A 17.5 mm aneurysmal dilatation of the proximal great saphenous vein

years. Combined treatments are generally required for endovenous ablation with either foam UGS or ambulatory phlebectomy. There are reports of thermal injury and thrombus extension into the common femoral and popliteal veins with potential for pulmonary embolus. So, for large varicose veins, no procedure has been available that is without potentially significant adverse effects.

Foam UGS, either alone or in combination with surgery or endovenous ablation techniques, has become an important treatment option for large varicose veins. However, patients need to be aware that with any treatment for large varicose veins there is a significant chance of recurrence, so that repeated treatments over the years may be necessary for long-term control. Once this is understood, patients are very accepting of the need for top-up treatments and serial observation if recurrent varicose veins or symptoms of chronic venous insufficiency break through. Given the relatively benign nature of foam UGS treatment (no requirement for general anesthesia, rapid return to work, high patient satisfaction and low side-effect profile),[9] foam UGS is proving to be an excellent alternative both for primary treatment of large veins and, in particular, for treatment of recurrences of large veins. Of course, any new technique must eventually be assessed against existing techniques with respect to efficacy and safety. Unfortunately, direct comparisons are currently not possible for large varicose veins as there are no long-term comparative studies documenting the efficacy of foam UGS, endovenous ablation or surgery specifically in varicose veins >10 mm in diameter.

Barrett et al.[10] have reported success at 2 years in both patient satisfaction and clinical efficacy for veins >10 mm in diameter, but 5-year studies have yet to be completed. Kanter[11] looked at the effects of age, gender and vein size and found that, regardless of gender and age, larger veins were more likely to recanalize but were not necessarily associated with clinical recurrence. Thibault,[12] reporting 5-year recurrence rates in 35 limbs with great saphenous vein (GSV) incompetence treated with UGS, found that when comparing his results with those of shorter-term studies, there was a slow but steady increase in cumulative recurrence with time. This is likely to be more pronounced with large varicose veins because the resultant thrombosclerotic process in large-diameter veins leads to slower fibrotic contraction and greater chance of recanalization. In the author's experience, recanalization leading to the appearance of recurrent varicosities can be delayed for many years following foam UGS.

The advent of ultrasound-guided foam sclerotherapy and its use in our clinic

Until the advent of foam, UGS had previously been thought of as useful only for saphenous veins with diameters <8 mm.[13] Veins of diameter >8 mm had been regarded as the domain of surgery, requiring ligation followed by stripping, sclerotherapy or ambulatory phlebectomy. The assumption had been that sclerosants were not powerful enough to cause sufficient sclerosis in large vessels because of significant dilution of sclerosant solutions by the blood in large-diameter veins. Foam sclerosants, however, allow maximum concentration of sclerosant at the surface of each microbubble, thus maximizing contact of the sclerosant at the endothelial surface, allowing more effective irritation and inflammation as precursors to sclerosis.[1,14–19]

Since September 2000, our clinic has treated over 6000 legs with foam UGS as the only form of treatment. A significant number of saphenous veins with diameters between 10 mm and 30 mm have been treated using this technique. Our general experience suggested there was equally high patient satisfaction in the larger-vein patients, and this was confirmed in a study[10] in which Barrett et al found little difference in the age, limb or characteristics of GSVs or small saphenous veins (SSVs) of diameter <10 mm compared with those >10 mm in diameter. Males were over-represented in the large-diameter group, however: 31% male for veins <10 mm and 37.5% male for veins >10 mm in diameter. The assumption made is that males are more accepting of their varicosities and therefore tend to present later for treatment. Occupation may also play a part, with more males participating in occupations involving repetitive straining, which may add to the raised venous pressures.

Symptoms of venous insufficiency in large varicose veins

Symptoms associated with large varicose veins cover the full spectrum from (surprisingly) no symptoms at all, through to severe aching, throbbing, heavy legs, burning, cramp, swelling, skin irritation in the form of itching, or frank varicose eczema and varicose ulcers. Large varicose veins tend to be associated with more symptoms such as swelling, varicose eczema and varicose ulcers compared with smaller veins, as a direct manifestation of the higher venous pressure and increased reflux times in association with increased leukocyte-activated inflammation.[20] In the author's experience, large varicose veins also have a greater association with superficial thrombophlebitis due to reduced flow rates in large veins. Varicose eczema, varicose ulcers and lipodermatosclerosis are the commonly recognized skin manifestations of chronic venous insufficiency, and these are over-represented in large veins. There are also many less common skin manifestations of venous insufficiency, such as those outlined by Parsi,[21] including purpuric dermatoses and acroangiodermatitis.

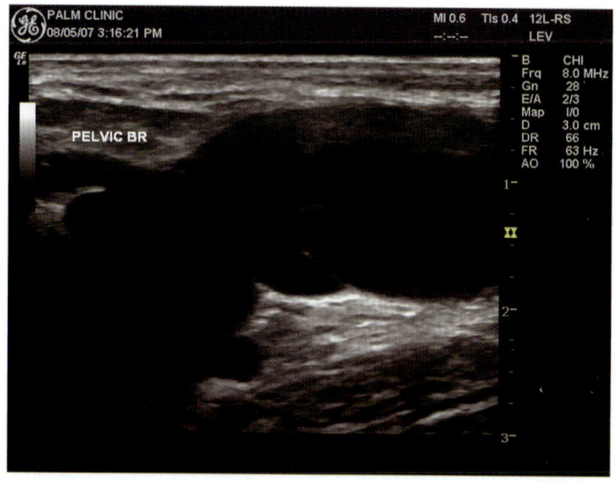

Figure 11.2 Pelvic branch of the great saphenous vein immediately distal to the saphenofemoral junction

Diagnosis

Treatment of large varicose veins is not in the domain of the casual sclerotherapist. An accurate diagnosis of all sources of reflux is mandatory. Diagnosis begins, as always, with a careful history and clinical examination (supplemented with Doppler), but for large varicose veins the required level of diagnostic accuracy is achieved with Duplex ultrasound. Whilst a hand-held Doppler may be useful for preliminary diagnosis at the initial consultation, it is no substitute for a complete analysis with duplex ultrasound by either an experienced phlebologist or a vascular sonographer.

Determining ultrasound characteristics of large veins

Varicose veins >10 mm in diameter are usually the result of incompetence at the SPJ in the case of the great GSV or at the SPJ in the case of the SSV. Incompetence of the GSV is seen more commonly than the SSV in a ratio of about four to one. The incompetent GSV typically has a diameter larger than that of the SSV. Occasionally, the proximal GSV or SSV will have an aneurysmal dilatation. Contributors to large varicose veins include large feeding veins from the pelvis (more common in females, often as a result of pregnancy) (Figure 11.2). In our initial series, the ratio of men to women presenting with varicose veins >10 mm in diameter was approximately one man for every two women. We have noticed an increase in men presenting in the last three years, possibly as a result of the wider awareness of nonsurgical techniques. The very large veins >12 mm diameter tend to be found in men. This may be because of late presentation or to occupations involving increased straining. Women characteristically present earlier for cosmetic reasons. Large incompetent perforators can be a precursor to large varicose veins. Commonly, a large mid-thigh perforator will render the distal GSV incompetent. A predominant feature of large varicose veins is an increased number and size of perforators seen on ultrasound, mainly in the calf (Figure 11.3). Such perforators may or may not be associated with skin manifestations such as lipodermatosclerosis or varicose ulceration. Although perforators have a typical location, it is important to follow large feeding veins to see if there is an incompe-

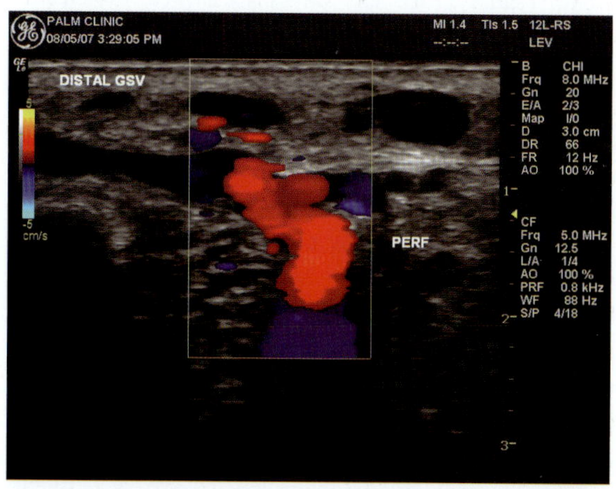

Figure 11.3 Perforator from the distal great saphenous vein

tent perforator responsible. Where there is a large incompetent perforator, there is usually a corresponding increase in vein diameter. Documentation of the location of these perforators is important to avoid injecting into or close to them. Where there is a perforator, there is generally an associated arteriole.

In patients who have had previous vein surgery, there is a further level of complexity, with possible absent segments, isolated segments, and/or neovascularization at the main junctions and previous incision sites. Such neovascularization at the site of ligation in the proximal GSV can form a large cluster of fragile veins that join to form a large incompetent remnant. This can also be seen in the popliteal fossa in relation to previous SSV ligation. For good control of distal reflux in these cases, the areas of neovascularization need to be meticulously injected with foam. The walls of such vessels are typically very thin, so extravasation is possible, but this rarely causes any problems in our experience. Large veins reflux, and although the reflux time does not always correlate with vein size, the reflux volume is typically much greater with a larger vein. This large refluxing volume can put pressure on the underlying deep veins and in some cases will cause incompetence in the deep veins themselves. Typically, such deep vein reflux improves or ceases after treating the incompetent superficial vein.

The valves of large varicose veins are generally easy to see on ultrasound, particularly the terminal and subterminal valves. The number of valves in the leg increases from proximal to distal, so that damage to the proximal valves has greater impact than isolated damage to distal valves. At the site of the damaged valve, there is often a localized increase in diameter of the vein around the valve (Figure 11.4). The valves are typically bicuspid, permitting unidirectional flow toward the heart. When damaged, the valves become fibrosed and fixed or floppy, allowing bidirectional flow.

Edema, lipodermatosclerosis and varicose ulcers associated with incompetent large varicose veins make scanning more difficult. The edematous or obese patient will have an increased calf circumference, making the scanning of the deep veins more technically challenging such that a change in frequency or transducer may be required (e.g., a curvilinear array transducer of 3.5–5 Hz can be useful in these situations) (Figure 11.5). Any fluid lakes associated with edema must be differentiated from incompetent veins (Figure 11.6).

Patients with lipodermatosclerosis are difficult to scan. They are often tender, particularly in the lower leg,

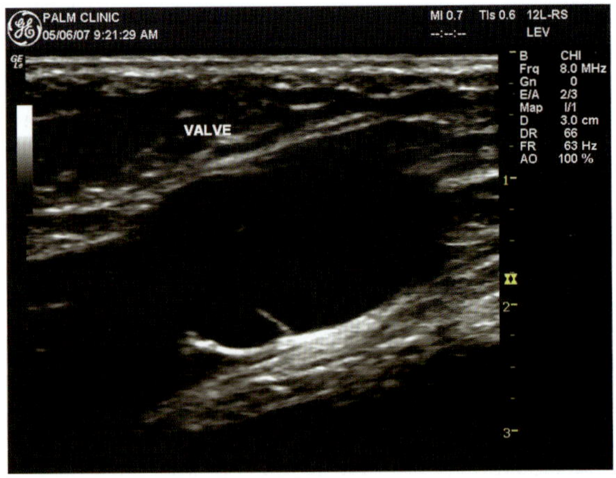

Figure 11.4 Valve in the great saphenous vein demonstrating common finding of dilatation around the incompetent valve

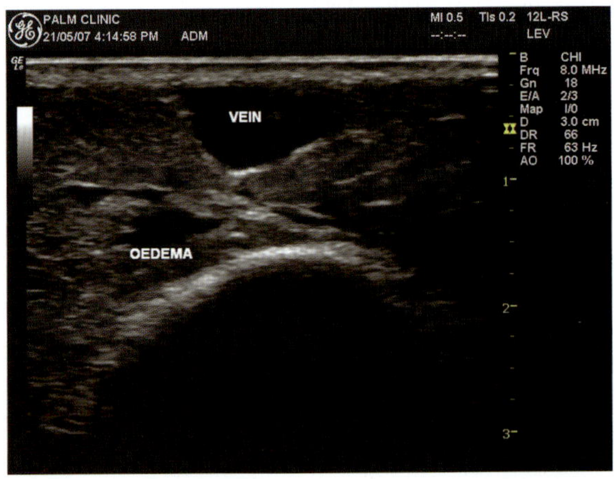

Figure 11.5 Peripheral edema associated with great saphenous vein incompetence

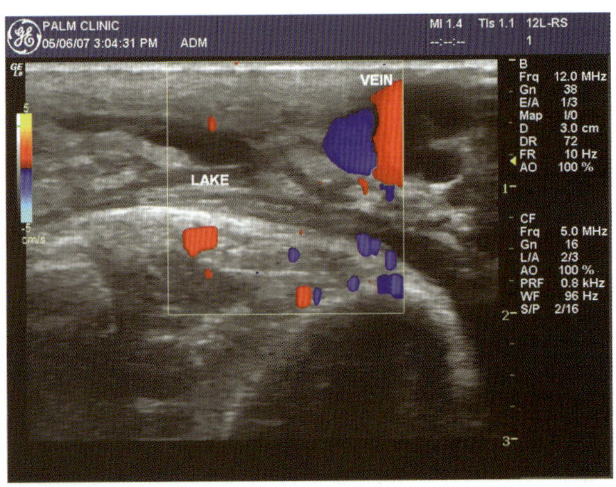

Figure 11.6 Fluid lake next to an incompetent distal great saphenous vein

making compression scanning and augmentation more difficult. Impaired acoustic transmission through the scarred and edematous tissue, even with low-frequency scanning, makes visualization of the deep veins suboptimal. Ulceration poses significant problems in relation to patient discomfort when attempting to identify the deep veins and the location of varicose veins and perforators. Dressings need to be removed, and a careful, clean scanning technique using sterile pads, covers or gel is required. If the ulcer is inconsistent with the venous abnormality, other causes for the ulceration must be considered. Larger veins have a greater tendency to develop superficial thrombophlebitis (STP), and this is a common finding during ultrasound mapping of large veins (Figure 11.7). The size and location of the STP is recorded and an assessment made as to whether this may be a recent event or longstanding. Generally, there will be clinical symptoms with an acute STP, but not always, and the extent of the STP often extends well beyond the area of clinical symptoms. This is often true of ascending superficial thrombophlebitis, where in the case of the GSV the clinical symptoms are often confined to the calf or distal thigh but ultrasound may reveal extension toward the SFJ or even flush with or extending into the common femoral vein. This requires urgent treatment with low-molecular-weight heparin. Significant common femoral vein extension of the thrombophlebitis may require a surgical sieve. In the case of an old STP, retraction of the thrombus is a feature on ultrasound. Later there are often fibrotic strands and calcification seen within the affected area of the vein. In the case of an acute STP, as well as conservative management with nonsteroidal anti-inflammatories and class 2 compression hosiery, serial ultrasound scans should be performed until it is evident that the STP is stable and not extending proximally.

Other lumps and bumps may mimic a large varicose vein, so scanning must aim to differentiate these. Lipomas and cysts can suggest large varicose veins clinically, but are easily distinguished on ultrasound because of their localized nature. Subfascial muscle hernias can present as a large focal bulge, but will be reducible on ultrasound. Baker's cysts on ultrasound can appear like large veins, but again are localized to the posteromedial aspect of the knee (Figure 11.8). They are usually tear-shaped and do not demonstrate color flow. An aneurysmal dilatation can be seen in arteries and in deep veins, particularly in the popliteal fossa. These need to be evaluated by tracing connections and using Doppler and/or color flow for arteries (Table 11.1).

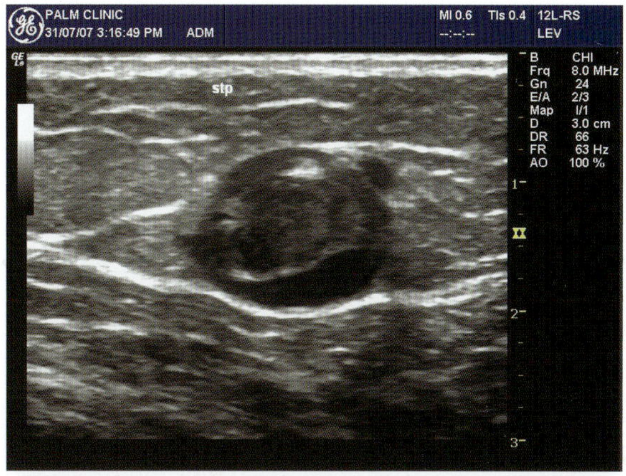

(a)

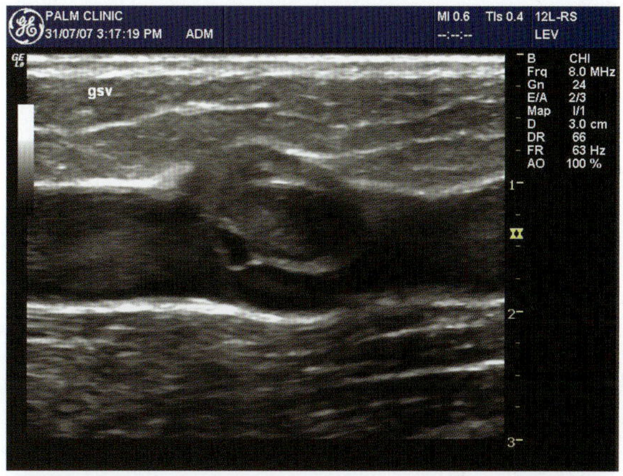

(b)

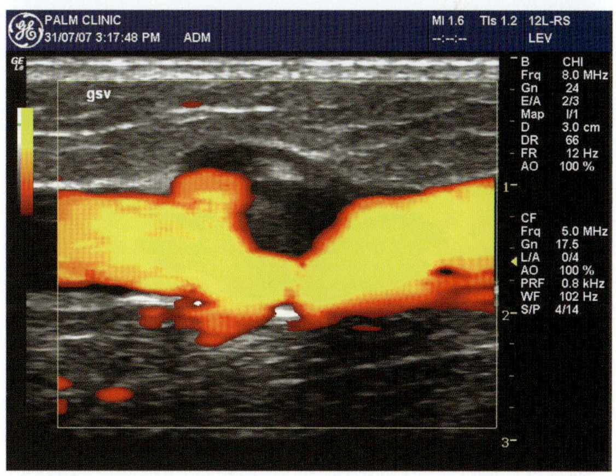

(c)

Figure 11.7 (a) Localized superficial thrombophlebitis demonstrated in a cross section of the great saphenous vein. (b) Localized superficial thrombophlebitis in a longitudinal section of the great saphenous vein. (c) Localized superficial thrombophlebitis in longitudinal section highlighted by absence of color flow

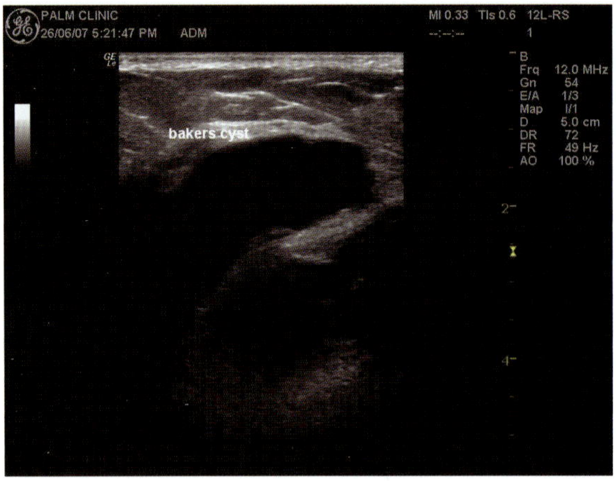

Figure 11.8 Baker's cyst mimicking a saphenous vein differentiated by site, shape and lack of color flow

Table 11.1 Ultrasound assessment of large varicose veins

1. To rule out underlying deep vein pathology, particularly reflux and deep vein thrombosis
2. To identify and map both normal and refluxing superficial veins, making note of vein size, location and any aneurysmal dilatation
3. To identify and record any abnormality in the superficial system such as superficial thrombophlebitis
4. To record perforator location and size, particularly those related to skin pathology
5. To document and where possible categorize incidental and potentially confusing pathology

Criteria for ultrasound-guided foam sclerotherapy

Patient selection

The only absolute contraindications to treatment of large varicose veins with foam UGS are previous anaphylaxis to the proposed sclerosant (in which case an alternative is generally available), acute DVT, pregnancy and breast-feeding. Relative contraindications include deep venous obstruction, peripheral vascular disease, documented thrombophilia, coexisting cancer as a risk factor for thrombophilia, inability to mobilize, acute superficial thrombophlebitis, oral contraceptives and hormone replacement therapy. Risks and benefits are discussed with the patient and modifications to the treatment plan are made where appropriate.

Because of the increased risk of recanalization in large varicose veins following foam UGS, some occupations involving heavy lifting and some lifestyle options such as weightlifting may need to be curtailed. Other treatment options may need to be explored, such as endovenous ablation with laser or radiofrequency, SFJ ligation followed by saphenous stripping, endovenous ablation, foam UGS, or ambulatory phlebectomy.

Age and co-morbidity are seldom contraindications to treatment with foam UGS, making this technique available to a much broader spectrum of patients than surgery.

Those patients with a past history or documented evidence of thrombophilia can be treated with low-molecular-weight heparin. Whilst oral contraception and HRT are relative contraindications, such medication can be continued, but close monitoring for DVT with duplex ultrasound is necessary for 2 weeks post-treatment. Warfarin is not a contraindication to treatment.

Where superficial thrombophlebitis is a concern, careful monitoring with duplex ultrasound will identify ascending STP. If the SFJ or SPJ is threatened, where appropriate, patients are prescribed low-molecular-weight heparin. Many cases of STP will fully recanalize over several months, and definitive treatment can be withheld until this occurs. For those cases of STP that have not resorbed after 6 months, treatment both proximally and distally to the STP is performed.

Foam volume

From our earliest forays with foam UGS in 2000, we have been concerned to limit the amount of foam injected on any one day to minimize the potential risk of deep vein sclerosis and/or thrombus. We are mindful of inadequate research as to the systemic effects of large volumes of foam on the pulmonary vasculature and/or cerebral blood flow through a patent foramen ovale (PFO). Such concern has been confirmed by Morrison's recent study[22] demonstrating significant flow of sclerosant foam into the heart and cerebral system through PFOs. On transthoracic echocardiography, bubbles were identified in the right side of the heart within 10–30 s after every injection of foam UGS (volumes limited to 1–3 mL of polidocanol 1%). A variety of bubble patterns from none to showers lasting several seconds were detected in the left heart via a PFO or possible pulmonary arteriovenous fistula. Hyperechoic, sharp, short-lived echoes associated with cerebral emboli were observed in the middle cerebral artery of four of the seven patients (detected by transcranial Doppler) who had bubbles in the left side of the heart.

Human studies are not available regarding pulmonary circulation effects, and it is not clear whether multiple treatments with small to medium daily volumes (up to 16 mL foam) will be any better in this regard than single treatment with large volumes greater than 16 mL. Until further studies can demonstrate the incidence and ramifications of foam in the pulmonary and cerebral circulation, it seems prudent to limit daily foam volumes. Such volume restrictions mean that large varicose veins will need multiple treatments, but we have not found patient resistance to this and it does allow for serial review to exclude and/or treat DVT should it arise. The very small number of patients in our clinic who have exhibited cerebral symptoms following foam UGS have had their treatment completed using sclerosant solution.

As previously stated, short- and long-term studies have shown effectiveness of foam UGS for small varicose veins but there are limited studies on long-term effectiveness of large veins. In 2004, we reported good success at 2 years,[10] but 5-year studies are yet to be completed. Anecdotally, we are aware that there is a significant failure rate in veins >10 mm in diameter at 5 years following foam UGS; however, patient satisfaction with the technique remains strong. Patients returning for further treatment often have minor recurrences of varicosities related to partial or complete recanalization of reduced diameter or new varicosities related to new areas of reflux such as an incompetent perforator.

With the advent of newer ablative techniques such as endovenous laser or radiofrequency ablation, we have reassessed our approach and developed new protocols for foam UGS.

Protocols for ultrasound-guided foam sclerotherapy in our clinic

(i) Veins suitable for combined treatment of endovenous laser ablation (EVLA) and foam UGS. In these cases we perform EVLA on the proximal straight segment of the saphenous vein and typically treat the distal segment and associated tributaries 5 days later with foam UGS. The advantage of this approach for large varicose veins is that less foam is used, the proximal segment is typically ablated with greater certainty, and resulting blood trapping and/or associated phlebitis in the distal tributaries tends to be less with this combined approach than after foam UGS alone. The initial EVLA of the proximal segment "turns the tap off" and over four or five days the tributaries reduce in diameter, requiring less foam sclerosant to complete the chemical ablation following foam UGS.

(ii) Veins suitable only for foam UGS. These are large varicose veins where the proximal saphenous vein is not straight enough to insert a laser fiber.

In our experience, following EVLA the treated saphenous vein forms a smaller cord of tissue, which is often not detectable on ultrasound a year later. Whilst this occasionally occurs in large vessels >10 mm in diameter following foam UGS alone, it is more typical to see a reduced diameter of vessel that is typically closed but occasionally remains partially or completely open requiring further treatment. For younger patients with large varicose veins, desirous of a more energetic lifestyle, we now feel the combined approach of proximal EVLA and distal foam UGS should be used where possible.

Using ultrasound-guided foam sclerotherapy for large varicosities in our clinic

Preparation of foam

Foam is prepared with the Tessari microfoam technique using 3% sodium tetradecyl sulfate (STS) in a ratio of 1 mL STS to 3 mL ambient air for saphenous trunks. Two 3 mL syringes are connected via a three-way tap. An aliquot of 1 mL of STS 3% solution is placed into one of the syringes along with 1 mL of air. In the other syringe, 2 mL of air are drawn up. The tap is aligned so that there is sufficient resistance to create the foam, which should look white with no evidence of individual bubbles macroscopically. Some phlebologists prefer an in-line filter. It is important to use the foam as soon as possible after preparation. Once macroscopic bubbles can be observed in the syringe, the foam should be discarded. The author uses 2 mL aliquots for each injection until the smaller tributaries are treated; then smaller volumes may suffice. Smaller tributaries are treated with varying concentrations of microfoam STS or polidocanol, depending on the size of the saphenous branches and associated varicosities as described below. STS 3% is used for saphenous trunks because of its greater potency, and varying concentrations of STS (0.5–1.5%) or polidocanol foam (1–2.5%) are used for visible varicosities. Some phlebologists prefer to use carbon dioxide rather than air, but there is currently no proof that this reduces the risk of potential cerebral incidents. Ambient air is quick, simple and efficient to use, making it a preferred gas for foaming.

Treatment techniques

Patients are treated supine with the treated leg slightly elevated and externally rotated at the hip. The knee is usually slightly flexed. The veins can be approached under ultrasound guidance from the transverse or longitudinal (sagittal) plane. The transverse approach is much easier ergonomically on the phlebologist as the longitudinal approach requires the phlebologist to rotate and flex the spine to approach the leg longitudinally, whereas the transverse approach only requires flexion. Sometimes it is helpful to have the patient roll toward the phlebologist in a semilateral recumbent position if the GSV is particularly medial.

The author uses the "closed technique" as described by Thibault.[23]

Small aliquots (typically 2 mL) are injected serially from proximal to distal. With volumes restricted to 12–16 mL per session there is less likelihood of significant flow of large volumes into the deep system. Injectate volumes are often reduced in the lower leg, and one needs to be sensitive to pressure changes during injection. If there is increasing resistance to injection, it is wise to withdraw and review the spread of the foam with ultrasound. The end-point of treatment is either noncompressibility of the treated vein/s or having reached the 16 mL maximum foam volume injected.

For large varicose veins, focus in the first treatment is to close the proximal saphenous trunk and any associated proximal tributaries contributing to reflux such as pudendal veins, abdominal wall veins or neovascularization secondary to previous surgery. Distal tributaries are generally treated at a subsequent visit or visits if constrained by foam volume limits on the first treatment.

Great saphenous vein: one leg

The first injection is typically started within 5 cm of the SFJ because of the larger capacity of a >10 mm diameter vein. The SFJ or SPJ will be protected by gentle probe pressure during the proximal injection. A volume of 2 mL of STS 3% foam is injected through a 25-gauge, 3.3 cm needle in the tangential plane. Depending on the diameter of the saphenous trunk, up to 16 mL of foam is injected in 2 mL aliquots, working from proximal to distal. Each subsequent injection is placed immediately beyond the last point of spasm. At this point, we are not concerned about closure of the varicose tributaries, but such tributaries may spasm as the foam flows into them.

On a second visit, closure of the saphenous trunk is confirmed, DVT is excluded, and further injections of 2 mL STS 3% foam are provided working proximal to distal to the varicose tributaries, again not exceeding 16 mL of foam for the treatment. With this approach, large varicosities can be treated in one to four treatment sessions, depending on the size and complexity of the veins. For smaller varicose tributaries, varying lower concentrations of STS or polidocanol foam are used.

Great saphenous vein: two legs

The great saphenous trunk of one leg will be treated as above, with the second leg being treated two days later. Subsequent treatments to visible varicosities and/or distal perforators of both legs are typically completed two days later, so for the majority of patients the treatment of two legs with large varicosities is completed in three to four visits spaced two days apart. We choose this protocol to minimize both treatment volumes and the time spent in compression hosiery.

Small saphenous vein: one leg

If an SSV is involved in isolation, the saphenous trunk and tributaries are typically treated in a single session because of the relatively small capacitance of the SSV and its tributaries. However, in these cases, foam volume is limited to 10 mL. Most small saphenous trunks >10 mm at the junction or mid-calf will close satisfactorily with 4–6 mL of foam, the rest being used for the tributaries and perforators. In our experience, all but one of the small number of DVTs that we have seen have occurred in the lower leg, usually in the medial gastrocnemius or soleal veins, with extremely rare involvement of the popliteal vein.

Small saphenous vein: two Legs

Because we limit our foam volume to 10 mL for the SSV and often achieve our end-point with 4–6 mL, we can often treat both legs on the same day, or alternatively treat both the GSV and SSV of one leg on the same day, provided we do not exceed 16 mL foam volume per patient per day.

Perforators

Where large veins are complicated by lipodermatosclerosis or venous ulcers, several perforators will often be implicated in the pathology, which require specific attention. Whilst it is technically possible to inject foam directly into the perforator, this is not necessary or desirable in most cases. By injecting 2–3 cm proximal or distal to the perforator, sufficient foam flows into the perforator whilst reducing the risk of any significant volume of foam flowing into the deep vein system.

Postoperative care

Good postoperative care emanates from the initial consultation, with a realistic explanation of the procedure, likely side-effects and expectations around the recovery period and expected long-term outcomes.

Occupations and lifestyles need to considered before the treatment to ascertain likely compliance with postoperative instructions and measures that may be taken to manage the period. Clearly, a manual laborer expected to lift heavy materials or a young man lifting weights at the gymnasium could be at greater risk of recanalization than a sedentary professional. However, the latter may have a greater risk of venous thromboembolism through inactivity.

Postoperative instructions following foam UGS are:

1. Class 2 compression hosiery worn from the beginning of treatment, continuing for 2 weeks after the last treatment. As most treatments are completed within a week, patients are advised that they will usually need to wear such hosiery for around three weeks. For large varicose veins, we insist on the hosiery remaining on 24 hours a day for the first week; thereafter they can be removed for a shower and overnight. For large veins, additional padding overlying the varicosities under the compression hosiery may be helpful in reducing blood trapping for the first 48 hours. Such padding can be in the form of foam or bubble-wrap covered with Tubigrip cut to the size and shape of the varicosities. This can often be uncomfortable for the patient and in our experience is not essential. We have never used bandaging postoperatively, but others find this useful.
2. Over the same 3-week period, we expect our patients to walk for an hour a day – this is described as a stroll rather than a power walk.
3. Over the same period, patients are asked to avoid significant straining or heavy lifting that would result in a Valsalva maneuver. We believe this is particularly important for large varicose veins, where a significant Valsalva maneuver could result in sufficiently high intra-abdominal pressures to cause early recanalization. For this reason, patients with occupations requiring heavy lifting should be advised to restrict activities to light duties. This can require significant forethought for young mothers, and carers for the elderly or disabled, as compliance will often require significant help from others.
4. Patients are advised to avoid long-haul travel greater than 4 hours (plane, train or car) for 1 month after treatment, to minimize the risk of DVT.

Postoperative review

Following completion of treatment, patients are reviewed at 3 months and 1 year. At each review, an assessment of the deep vein system is performed, and a complete assessment of the superficial system is carried out including the degree of sclerosis, any areas of recanalization, new incompetent perforators and other sources of potential reflux.

Recanalization can occur with large varicose veins because of the significant thrombus formation that predates the thrombosclerotic process. Careful attention to aspiration of trapped blood may minimize this process (Figure 11.9a, b). Treatment of areas of recanalization is performed if necessary at the 3-month and 1-year reviews. Occasionally, recanalization can present late. One would expect that the fibrotic process would render further sclerotherapy difficult, but in our experience this does not diminish results with subsequent treatment. Such areas of recanalization in the saphenous trunks do not always lead to repeat varicose veins.

Patients with large varicose veins in CEAP categories C_3 to C_6 are advised that they will need ongoing review for the rest of their life. In particular, patients with lipodermatosclerosis, atrophie blanche, venous ulcers or other significant skin manifestations of chronic venous insufficiency should be monitored on a regular basis. Early treatment of recurrences visible on ultrasound will minimize further complications.

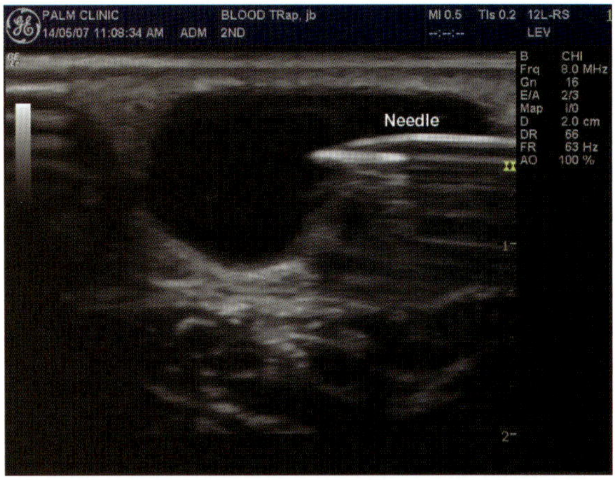

(a)

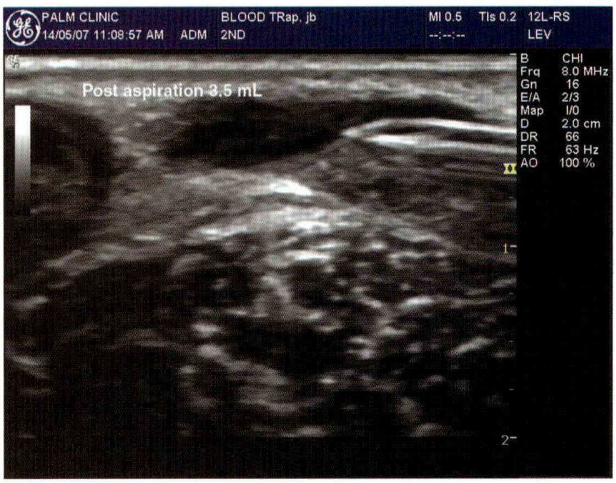

(b)

Figure 11.9 (a) Needle in area of trapped blood immediately before aspiration. (b) After aspiration of 3.5 mL of trapped blood

Ultrasound-guided foam sclerotherapy techniques used for large varicosities by other practitioners

Other phlebologists such as Pascarella and Bergan[24] cannulate a peripheral varicosity under direct vision, and inject foam into the SFJ or SPJ under ultrasound monitoring. These authors note a very low incidence of DVT with this technique. To achieve filling of large varicose veins >10 mm in diameter, however, would generally require significant volumes of foam. Once a large saphenous vein is in spasm, one assumes that a significant amount of foam could reach the deep vein system in large veins treated in this manner.

The ELLE technique, first described by Parsi in 1997[25] and later reported by Min and Navarro,[26] has been documented in detail by Parsi and Lim.[27] The technique describes the cannulation and catheterization of the GSV or SSV to allow small aliquots of solution or foam to be injected into an empty vein as the catheter is withdrawn. The leg is elevated to a 30°–45° angle to empty the vein, which theoretically allows for better contact of the sclerosant with the venous endothelium in large varicose veins. The technique has largely been abandoned, as the very veins that are suitable for the ELLE technique are those suitable for EVLA or RFA. The ELLE technique cannot be used in large tortuous veins because of technical issues in advancing the catheter.

External compression provided by saline injections into the saphenous eye to compress the saphenous trunk is described by Thibault.[28]

Adverse reactions using ultrasound-guided foam sclerotherapy techniques in our clinic

The use of foam UGS for the treatment of large varicose veins has a high safety profile under the protocols outlined above and in our previous study.[10] The only serious adverse reactions in over 6000 legs treated by foam UGS has been one pulmonary embolus and one major DVT. Minor DVTs involving small muscle veins such as the medial gastrocnemius occur from time to time, but these resolve with compression hosiery and nonsteroidal anti-inflammatories.

Expected sequelae include blood trapping and hemosiderin staining in a significant proportion of patients, which is typically proportional to the size of the vein, thus being over-represented in large varicose veins. Blood trapping typically takes 3–6 months to resolve and can be associated with a hard, ropey feeling along the affected vein. Aspiration of trapped blood where possible is necessary on some occasions, particularly where there is a feeling of pressure reported by the patient. Such aspiration is usually performed with an 18-gauge needle attached to a 3 mL Luer lock syringe and gentle vacuum applied (Figure 11.9). This can be performed under direct vision, but the best results are obtained under ultrasound control, as some of the affected areas are not obvious on the skin surface. Once the initial aspiration has been performed, it is best to massage the affected vein gently from distal and proximal approaches to milk any further trapped blood through the incision site. Aspiration of trapped blood can be attempted at any time after treatment, but effectiveness diminishes beyond 4–6 weeks after treatment as the sclerotic process replaces the thrombus.

Occasional phlebitis associated with trapped blood can occur in the immediate postoperative period and occasionally at around 4–6 weeks after treatment. Such phlebitis usually responds rapidly to nonsteroidal anti-inflammatories and/or aspiration. Chemical phlebitis can be a result of an overly strong reaction to the sclerosant following foam UGS and will result in inflammation, redness and induration on the skin surface. Ultrasound findings demonstrate a hyperechoic area in the fat space around the treated vein This may be the result of unnecessarily strong concentrations of STS or polidocanol for the size of vessel treated. This is seldom an issue with large varicose veins, but if it occurs will usually settle rapidly with nonsteroidal anti-inflammatories.

Hemosiderin staining typically takes 6–12 months to resolve, with rare cases of staining persisting beyond a year. Such hemosiderin staining is more likely with significant amounts of trapped blood, making aspiration of trapped blood the primary preventative treatment. A large anterior thigh varicosity in a young woman is often associated with hemosiderin staining, and such patients need to be well advised of this possibility ahead of treatment. We find it useful to show patients a photograph of staining. Patients who are not fully aware of this possibility before treatment will be unimpressed if it occurs. Ferritin levels may be measured and unnecessary iron tablets avoided where applicable. Ulceration secondary to extravasation of the sclerosant is a known potential complication, but we have not seen this in our practice. Nor have we experienced skin or muscle necrosis from inadvertent arterial injection.

Bruising is variable and when apparent does not present any issues for the patient. Patients are advised to stop nonsteroidal anti-inflammatories or aspirin where possible for at least 10 days before treatment unless prescribed by their primary physician.

Telangiectatic matting can result from treatment of varicose veins, but often there will be an underlying source of pressure that has been missed – either from a direct perforator or from a reticular vein.

Summary

- Foam UGS has proven to be a safe, effective alternative for treatment of large varicose veins >10 mm in diameter, either on its own or in combination with SFJ ligation or endovenous ablation.
- With the treatment protocols outlined above, patients have excellent outcomes without the need for general or local anesthesia. In our experience, patients appreciate the simplicity of the technique and are not concerned about the need for repeat visits, provided they have been well informed at the initial consultation.
- It is acknowledged that long-term studies on large varicose veins remain to be conducted and issues around potential cerebral embolism and pulmonary fibrosis need to be more accurately documented in human studies. In the meantime, current safety data suggest that foam UGS, either alone or in combination with SFJ ligation or endovenous ablation, is an excellent treatment for large varicose veins.

Acknowledgements

Thanks are due to Dr Bruce Allen, Dr David Jenkins and Dr Paul Thibault for assistance in developing protocols and Jenny Weeks ACBDR, DMU for her assistance with “Determining Ultrasound Characteristics of Large Veins.”

References

1. Cabrera J, Cabrera J Jr, Garcia-Olmedo MA. Treatment of varicose long saphenous veins with sclerosant in microfoam form: long term outcomes. Phlebology 2000; 15: 19–23.
2. Van Rij AM, Jiang P, Solomon C, et al. Recurrence after varicose vein surgery: a prospective long-term clinical study with duplex ultrasound scanning and air plethysmography. Vasc Surg 2003; 38: 935–43.
3. Blomgren L, Johansson G, Dahlberg-AKerman A, et al. Recurrent varicose veins: incidence, risk factors and groin anatomy. Eur J Vasc Endovasc Surg 2004; 27: 269–74.
4. Bounameaux H, Huber O. Postoperative deep vein thrombosis and surgery for varicose veins. Letter to Editor. BMJ 1996; 312: 1169.

5. Sam RC, Silverman SH, Bradbury AW. Nerve injuries and varicose vein surgery. Eur J Vasc Endovasc Surg 2004; 27: 113–20.
6. Wellwood JM, Cox SJ, Martin A et al. Sensory changes following stripping of the long saphenous vein. J Cardiovasc Surg 1975; 16: 123–4.
7. Holme J B, Skajaa K, Holme K. Incidence of lesions of the saphenous nerve after partial or complete stripping of the long saphenous vein. Acta Chir Scand 1990; 156: 145–8.
8. Ramsheyl A, Soury P, Saliou C, et al. Inadvertent arterial injury during saphenous vein stripping: three cases and therapeutic strategies. Arch Surg 1998; 133: 1120–3.
9. Barrett JM, Allen B, Ockelford A, Goldman MP. Microfoam ultrasound guided sclerotherapy of varicose veins in 100 legs. Dermatol Surg 2004; 30: 6–12.
10. Barrett JM, Allen B, Ockelford A, Goldman MP. Microfoam ultrasound guided sclerotherapy treatment for varicose veins in a subgroup with diameters at the junction of 10 mm or greater compared with a subgroup of less than 10 mm. Dermatol Surg 2004; 30: 1386–90.
11. Kanter A. Clinical determinants of ultrasound guided sclerotherapy outcome. Part 1: The effects of age, gender and vein size. Dermatol Surg 1998; 24: 131–5.
12. Thibault PK. "5 year" follow-up of greater saphenous incompetence treated by ultrasound guided sclerotherapy. Austr NZ J Phlebol 2003; 7: 5–8.
13. Kanter A, Thibault P. Saphenofemoral incompetence treated by ultrasound guided sclerotherapy. Dermatol Surg 1996; 22: 648–52.
14. Cavezzi A, Frullini A. The role of sclerosing foam in ultrasound guided sclerotherapy of the saphenous veins and of recurrent varicose veins: our personal experience. Austr NZ J Phlebol 1999; 3: 49–50.
15. Cavezzi A. The use of sclerosant foam in sclerotherapy: possibilities and limits. Austr NZ J Phlebol 2000; 4: 100–1.
16. Tessari L, Cavezzi A, Frullini A. Preliminary experience with a new sclerosing foam in the treatment of varicose veins. Dermatol Surg 2001; 27: 58–60.
17. Tessari L, Cavezzi A, Frullini A. New sclerosing foam. Phlebol Digest 2001; 14(4): 18–9.
18. Frullini A, Cavezzi A. Sclerosing foam in the treatment of varicose veins and telangiectases: history and analysis of safety and complications. Dermatol Surg 2002; 28: 11–15.
19. Cavezzi A, Frullini A, Ricci S, Tessari L. Treatment of varicose veins by foam sclerotherapy: two clinical series. Phlebology 2002; 17: 13–18.
20. Takase S, Schmid-Schonbein G, Bergan JJ. Leukocyte activation in patients with venous insufficiency. J Vasc Surg 1999; 30: 148–56.
21. Parsi K. Dermatological manifestations of venous disease: Part 1. Austr NZ J Phlebol 2007; 10: 11–19.
22. Morrison N, Neuhardt DL, Hansen K, et al. Tracking foam to the heart and brain following ultrasound-guided sclerotherapy of lower extremity veins. Austr NZ J Phlebol 2007; 10: 6–10.
23. Thibault P. Sclerotherapy and ultrasound guided sclerotherapy. In: Bergan JJ, ed. The Vein Book San Diego: Elsevier Academic Press, 2006: 189–99.
24. Pascarella L, Bergan J. Ultrasound Guided Catheter and Foam Therapy for Venous Insufficiency. In: Bergan JJ, ed. The Vein Book San Diego: Elsevier Academic Press, 2006: 219–26.
25. Parsi K. Extended long line echosclerotherapy. News Bulletin of the Sclerotherapy Society of Australia 1997; 1: 10–12.
26. Min RJ, Navarro L. Transcatheter duplex ultrasound guided sclerotherapy for treatment of greater saphenous vein reflux: Preliminary report. Dermatol Surg 2000; 26: 410–14.
27. Parsi K, Lim AC. Extended long line echosclerotherapy. Austr NZ J Phlebol 2000; 4: 6–10.
28. Thibault PK. Internal compression (perivenous compression) following ultrasound guided sclerotherapy to the great and small saphenous veins. Austr NZ J Phlebol 2005; 9: 29–32.

12 Transition from alcohol to foam sclerotherapy for localized venous malformations with high risk

BB Lee and John Bergan

Introduction

The study reported by Orbach in 1944 provided early evidence that adding air to liquid sclerosants enhanced their efficacy in treating varicose veins. This is referred to elsewhere in this volume. However, Orbach's concept received little attention until about a decade ago when clinicians showed that sclerotherapy with foam was more effective than treatment with liquid sclerosants, particularly under ultrasound guidance.[1–8] Many reports are now available, mostly based on polidocanol or sodium tetradecyl sulfate. Typical of these is the study reported by Darke and Baker[4] on complete venous occlusion in 91% of legs with varicose veins done safely under ultrasound-guided foam sclerotherapy.

It was Cabrera in Granada who rekindled interest in the new role of foam sclerotherapy in venous insufficiency and in vascular malformations as well.[9,10] He reported a retrospective study on the efficacy and safety of sclerosant in microfoam form in treating congenital venous malformations based on 19 patients with limited venous malformations, 16 with infiltrating venous malformations and 15 with Klippel–Trenaunay (KT) syndrome (mean follow-up, 30 months). He used direct injection of 0.25–4% polidocanol microfoam under duplex ultrasonographic guidance with no major adverse effects.

Subsequently, Bergan confirmed the efficacy of foam therapy in venous angiomas and the KT syndrome,[11,12] in addition to varicose veins, using 1–3% polidocanol with the Tessari technique. He clearly set the treatment goals not for the "cure" of these unique conditions, but for the "control of the lesions with minimum or no complications or morbidity." Thus foam therapy showed new advantages of no disability, no down-time, and no need for analgesics or sedation, all done in much less time than equivalent surgical or alcohol techniques, and not requiring general or regional anesthesia.[12,13]

For the proper application of foam sclerotherapy to venous malformation (VM) treatment, basic knowledge of the characteristics of various congenital vascular malformations (CVMs) is mandated in order to predict the role of foam and the risks involved in its use.

VMs are the most common form of CVM and comprise some 80% of those presenting for therapy.[14–16] They are low-flow lesions affecting the venous system as inborn errors throughout the body.

They come with a wide range of clinical presentations in both extent and severity. They take an unpredictable clinical course and by nature have shown erratic responses to treatment. Their record of high recurrence gives them a notorious reputation.[17] But now, with more advanced knowledge and experience in the last few decades, three critical aspects of CVMs are better understood.

First, the CVMs are different from true infantile/neonatal hemangiomas, which are vascular tumors.[18,19] Hemangiomas are mostly postnatal developments and are rapidly growing tumors. In contrast, VMs are clearly visible at birth and are an embryonic tissue remnant.

Hemangiomas have a distinctive initial proliferating phase with rapid growth followed by an involutional phase of slow regression. This occurs usually before the patient reaches the age of 7 years. But vascular malformations never disappear. Their steady growth is commensurate with body growth.

Second, many different kinds of CVMs affect the entire vascular system: arterial, venous, lymphatic and capillary. This is as a natural outcome of vascular defects caused by developmental arrest in various stages of angiogenesis/vasculogenesis.[20,21] There are VMs, lymphatic malformations (LMs),[22,23] arterial malformations (AMs),[24,25] arteriovenous malformations (AVMs),[26,27] and capillary malformations (CMs).[28,29] All of these occur either alone or together.[30,31] Most importantly, not all CVMs are the same. For example, VMs are different from AVMs, and this fact in particular cannot be overemphasized. This is of critical value in the clinical management of these two different conditions.[32]

Third, not all the VMs are the same: the "extratruncular" subtype, for example, can be blamed as the cause of bad results in treating some cases: this subtype can recur because of its embryologic characteristics.[17]

These three critical facts have led to substantial changes in the concept of CVMs and their management.

This chapter is mainly dedicated to one unique group of extratruncular VMs and their management with foam sclerotherapy. There are two different types of VMs, classified on the basis of their embryonic stage of developmental arrest. These are the extratruncular and the truncular types.[33–35] The extratruncular VMs are embryonic tissue remnants from early stages of embryogenesis. They possess mesenchymal cell characteristics of growth. The truncular VM does not have potential for independent growth as it is the outcome of developmental arrest in the late stages of embryogenesis.

Therefore, in the past, this extratruncular VM has remained an enigma to clinicians due to its apparently totally unpredictable behavior. For example, it grows rapidly when stimulated by various conditions such as hormonal changes, menarche, pregnancy, trauma and surgery.

The extratruncular type is a diffusely infiltrating condition that exerts its own hemodynamic impact on the venous circulation and also produces mechanical compression on the surrounding tissues and organs. This results in many bizarre symptoms, each with its impact on the quality of life (QoL).[36]

In general, the VM rarely becomes a limb- or life-threatening condition. Exceptions include a few unique conditions with proximity to vital organs and threat to vital functions (seeing, breathing, eating and hearing) or trauma-prone locations, which might cause joint compromise such as hemarthrosis.[37] Therefore, the VM is strikingly different from AVMs that are potentially limb-, if not life-, threatening.[26,38]

Before these critical facts were adequately understood, extratruncular VMs often became frequent targets for surgeons to perform radical control with extensive and often deforming surgery. Such an indiscriminate approach across all the varieties of CVMs was based on limited knowledge and often resulted in a disastrous outcome with severe complications and morbidity. Eventually, VMs together with other CVMs were abandoned by surgeons, as a disease condemned by intolerably bad results.[39]

Therefore, throughout the last half of the 20th century, sclerotherapy with various liquid agents gained momentum as a potential substitute for traditional surgical therapy. But the results of early experience with sclerotherapy of CVMs were disappointing, with high recurrence rates.

In the 1990s ethanol was introduced to the sclerotherapy of CVMs,[40,41] as it gave the best outcome with the least recurrence rate. Unfortunately, ethanol sclerotherapy had an extremely high rate of complications and morbidity, which could hardly justify its use in VM management.[14,16] At present, the risk involved in ethanol therapy of VMs remains controversial because the VM is potentially neither a limb- nor life-threatening condition, unlike AVMs.[38]

Despite careful exercise of necessary precautions to reduce the morbidity and complications involved in ethanol therapy, the VM lesion with transdermal extension to the skin or mucosa has been known to be an extreme risk for skin or mucosal necrosis[14,16] (Figure 12.1).

This complication along the tongue, lip, and gum/oral mucosa, and the skin of finger, palm, toe and sole has had tremendous morbidity, especially following skin grafting (Figure 12.2).

We therefore tried foam sclerotherapy using polidocanol for these special conditions that were vulnerable to skin, or mucosal damage by ethanol-based sclerotherapy. Some of the candidates for foam therapy were already the victims of unwanted complications of ethanol sclerotherapy to other adjacent VM lesions. After all, the objective of foam therapy is adequate palliation without complications rather than a cure with its hefty payments of complications and morbidity.[11]

There is no doubt that ethanol will remain a main sclerosing agent across all varieties of CVMs, especially the AVMs. Ethanol has the best chance for cure – at least

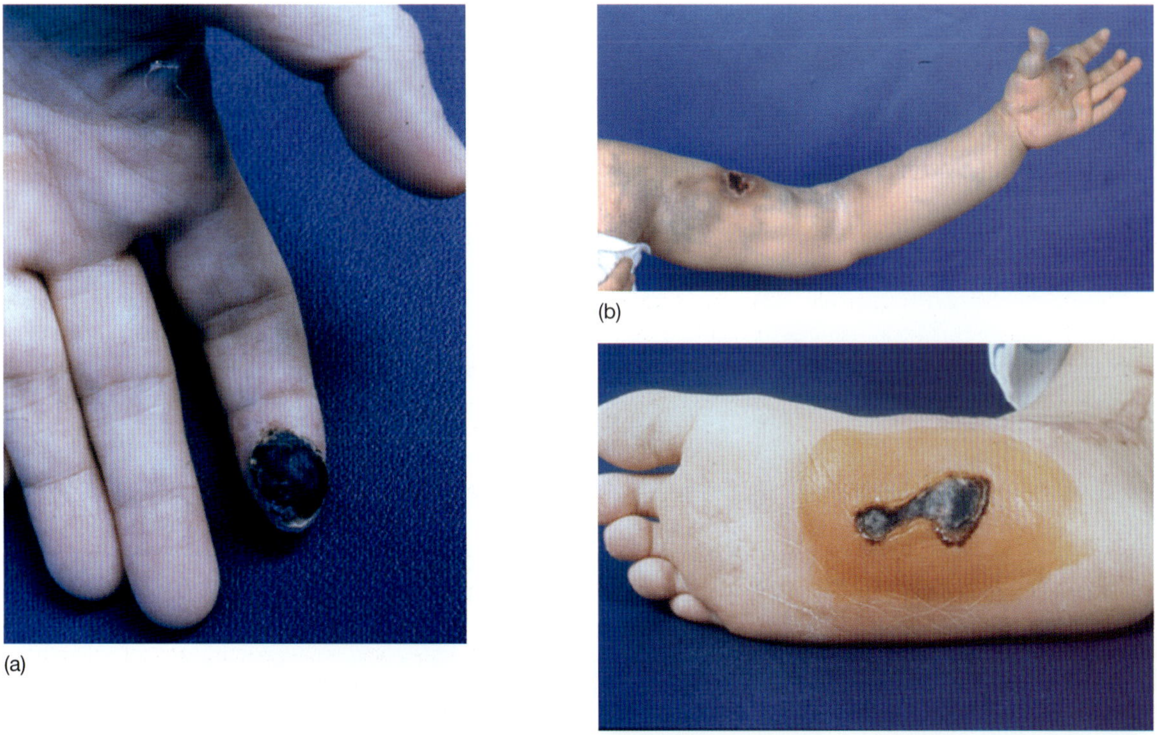

(a) (b) (c)

Figure 12.1 Complications of ethanol sclerotherapy. (a) This shows full-thickness skin necrosis on the volar aspect of the index finger following ethanol sclerotherapy to a venous malformation (VM) in close proximity to the skin. The lesion required a skin graft, but the sensory/tactile function was never fully regained. (b) This shows similar results of skin necrosis caused by ethanol along the upper arm. The treated lesion had transdermal extension that made the skin more vulnerable to damage by the alcohol. (c) This shows full-thickness skin damage causing significant morbidity on the plantar surface of the foot, which required a skin graft

equal to that of radical surgical excision.[42] But the particular group of VMs with unique conditions of low-risk certainly deserves to have a chance for better control with minimum morbidity. Recurrence, after all, can be controlled with repeated foam therapy if indicated.

Clinical experience

Among the 1203 CVM patients in the CVM Clinic of the Samsung Medical Center, SungKyunKwan University in Seoul, Korea during the years 1994–2004, 453 were proven to have independent or predominant VMs. Of these, 186 had indications for treatment.

Earlier experiences with complications and morbidity of the ethanol therapy to VMs through $N = 434$ sessions in $N = 166$ patients had shown too high an incidence of skin/mucosa necrosis among the lesions in unique locations such as the lip, tongue, gum/oral mucosa, plantar surface of toes and sole, and volar surface of fingers and palm. Full debridement and skin/mucosal grafts did not relieve treatment-induced intense pain, even after complete healing. Often, tactile sensation was permanently hampered, especially in the skin-grafted area.

Therefore, we concluded that ethanol was no longer the first choice for this unique group. We looked for another sclerosing agent with fewer complications and lower morbidity.

Among the 186 patients with VMs, we selected $N = 17$ (7 male, 10 female; mean age 21.4 years) with the localized type of VM as candidates for polidocanol foam sclerotherapy to avoid the risk of complications (e.g.,

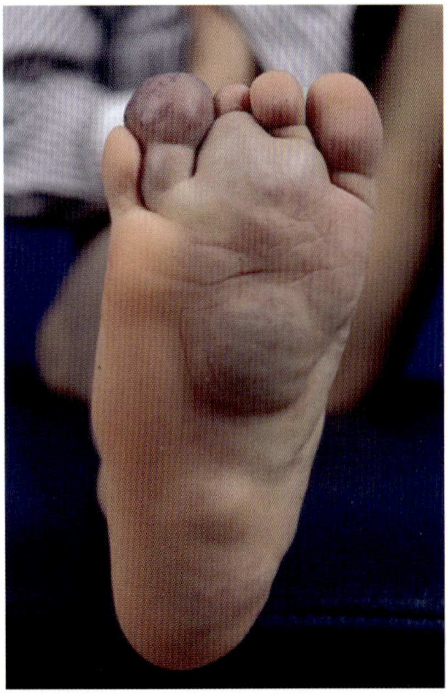

(a)

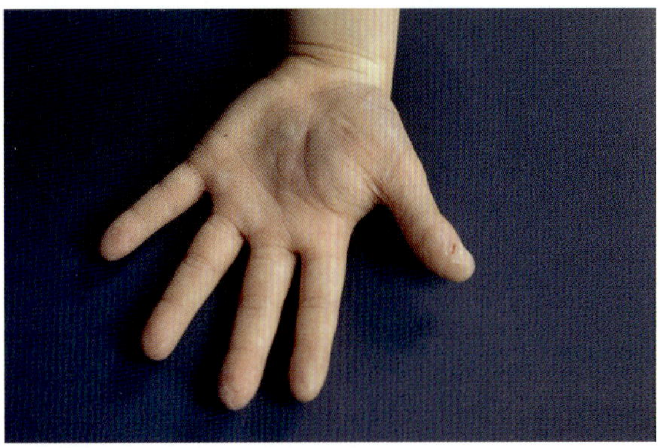

(b)

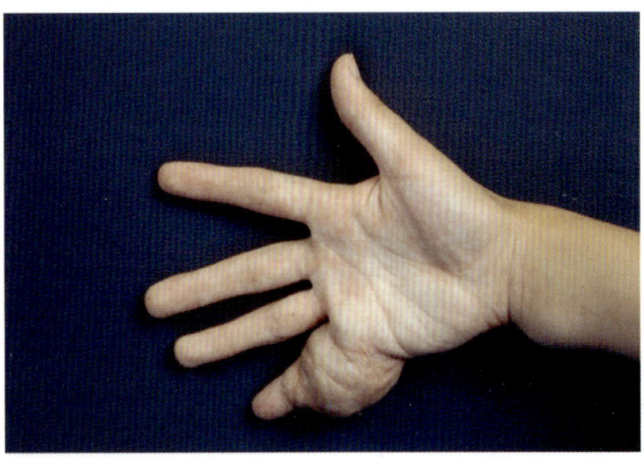

(c)

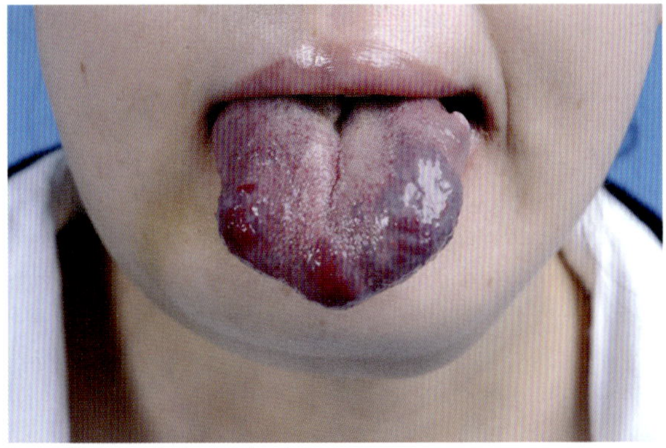

(d)

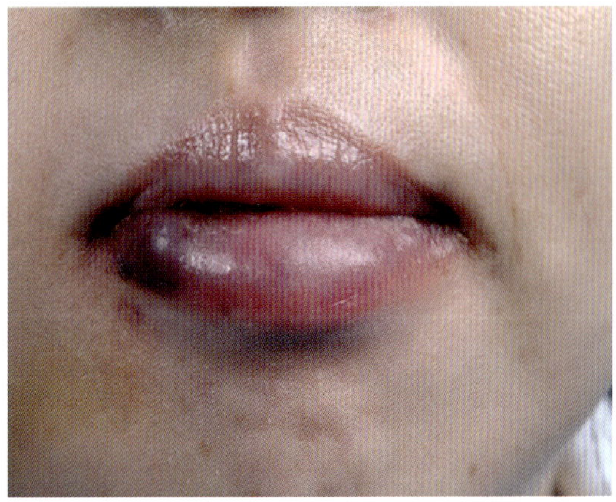

(e)

Figure 12.2 These are typical localized VM lesions affecting skin and mucosa. Variations of VM lesions are depicted affecting toes and sole of the foot (a), palm (b), finger and wrist (c), tongue (d) and lip (e). The lesions in these locations connote serious risks of complications such as full-thickness skin necrosis and the morbidity of pain and sensory loss, which is more serious than for VMs in other locations full-thickness skin necrosis) and morbidity (e.g., pain and dysfunction of finger or tongue). Selection was by their unique conditions (e.g., transdermal extension) or their location.

All the candidates for foam therapy had the same standard evaluation as CVM patients. First was duplex ultrasonography[43] (Figure 12.3), and then MRI.[44] This was followed by a more specific study such as a whole body blood pool scintigraphy (WBBPS).[45] Every effort was exerted to rule out the arterial component with every possible means, including transarterial lung perfusion scintigraphy (TLPS),[46,47] in order to confirm the independent status of the VM. Finally, an additional evaluation for the cardiopulmonary and neurologic status was added to this foam therapy group. This was mainly to clear the theoretical risk of paradoxical foam particulate embolization.[48–50] An echocardiogram was not included routinely.

The lesions treated with foam were with transdermal extension to the skin ($N = 3$) or proximity to the skin ($N = 7$): the fingers = 3, palm = 3, toes = 2 and sole = 2, and also submucosal lesions ($N = 7$): lips = 2, tongue = 2, gum/oral mucosa = 2 and penile glans = 1 were part of this group.

All the lesions were treated with 1% polidocanol foam made up by the Tessari method and used in an average amount of 2.3 mL (0.7–3.2 mL) in each session through an average of 1.8 sessions (1–5 sessions) with a minimum of 3 weeks interval between sessions.

Initially, the foam therapy ($N = 6$) was done in the radiology suite, but subsequently all procedures were done in the outpatient clinic using ultrasonographic guidance. The initial four cases were done with patients under general sedation and closely monitored for a minimum of 8 hours following the procedures. Subsequently, the rest of the procedures ($N = 13$) were done with minimum local or no anesthesia and patients discharged from the clinic within 2 hours after the procedure, except one patient who was kept overnight for the observation of transient disorientation.

No sedation was given, as these were all outpatient procedures. Compression dressings were not allowed to accommodate swelling for the first 48 hours. Analgesics were recommended for control of pain on discharge.

Following the therapy, $N = 3$ of five patients with transient symptoms during or shortly after the procedure had an electrocardiogram ($N = 1$) for chest tightness, echocardiogram ($N = 1$) for visual disturbance, and MR cerebral perfusion/diffusion scans ($N = 1$) to clarify cause of the disorientation after the procedures.

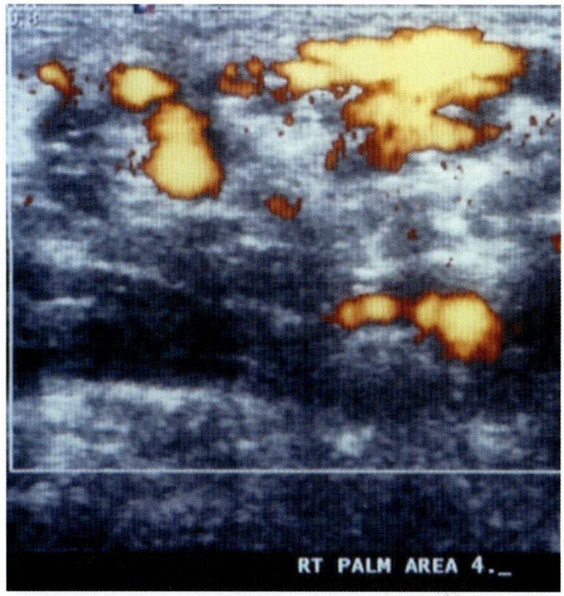

(a)

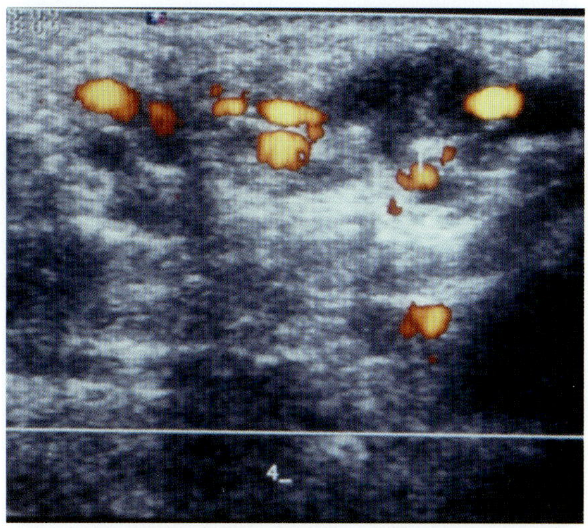

(b)

Figure 12.3 Duplex ultrasonographic evaluation of VM lesions before and after the foam sclerotherapy. (a) This shows the baseline duplex scan finding of a VM lesion in the right palm before foam sclerotherapy was started. (b) This shows the results of therapy, with near complete disappearance of the lesion following two consecutive sessions of foam sclerotherapy

Interim results of treatment were assessed with a duplex scan on days 3 and 7 and at 2 weeks, 1 month and then 3-month intervals until 24 months.

Results

All patients ($N = 17$) tolerated the procedures very well with minimal to moderate pain ($N = 13$), which was easily controlled with analgesics. None required narcotics. Among the 17 patients, transient symptoms were noticed in 5: dry cough in 2, chest tightness in 1, visual disturbances in 1, and disorientation in 1.

Subsequent investigation failed to prove any paradoxical air embolization as the cause of symptoms. The patient with the dry cough was found to have a potential patent foramen ovale.

Fifteen patients had excellent to good immediate outcomes following completion of multisessions. All had clinical and duplex scan follow-up assessments. Fifteen had good initial responses showing complete disappearance of lesions ($N = 8$) or near complete disappearance ($N = 4$) (Figure 12.4). A substantial reduction in size of over 50% of initial size ($N = 3$) was documented on periprocedural mapping of the lesion (Figure 12.2).

Two patients had less than 30% reduction in size of the lesions. One patient refused to have a third session after the experience with disorientation and another refused for a nonmedical reason following two sessions.

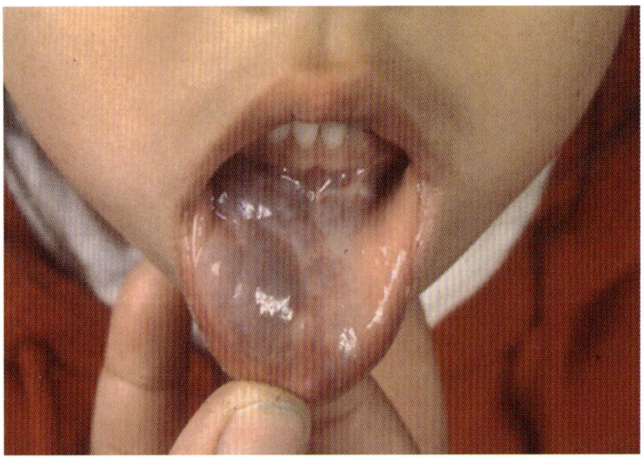

(a)

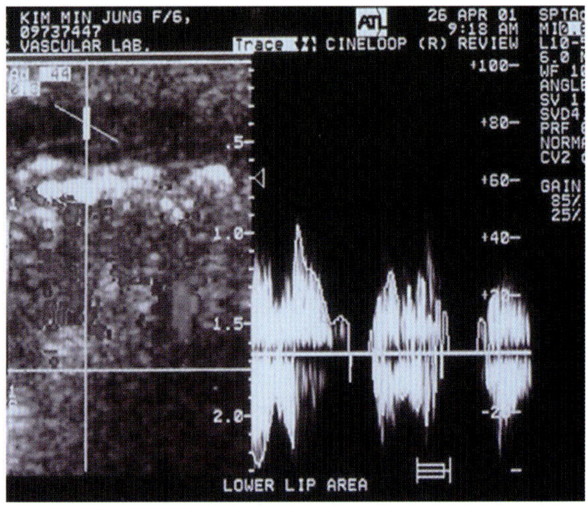

(b)

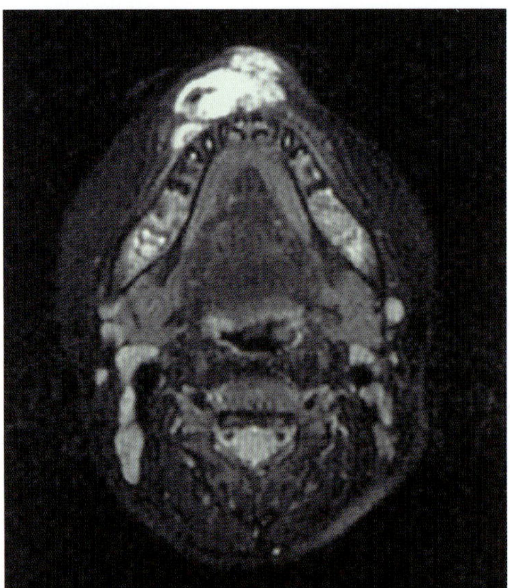

(c)

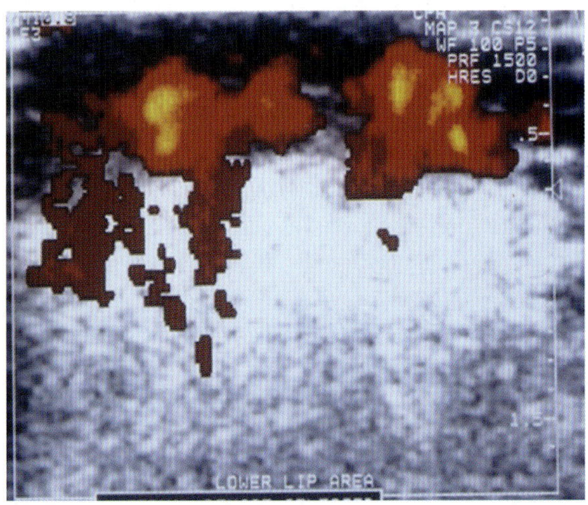

(d)

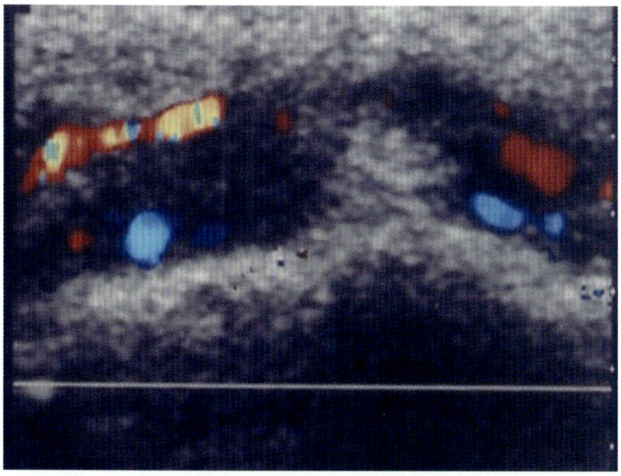
(e)

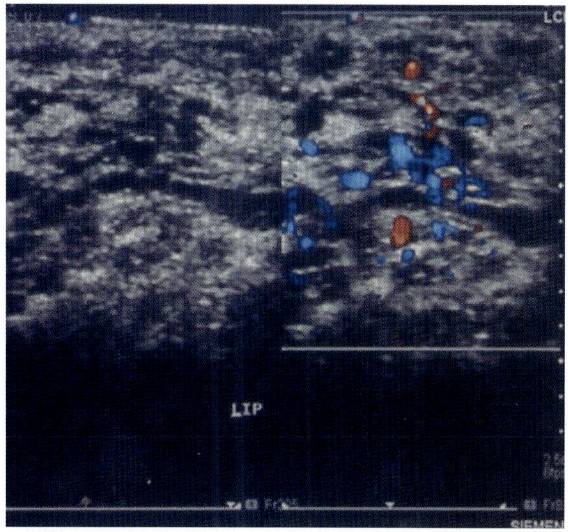

(f)

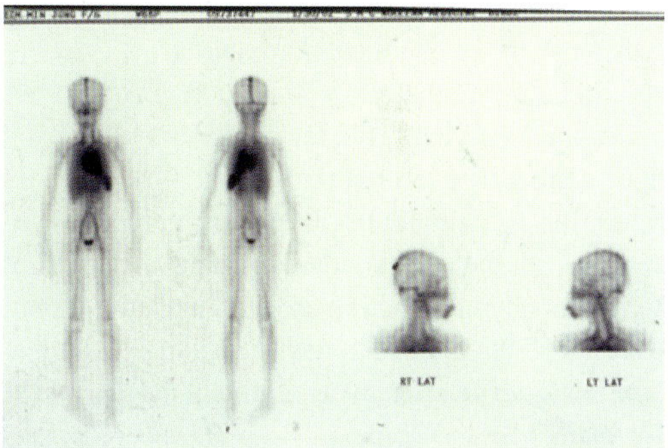

(g)

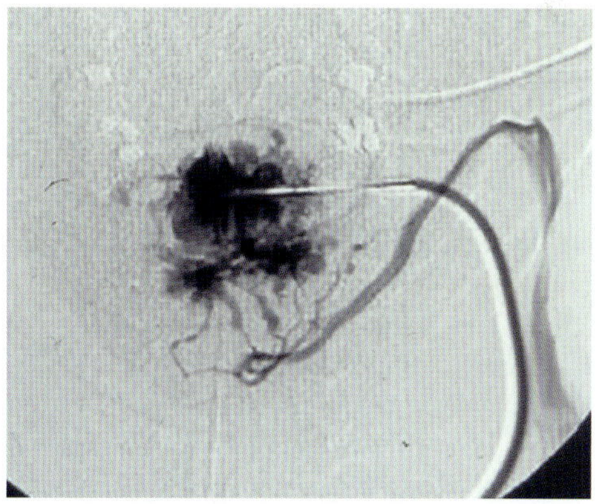
(h)

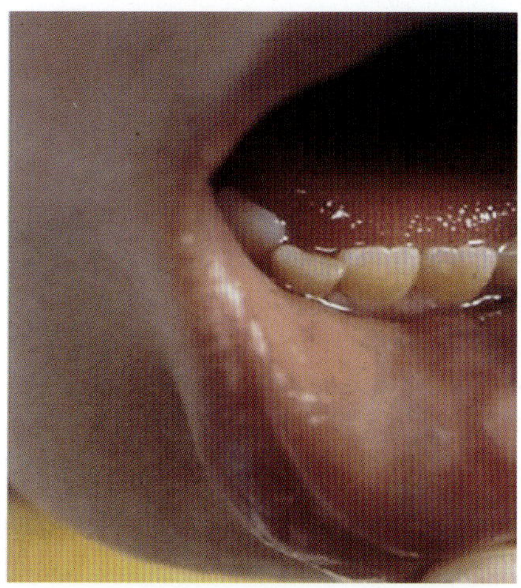
(i)

Figure 12.4 Clinical and laboratory findings of a VM lesion in the oral mucosa. (a) This shows the clinical appearance of a slow but steadily growing VM lesion affecting the oral mucosa of right lower lip. It had a history of recurrent swelling with pain causing a significant decrease in QoL. The duplex ultrasonographic findings in (b) depict a low-flow VM along the lower lip. MRI (c) confirmed the Duplex findings. Finally, the duplex scan was used for the assessment of the results of treatment: (d) shows the color Doppler findings of another VM before the therapy, and (e) shows the findings immediately after completion of three sessions of foam therapy. (f) is the follow-up scan at the 24-month final follow-up. (g) shows the whole body blood pool scintigraphy (WBBPS) findings of abnormal blood pooling along the lower lip, which is more clearly seen in the close-up view (right image). The WBBPS is an excellent technique for documenting follow-up and avoiding MRI expense, especially when combined with duplex scans. (h) shows the direct puncture percutaneous phlebography findings of the draining vein of the VM lesion affecting lower lip. (i) shows the clinical appearance of a completely controlled VM lesion of the oral mucosa after foam therapy

Among the 17 patients, 3 had mild sloughing of overlying skin or mucosa; they then had slow healing with minimal interference with function. One patient developed skin necrosis less than 0.5 cm in diameter following the third session, but healed without additional treatment.

The recurrence rate during the follow-up period of 24 months was in 23.5% (4 of 17) within 12 months and reached to 35% (6 of 17) in 24 months. However, the recurrent lesions were less than one-third of the original size in the majority (4 of 6). But, by protocol, we withheld further foam therapy until we reached the end-point of 24 months for each patient.

All patients with very well sustained initial success during this limited follow-up period ($N = 15$) had improved their QoL substantially, and the lesions remained stable on repeated evaluation with Duplex ultrasound.

Discussion

We intentionally limited the candidates for foam sclerotherapy only to this particular group of VM with the unique conditions explained above because there had not been any convincing data on foam therapy for VMs up to the year 2002; Then, after the unique opportunity to make a personal review of Cabrera's data, we decided to start a small pilot project as Bergan had advised.

Following an intense review of various issues related to potential risks of foam particle embolization, the study was limited to 24 months' follow-up to evaluate the efficacy of foam therapy.

Our experiences were, therefore, limited to this group, which could not tolerate ethanol therapy. It was our first experience and occurred in the midst of much controversy, especially on the physical characteristics of the air used to make foam.[3,6] We selected only 17 cases among 29 with similar conditions. Also we decided to use the lowest possible concentration of sclerosant despite an anticipated higher recurrence rate. However, we took the advantage of the unique physical property of foam. Its mechanism of disrupting the endothelium is different from that of ethanol. The detergent has a strong affinity, which allows the chemical to have a longer and undiluted contact, which penetrates to the cell membranes, causing an effective disruption of cellular proteins.

Foam sclerotherapy is now widely accepted in the management of varicose veins and saphenous veins, as detailed elsewhere in this book, with excellent interim results.[1–8] Recurrence of lesions is not a serious issue, as the risk involved in dealing with recurrence is not substantial.

Recurrence has an entirely different meaning with regard to well-matured cells of varicose veins and to immature VM cells. Recurrence in saphenous veins and varicose veins is the result of recanalization following incomplete thrombosis and cellular damage. Therefore, in the worst scenario, the condition goes back to the original state and no more.

But the recurrence of the VM causes different results because of its embryologic characteristics originating from mesenchymal cells. The surviving cells of VMs that withstand the chemical attack could theoretically rebound to grow worse than their original state as a natural response to the chemical stimulation.

We should be aware that the VM is not a varicose vein or even a saphenous vein. This fact is so crucial that its importance cannot be overemphasized.

However, the foam modality has a distinctive advantage due to its unique dual conditions of physical action as foam and its chemical action at the same time. Foam therapy seems to have more meaning in its treatment of VMs. The long-term efficacy is unlikely to be established for many years to come.

Ethanol sclerotherapy still remains a mainstay of sclerotherapy across all the varieties of CVMs, including the VMs.[40,41,51] Although it has a very high risk of complications and morbidity,[14,16] there is no better replacement in the foreseeable future.[36]

Our 17 patients were initially ruled out as poor candidates for ethanol therapy due to the increased risk of skin/mucosal necrosis; 4 among them (palm = 2, sole = 2) had experienced actual damage to their skin from previous ethanol therapy to nearby lesions with similar characteristics. These lesions were relatively well localized and extended through or very close to the skin/mucous membranes on duplex study, and showed clinical findings of bluish color extending to the epidermis.

Therefore, the foam sclero-agent seems to be an ideal substitute for ethanol with minimum complications and morbidity. It may replace the too powerful and risky ethanol to treat the relatively benign VM condition.

Although 35% recurrence within 24 months with foam is inferior to results with ethanol, it was totally anticipated that the lowest possible concentration of polidocanol could avoid collateral damage to local tissue. We deliberately planned to repeat the therapy to continue to control the lesion whenever it recurred.

The best aspect of ethanol sclerotherapy is, however, its lowest recurrence rate among all the sclero-agents. The worst aspect is its very high complication rate.

Lesions such as AVMs will all become limb-, if not life-threatening eventually if neglected for long enough. Therefore, recurrence could become a major issue for AVMs in long-term care. A high complication/morbidity rate could be accepted for a chance of cure.

However, VMs never become life- or limb-threatening conditions except for a few exceptional lesions as mentioned above. Therefore, we selected and advocate foam sclerotherapy for functionally sensitive areas such as the palm, fingers and tongue, which often have augumented morbidity following their treatment. These deserve to have minimal morbidity, and it is possible to repeat the therapy to the recurrent and incompletely controlled lesion as necessary.

So far there is no sclero-agent for which there is no risk of recurrence or morbidity.

We therefore recommend this lesser evil for VMs, especially in the specialized conditions for which we used it.

Conclusion

Foam sclerotherapy with 1% polidocanol is an excellent substitute for ethanol, especially in high-risk, localized VM lesions.

Localized lesions on the lip, tongue and gum/oral mucosa, as well as those on the finger, toe, palm and sole with or without transdermal extension, are excellent candidates for foam, although the recurrence rate up to a 2-year follow-up is high. This is an acceptable price to pay for no complication or morbidity, especially since the therapy can be repeated with no increased risk.

After all, the aim of the treatment of this particular group of VM is palliation without complication.

References

1. Yamaki T, Nozaki M, Fujiwara O, Yoshida E. Duplex-guided foam sclerotherapy for the treatment of the symptomatic venous malformations of the face. Dermatol Surg 2002; 28: 619–22.
2. Yamaki T, Nozaki M, Iwasaka S. Comparative study of duplex-guided foam sclerotherapy and duplex-guided liquid sclerotherapy for the treatment of superficial venous insufficiency. Dermatol Surg 2004; 30: 718–22.
3. Barrett JM, Allen B, Ockelford A, Goldman MP. Microfoam ultrasound-guided sclerotherapy of varicose veins in 100 legs. Dermatol Surg 2004; 30: 6–12.
4. Darke SG, Baker SJ. Ultrasound-guided foam sclerotherapy for the treatment of varicose veins. Br J Surg 2006; 93: 969–74.
5. Frullini A, Cavezzi A. Sclerosing foam in the treatment of varicose veins and telangiectases: history and analysis of safety and complications. Dermatol Surg 2002; 28: 11–15.
6. Alos J, Carreno P, Lopez JA, et al. Efficacy and safety of sclerotherapy using polidocanol foam: a controlled clinical trial. Eur J Vasc Endovasc Surg 2006; 31: 101–7.
7. De Waard MM, der Kinderen DJ. Duplex ultrasonography-guided foam sclerotherapy of incompetent perforator veins in a patient with bilateral venous leg ulcers. Dermatol Surg 2005; 31: 580–3.
8. Coleridge Smith P. Saphenous ablation: sclerosant or sclerofoam? Semin Vasc Surg 2005; 18: 19–24.
9. Cabrera J, Cabrera J Jr, Garcia-Olmedo MA, Redondo P. Treatment of venous malformations with sclerosant in microfoam form. Arch Dermatol 2003; 139: 1409–16.
10. Cabrera J, Redondo P, Becerra A, et al. Ultrasound-guided injection of polidocanol microfoam in the management of venous leg ulcers. Arch Dermatol 2004; 140: 667–73.
11. Bergan J, Pascarella L, Mekenas L. Venous disorders: treatment with sclerosant foam. J Cardiovasc Surg (Torino) 2006; 47: 9–18.
12. Pascarella L, Bergan JJ, Yamada C, Mekenas L. Venous angiomata: treatment with sclerosant foam. Ann Vasc Surg 2005; 19: 457–64.
13. Coleridge Smith P. Saphenous ablation: sclerosant or sclerofoam? Semin Vasc Surg 2005; 18: 19–24.
14. Lee BB, Kim DI, Huh S, et al. New experiences with absolute ethanol sclerotherapy in the management of a complex form of congenital venous malformation. J Vasc Surg 2001; 33: 764–72.
15. Lee BB. Current concept of venous malformation (VM). Phlebolymphology 2003; 43: 197–203.
16. Lee BB, Do YS, Byun HS, et al. Advanced management of venous malformation with ethanol sclerotherapy: mid-term results. J Vasc Surg 2003; 37: 533–8.
17. Lee BB. Critical issues on the management of congenital vascular malformation. Ann Vasc Surg 2004; 18: 380–92.
18. Mulliken JB, Glowacki J. Hemangiomas and vascular malformations in infants and children: a classification

based on endothelial characteristics. Plast Reconstr Surg 1982; 69: 412–20.

19. Mulliken JB. Cutaneous vascular anomalies. Semin Vasc Surg 1993; 6: 204–18.
20. Folkman J. Toward a new understanding of vascular proliferative disease in children. Pediatrics 1984; 74: 850–6.
21. Leu HJ. Pathomorphology of vascular malformations: analysis of 310 cases. Int Angiol 1990; 9: 147–55.
22. Lee BB, Kim YW, Seo JM, et al. Current concepts in lymphatic malformation (LM). J Vasc Endovasc Surg 2005; 39: 67–81.
23. Lee BB: Lymphedema–angiodysplasia Syndrome: a prodigal form of lymphatic malformation (LM). Phlebolymphology 2005; 47: 324–32.
24. Zhang YJ, Barrow DL, Day AL. Extracranial–intracranial vein graft bypass for giant intracranial aneurysm surgery for pediatric patients: two technical case reports. Neurosurgery 2002; 50: 663–8.
25. Kan P, Liu JK, Couldwell WT. Giant fusiform aneurysm in an adolescent with PHACES syndrome treated with a high-flow external carotid artery–M3 bypass. Case report and review of the literature. J Neurosurg 2007; 106(6 Suppl): 495–500.
26. Lee BB, Do YS, Yakes W, et al. Management of arterial–venous shunting malformations (AVM) by surgery and embolosclerotherapy. A multidisciplinary approach. J Vasc Surg 2004; 39: 590–600.
27. Lee BB. Arteriovenous malformation. In: Zelenock GB, Huber TS, Messina LM, Lumsden AB, Moneta GL, eds. Mastery of Vascular and Endovascular Surgery. Philadelphia, PA: Lippincott, Williams & Wilkins, 2006: 597–607.
28. Berwald C, Salazard B, Bardot J, et al. Port wine stains or capillary malformations: surgical treatment. Ann Chir Plast Esthet 2006; 51: 369–72.
29. Goldman MP, Fitzpatrick RE, Ruiz-Esparza J. Treatment of port-wine stains (capillary malformation) with the flash lamp-pumped pulsed dye laser. J Pediatr 1993; 122: 71–7.
30. Belov St. Anatomopathological classification of congenital vascular defects. Semin Vasc Surg 1993; 6: 219–24.
31. Rutherford RB. Classification of peripheral congenital vascular malformations. In: Ernst C, Stanley J, eds. Current Therapy in Vascular Surgery, 3rd edn. St Louis, MO: Mosby, 1995: 834–38.
32. Lee BB. Critical issues on the management of congenital vascular malformation. Ann Vasc Surg 2004; 18: 380–92.
33. Woolard HH. The development of the principal arterial stems in the forelimb of the pig. Contrib Embryol 1922; 14: 139–54.
34. Bastide G, Lefebvre D. Anatomy and organogenesis and vascular malformations. In: Belov St, Loose DA, Weber J, eds. Vascular Malformations. Reinbek: Einhorn-Presse Verlag, 1989: 20–2.
35. Belov St. Classification of congenital vascular defects. Int Angiol 1990; 9: 141–6.
36. Lee BB. Status of new approaches to the treatment of congenital vascular malformations (CVMs) – single center experiences [Editorial Review]. Eur J Vasc Endovasc Surg 2005; 30: 184–97.
37. Lee BB, Bergan JJ. Advanced management of congenital vascular malformations: a multidisciplinary approach. Cardiovasc Surg 2002; 10: 523–33.
38. Lee BB. Vascular surgery; cases, questions and commentaries. In: Geroulakos G, van Urk H, Hobson II RW, Calligaro K, eds. Congenital Vascular Malformation. London: Springer-Verlag, 2003: 315–23.
39. Szilagyi DE, Smith RF, Elliott JP, Hageman JH. Congenital arteriovenous anomalies of the limbs. Arch Surg 1976; 111: 423–9.
40. Yakes WF, Haas DK, Parker SH, et al. Symptomatic vascular malformations: ethanol embolotherapy. Radiology 1989; 170: 1059–66.
41. Yakes WF, Parker SH, Gibson MD, et al. Alcohol embolotherapy of vascular malformations. Semin Intervent Radiol 1989; 6: 146–61.
42. Lee BB. Management of arteriovenous malformation. In: Fast Facts – Vascular Surgery Highlights 2006–07. Abingdon, UK: Health Press, 2007: 42–50.
43. Lee BB, Mattassi R, Choe YH, et al. Critical role of duplex ultrasonography for the advanced management of a venous malformation (VM). Phlebology 2005; 20: 28–37.
44. Lee BB, Choe YH, Ahn JM, et al. The new role of MRI (magnetic resonance imaging) in the contemporary diagnosis of venous malformation: Can it replace angiography? J Am Coll Surg 2004; 198: 549–58.
45. Lee BB, Mattassi R, Kim BT, et al. Contemporary diagnosis and management of venous and AV shunting malformation by whole body blood pool scintigraphy (WBBPS). Int Angiol 2004; 23: 355–67.
46. Lee BB, Kim HH, Mattassi R, et al. A new approach to the congenital vascular malformation with new concept – Seoul Consensus. Int J Angiol 2003; 12: 248–51.
47. Lee BB, Mattassi R, Kim BT, Park JM. Advanced management of arteriovenous shunting malformation with transarterial lung perfusion scintigraphy (TLPS) for follow up assessment. Int Angiol 2005; 24: 173–84.
48. Eckmann DM, Kobayashi S. Microvascular embolization following polidocanol microfoam sclerosant administration Dermatol Surg 2005; 31: 636–43.
49. Forlee MV, Grouden M, Moore DJ, Shanik G. Stroke

after varicose vein foam injection sclerotherapy. J Vasc Surg 2006; 43: 162–4.

50. Morrison N, Cavezzi A, Bergan J, Partsch H. Regarding "Stroke after varicose vein foam injection sclerotherapy." J Vasc Surg 2006; 43: 162–4.

51. Lee BB. Congenital vascular malformation. In: Geroulakos G, van Urk H, Hobson II RW, Calligaro K, eds. Vascular Surgery: Cases, Questions and Commentaries, 2nd edn. London: Springer-Verlag, 2005: 377–92.

13 Treatment of telangiectasias by sclerosing foam

Philippe Kern

Introduction

Sclerotherapy still represents the first choice of treatment for cosmetically unacceptable telangiectasias, despite its long history. Recently, sclerotherapy has attracted new interest internationally with the advent of foam. Whereas the use of foam has markedly improved sclerotherapy efficacy for the treatment of varicose veins, for the treatment of telangiectasias the superiority of foam compared with a standard solution is less obvious. Indeed, increased benefit seems to be negatively counterbalanced by an increase in side-effects. Therefore, the initial enthusiasm related to the use of foam for the treatment of telangiectasias has gradually faded with time.

The advantage of foam over a standard solution for sclerotherapy is thus less convincing for treatment of telangiectasias. Pretreatment investigations, treatment strategy, methods and contraindications for the use of foam do not differ from those of conventional liquid sclerotherapy. There are no specific foam-related side-effects, but those that do occur are more frequent than with liquid solutions. Comparative studies between foam and solutions in specific clinical settings are still scarce, and, therefore, definitive conclusions about foam efficacy are still lacking.

Definition, clinical presentation and epidemiology

Telangiectasias are intradermal dilatations of the subpapillary venous plexus.[1,2] They cannot be strictly regarded as varicose veins and they are not capillaries. In the CEAP classification, they are classified as C_1.[3] Telangiectasias are less than 1 mm in diameter. The smallest (0.1–0.2 mm) are frequently red, whilst the larger ones are usually blue. They can occur as isolated features or as starbursts, or as arborizing patterns. Their distribution is mostly symmetrical. Telangiectasias are frequently a consequence of an incompetent feeding reticular vein, a saphenous or nonsaphenous varicose vein, or an incompetent perforating vein, or are a clinical sign of deep venous insufficiency. On the medial malleolus, they can take on the characteristic appearance of the corona phlebectactica paraplantaris. This is a clinical sign that strongly correlates with the clinical severity and the hemodynamic disturbances of chronic venous insufficiency.[4]

The prevalence of telangiectasias in the general population is about 50–70%.[5] They affect women more often than men (M/F ratio: 3/4) and their frequency increases with age. Patients with class C_1 venous insufficiency often present a sensation of edema, muscular cramps, and restless legs more often than those with class C_0,[6] although this is still a matter of debate. Indeed, in the Edinburgh study,[7] a significant difference in symptoms, namely, sensation of lower limb heaviness and edema, was found only in women. In the San Diego study,[8] there was no difference in symptom frequency between patients in classes C_0 and C_1. Moreover, the class C_1 patients presented no more color flow duplex imaging (CFDI) abnormalities of the veins than did those in class C_0.[9] Nevertheless, reflux on CFDI is detected in as many as 46% of patients with telangiectasias.[10] Physical and mental quality of life scores in women seeking treatment for telangiectasias are similar to those of a healthy control population.[11]

Basis and objectives of treatment

Foam sclerotherapy is based on intravenous injection of a corroding agent that provokes fibrous involution of the telangiectactic vein and ultimately its visual disappearance.

Investigations prior to treatment

Investigations prior to treatment do not differ between foam and conventional liquid sclerotherapy. The diagnosis of telangiectasias is made clinically. Most patients with telangiectasias consult the phlebologist with mainly an aesthetic concern. The treatment efficacy relies not only on their visual disappearance, but also on the elimination of the reflux from feeding reticular veins. The persistence of reflux after treatment can be responsible for short-term relapse or even the occurrence of unaesthetic side-effects such as pigmentation or matting (neotelangiectasias).[2] Therefore, the presence of axial reflux is a contraindication to treatment of telangiectasias unless the reflux itself is corrected. This is why a precise diagnosis of the extension of the venous disorder and mapping of reflux patterns is mandatory. A recent study[10] showed that in symptomatic and asymptomatic women with class C_1 (telangiectasias and reticular veins), as many as 5% had reflux in both great (GSV) and short (SSV) saphenous veins, 39% had GSV reflux and 2% had SSV reflux on CFDI. Unfortunately, sensitivity and specificity of a clinical diagnosis of saphenous reflux is poor in comparison with CFDI.[12] The association of clinical examination and hand-held Doppler (HDD) improves the diagnostic precision, but is still far less efficient than CFDI. The sensitivity and specificity of HDD for the saphenofemoral junction are 85% (71–95%) and 83% (68–100%), respectively; for the saphenopopliteal junction they are 71% (36–92%) and 82% (53–93%).[5,13–18] We do not have data for patients with telangiectasias, who represent a different cohort from patients with varicose veins who need operation. But if we look to trials studying HHD accuracy prior to intervention, only 61–90% of the patients would have an appropriate intervention in comparison with those diagnosed with CFDI.[13–16,19]

This reflects the limitation of the diagnosis and treatment strategy based only on clinical examination and HDD.

We recommend performing at least an HHD examination, but better a CFDI, prior to treatment, especially if the telangiectasias are located in saphenous or perforator territories.

Principle and methods

The intravenous injection of a sclerosing agent damages the endothelium, provoking desquamation of the intima and exposing the underlining collagen fibers. The repair process (platelet aggregation, coagulation activation and invasion of fibroblasts) induces fibrosis of the vein and its visual disappearance.[2,5] Thrombus formation cannot be entirely prevented; however, it should be as little as possible. This avoids development of (1) an inflammatory reaction, which may promote angiogenesis and matting (formation of new telangiectasias), and (2) subsequent recanalization, which represents treatment failure. Moreover, thrombus degradation may induce skin pigmentation due to hemosiderin deposits and melanogenesis. Thrombus size increases when the sclerosing agent is too powerful, the concentration is too strong, or if a too large amount is injected. Therefore, it is recommended to use the minimal effective volume and concentration.[5]

Foam sclerosing agents

Two sclerosing agents commonly used for the treatment of telangiectasias have tensioactive properties and can be made into foam. Polidocanol and sodium tetradecyl sulfate are both corroding agents, and are used at low concentrations for this indication (0.25–1%). Several trials have been published on treatment with polidocanol foam,[20–25] but none on sodium tetradecyl sulfate foam. One explanation for this could be that most publications come from France and Switzerland, where polidocanol is one of the most popular sclerosing agents for treatment of telangiectasias, whereas sodium tetradecyl sulfate is rarely used in those countries for this indication.

The foam is obtained by mixing 1 part of the sclerosing agent with 3 parts of air. The sclerosing agent is concentrated on small foam bubbles (micelles). After intravenous injection, foam stagnates within the vessels and does not mix with blood, while the various solutions are quickly diluted in the blood stream. Moreover, foam microbubbles remain in tight contact with the venous wall. Therefore, foam is much more powerful than sclerosant solutions: its efficiency is superior at a lower concentration.

There are several different methods for producing foam. These are described elsewhere in this book. Foam sclerotherapy for telangiectasias was first employed using the Monfreux technique[26] with glass syringes. However, these produce an inhomogeneous foam composed of both small and large bubbles. Nowadays, Monfreux's technique has been largely replaced by the Tessari technique[27] or the double-syringe system technique (DSS).[28] This has the advantage of using plastic syringes, thus avoiding sterilization concerns. These induce a more homogenous and viscous foam with smaller microbubbles (<100 μm). Due to its properties, Tessari foam is certainly more powerful than Monfreux foam, but for telangiectasias this could be a disadvantage, as it may enhance side-effects such as formation of microthrombi.

Injection technique

Sclerotherapy for telangiectasias necessitates the use of very small needles (30-gauge ½-inch [0.3 mm diameter], or even 32-gauge ½-inch), because of the small size of the vessels. However, Ferrara[24] showed that foam loses its homogeneity and its efficiency when injected through a 0.3 mm diameter needle. This is not the case when larger needles are used; nevertheless, these larger needles are not always appropriate for telangiectasias smaller than 0.4 mm in diameter.

The principle of treatment technique is to inject the nourishing reticular veins first and the telangiectasias subsequently within the same session. Injections are made in a supine position through a direct needle puncture of the vein. Aspiration of the piston is performed to confirm blood reflux and an intravenous puncture (reticular veins). As the half-life of foam is only about 2.5 minutes, it cannot be prepared in advance, and the injection technique needs to be performed very quickly by skilled and trained physicians. If not, there will be more liquid than foam in the syringe for the last vessels treated. As far as possible, a needle greater than 30-gauge is used, to avoid destroying foam. A small angulation of the needle at its base, stretching of the skin and the use of magnifying glasses can facilitate the injection. Injection of very small volumes (0.1–0.2 mL for telangiectasias) of foam, treating a surface of telangiectasias not greater then 2 cm^2 per injection, has the advantage of limiting side-effects in case of accidental extravasation. Fewer microthrombi will form, and less pigmentation and matting will occur because of the limited intravascular pressure used. With this technique, we perform between 60 and 100 injections per session. Injection can be followed by vasospasm and a papule, which has to be differentiated from an allergic reaction and paravasal injection (histamine release from perivascular mast cells).

Postprocedural care

Immediately after the treatment, the leg can be cleaned and blood removed either with cold water or even better with peroxide (H_2O_2 3%).

Compression?

The use of compression following sclerotherapy for telangiectasias varies a great deal between countries,[29] and its utility has been a matter of controversy for half a century. If applied, different modalities of compressions are used, and the duration of compression varies among phlebologists: from 24 hours to 3 weeks. Compression modalities include medical compression stockings (20–40 mmHg) and various forms of compression bandages. Some phlebologists use local exocentric compressive pads in addition. The great diversity of methods used reflects personal experience and a lack of evidence of postsclerotherapy compression efficacy. Moreover, patients are often reluctant to use compression. Goldmann[30] showed that compression was effective for telangiectasias larger than 0.5 mm. In the study by Weiss,[31] the best effect was observed in patients wearing compression stockings (20–30 mmHg) for 3 weeks. Compression is thought to enhance sclerotherapy efficacy by reducing the formation of postsclerotherapy thrombi, as well as pigmentation and matting by minimizing inflammation and angiogenesis.[2] However, the efficacy of a 23–32 mmHg compression stocking is debatable, since emptying of blood from telangiectasias requires a pressure of about 80 mmHg. For instance, at the thigh level, compression stockings usually exert only 41–74% of the pressure exerted at the ankle.[2] Therefore, compression stockings of 23–32 mmHg would only exert approximately 10–18 mmHg of pressure at the thigh.

As the practitioner is often confronted with patients presenting with telangiectasias in the thigh, Kern et al.[11] designed a prospective randomized open-label trial to determine the relative efficacy of 3 weeks' use of compression stockings (23–32 mmHg) following sclerotherapy of telangiectasias and reticular veins of the thigh. If compression enhances vessel disappearance at the thigh, it is probably also true for the calf, but the contrary might not be true. As it was not possible to perform a power calculation on the previous compression studies,[30,31] because of either the lack of statistics or a different statistical methodology, the sample size required for this trial was calculated on the basis of Kern's previous similar methodological sclerotherapy study, which compared different sclerosing agents[23] and could demonstrate a statistically significant difference between the agents. Precalculation of the required sample size showed that to detect a true difference of half a standard deviation at a one-sided 5% significance level with a power of 80%, exactly 100 patients are required, 50 in each group. Therefore, 100 consecutive female patients with primary telangiectasias and reticular veins on the lateral surface of the thigh ($C_{1A\ or\ S}E_PA_{S1}P_N$) were included in the study. Main outcome (visual vessel disappearance) was assessed by a visual quantitative evaluation of photographs taken before and after 52 days on average after a single sclerotherapy session. Photographs were evaluated by two blinded expert reviewers. Data from 96/100 randomized patients could be evaluated. Patients' satisfaction with the outcome of treatment was similar in the two groups (compression vs no compression). Objective assessment of clinical vessel disappearance revealed a significant ($P = 0.026$) benefit of compression stockings (mean score 7.05 ± 1.7) compared with no compression (6.28 ± 2.1). This corresponds to a number needed to treat (NNT) of 4.7 patients to get a vessel disappearance score higher than 6. Inter-observer agreement was very high (intraclass correlation coefficient = 0.93). Compression was well tolerated with a low rate of discomfort (mean 17.5%). Microthrombi were rarely observed in either group, but were still less prevalent in the compression group. The rate of pigmentation and matting was low and did not differ significantly between the two groups.

In conclusion, 3 weeks of daily wearing of compression stockings (23–32 mmHg) after sclerotherapy of telangiectasias and reticular veins improved the objectively assessed skin appearance at 52 days from treatment. Even if the sclerosing agent (chromated glycerin) used in this study was not foam, these results can certainly be extrapolated to foam sclerotherapy of telangiectasias. The positive effect of compression could even be more significant with foam, as the latter produces generally more microthrombi and matting. This study showed that postsclerotherapy compression is effective and enhances treatment efficacy. However, the underlying mechanisms still remain to be elucidated. It may be that compression exerts an anti-inflammatory action in the perivenous space. Compression stockings are classified according to the pressure exerted at the ankle at rest. Their behavior during exercise may be different, including variation of pressure and the massage effect. Compression stockings could also reduce the blood flow from the feeding reticular veins and therefore enhance clinical disappearance of telangiectasias.

Time interval to control and new treatment

After one session, we wait about four weeks before treating the same area again. This time interval allows us to analyze the individual reaction and side-effects, and to avoid over-treatment of the surfaces. (Clinical response to sclerotherapy is generally not analyzable any earlier.) Some patients report a visual improvement of the treated area several weeks beyond the treatment session. After one session, about 60% of the telangiectasias disappear on visual examination;[11,23] two or three sessions are needed to have a complete result. In our experience, it is not too late to perform a microthrombectomy at 4 weeks. This method reduces significantly the postsclerotherapy pigmentation, but has no impact with regard to reticular vein thrombi.[32]

Indications for foam sclerotherapy

Since foam is more powerful than solutions at similar concentrations, the indication for use of foam is generally a lack of response to increasing concentrations of solution. The expert consensus meeting held at Tegernsee in 2006 proposed trying foam sclerotherapy with polidocanol 0.25% at a liquid/air ratio of 1/4 (Tessari or DSS) should there be a lack of response to liquid sclerotherapy with polidocanol at 0.25% and 0.5%.[33] Sclerotherapy is still the first-choice method for the treatment of telangiectasias, as it has the advantage of treating not only the telangiectasias themselves, but also the feeding veins. It is cheap and its rate of side-effects is small in trained hands. Comparative studies with laser (see below) confirm this.

Classic indications for sclerotherapy of telangiectasias are:

- aesthetic concern
- symptomatic telangiectasias (itching, etc.)
- bleeding from telangiectactic vein blebs
- matting postphlebectomy or stripping.

Contraindications to foam sclerotherapy of telangiectasias are the same as for liquid sclerotherapy:

- allergy to one of sclerosing agents
- recent thromboembolic event
- pregnancy
- local or general infection
- critical ischemia of the lower limbs
- known symptomatic patent foramen ovale.

Results

The first publications about the use of foam in the treatment of telangiectasias appeared in France. Henriet reported his one (1997)[34] and three-year (1999)[22] experience with foam. He employed Monfreux's technique using a 3 cm^3 glass syringe with diluted polidocanol (0.1–0.2% for telangiectasias, 0.3–0.4% for reticular veins). The liquid/air ratio was 1/5. With this technique, microbubbles are large, and their median size varies between 0.6 and 1.3 mm (in comparison, microbubbles with the DSS technique measure 0.07 mm). Injections were made through a 30-gauge ½-inch or 26-gauge ½-inch needle. More than 10 000 patients were treated over this period with about 70 000 injections. Results seemed to be comparable to use of solutions. Henriet claimed the following advantages of foam:

- Very low concentrations can be used.
- The injection is easy and the pressure applied on the piston during the injection is weak.
- There is a triple control during injection: the eye can see the replacement of blood in the telangiectasias by foam, the ear can hear crepitation during injection, and fingers placed over the vein can feel foam passing through the vein.
- There is less bleeding after extraction of the needle.
- The total volume of injection is less.
- Extravasation of injection is immediately visible due to the composition of foam.
- The risk of paravasal injection is reduced due to the low concentration and volume of the sclerosing agent.
- The cost is lower, as less sclerosing agent is required (3 mL of foam is produced by only 0.5 mL of agent).

Benigni et al presented a pilot study in 1999, whereby they compared 0.25% polidocanol foam (Monfreux technique) with liquid in a multicenter prospective study in the treatment of telangiectasias and reticular veins of the lateral aspect of the thigh.[20] The study involved 20 patients; one thigh was treated with foam whilst the other was treated with liquid. Saphenous insufficiency on CFDI was an exclusion criterion. Five sclerotherapy sessions were performed at intervals of 15 days. The treating physician, using an analog visual scale ranging from 0 to 10, made visual evaluations before each session and 2 weeks after the last session. The patients reported their satisfaction on an analog visual scale (0–10). For the physician, the visual improvement for telangiectasias increased from 3.4/10 to 5.2/10 (liquid) and from 3.6/10 to 7.3/10 (foam). Visual improvement for reticular veins increased from 3.6/10 to 5.1/10 (liquid) and from 3.6/10 to 8.01/10 with foam. Satisfaction of patients was also greater with foam. Therefore, after five sessions, foam achieved an efficacy of about 80%, in comparison with about 60% with liquid.

On the basis of the results obtained from these preliminary experiences, Kern et al[23] designed a prospective single-blind randomized study comparing liquid with foam. It was not possible to perform a double-blinded study, as the treating physician feels the different composition and the viscosity of foam versus liquid at the time of injection, and can see the foam in the injected telangiectasias.

Benigni encountered twice as many microthrombi with 0.25% polidocanol foam than with solution; Henriet obtained good results even with very low concentrations (0.10–0.20% polidocanol); Sadoun and Benigni proposed to use 0.20% polidocanol foam in the future,[21] and, because of Kern's personal experience of too many microthrombi with 0.5% foam, they decided to compare 0.25% foam to 0.25% liquid polidocanol. The principal objective of the study was to compare the efficacy of polidocanol foam versus liquid and not to find out the best sclerosing agent, as the authors knew from Norris' study[35] that liquid polidocanol at 0.25% is less effective than 0.5% in the treatment of telangiectasias.

Foam was also compared to another weak sclerosing agent: chromated glycerin.[2] In an experimental model, its sclerosing effect was similar to polidocanol 0.25%.[2] Foam was produced according to Monfreux's technique using a liquid/air ratio of 1/4. Chromated glycerin (composed of glycerin 72%, chromium alum 0.8%) was injected at 100% concentration. The study included 150 patients presenting with telangiectasias and reticular veins of the lateral aspect of the thigh and normal CFDI ($C_{1A \text{ or } S}E_PA_{S1}P_N$). Assessment was performed 5 weeks after a single sclerotherapy session, by two independent blinded experts comparing digital photographs taken before treatment and again at the 5-week control, using an "a priori" analog visual scale from 0 to 10. This assessment method could be validated: there was a highly significant correlation coefficient ($P < 0.001$) between the experts and the reproducibility of the results was excellent (significant correlation coefficient, $P < 0.001$). Patients were asked about their satisfaction, using a visual scale ranging from negative results to great satisfaction (scale 0–100).

For the blinded experts, there was no significant difference between the efficacy of foam in comparison with liquid polidocanol injected at the same concentration (0.25%) (Figure 13.1). In comparison with chromated glycerin, foam was actually less efficient (Figure 13.2). However, there was no difference in the patient satisfaction scores. Chromated glycerin had the disadvantage of provoking significantly more pain at injection than polidocanol, either as foam or liquid (the pain score was 35 for chromated glycerin and 20 for polidocanol, using an analog visual pain scale ranging from 0 to 100). One can argue that polidocanol foam at 0.25% was a too low concentration for telangiectasias and reticular veins, in comparison with chromated glycerin. In this case, if the power and effectiveness of foam were lower than those of chromated glycerin, the side-effects of foam should have been lower too. But, in fact, foam provoked more complications than chromated glycerin (Table 13.1).

Benoit reported results from an open trial on 22 patients presenting symmetric telangiectasias and reticular veins of the thighs.[25] One thigh was treated by polidocanol 0.5% foam (Tessari technique) and the other was treated with chromated glycerin at a 100% concentration. Injections were performed with a 27-gauge ½-inch needle. The same physician performed a blinded assessment 3 weeks later. Efficacy was assessed by comparing the visual disappearance of telangiectasias of one thigh versus the other thigh. The physician considered efficacy to be better with chromated glycerin than polidocanol foam in 10 patients; the latter was better in 3 patients and the results were equivalent in 9 patients. Patients' analysis of vessel disappearance produced similar results. Although no statistical analysis was performed and the power of the study was too low, chromated glycerin seemed to achieve better results than polidocanol 0.5% foam with the Tessari technique. Therefore, once again, foam in this indication did not seem to give better visual results than conventional liquid sclerotherapy, albeit with a higher concentration of foam sclerosant and different technique of foam production.

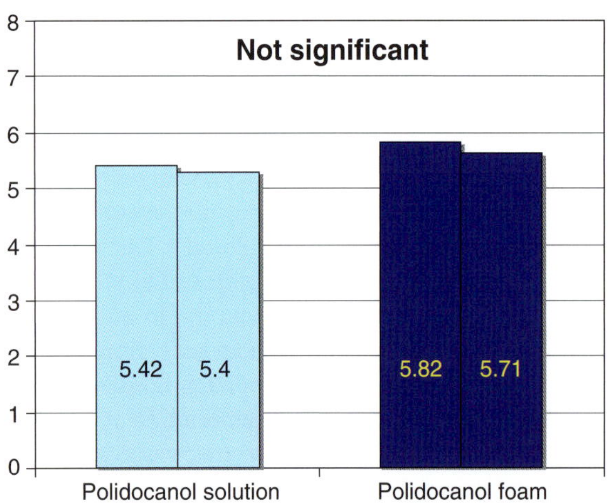

Figure 13.1 Polidocanol 0.25% foam versus polidocanol 0.25% solution for experts 1 and 2: there is no significant difference of the vessel disappearance score between polidocanol solution and polidocanol foam, for expert 1 as well as for expert 2 (From Kern et al[23])

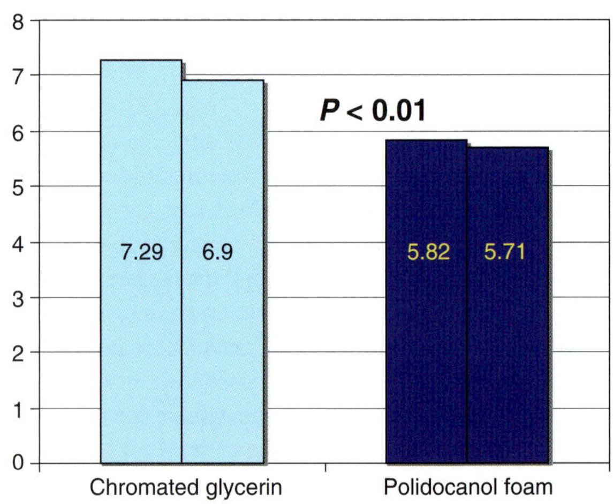

Figure 13.2 Chromated glycerin versus polidocanol 0.25% foam for experts 1 and 2: the vessel disappearance score was significantly higher with chromated glycerin than with polidocanol foam, for expert 1 as well as for expert 2 (From Kern et al[23])

Table 13.1 Comparison of side-effects

	Chromated glycerin (*n* = 51)	Liquid polidocanol 0.25% (*n* = 48)	Polidocanol 0.25% foam (*n* = 51)
Microthrombi	7	5	9
Thrombus in reticular vein	1		
Pigmentation		2	1
Matting		1	3
Transient visual disturbance			3

Adapted from Kern et al.[23]

Ferrara[24] evaluated the efficacy of polidocanol foam with different sized needles. Foam was produced according a personal method, connecting two glass syringes with a short catheter. The mixture consisted of 1 mL polidocanol 0.20% and 4 mL air. This gave a good-quality, compact, stable and viscous foam with homogenous small bubbles. The quality of foam was not altered when it was injected through a 26-gauge needle, but the author observed that foam losed its quality when injected through a small-diameter needle of 30-gauge: the foam immediately became unstable and inhomogeneous, containing several macrobubbles. This can be explained by the fact that microbubbles are destroyed when they pass through a small-diameter needle, as the bubbles rub against the needle wall. A microscopic examination showed that foam was not altered when a needle diameter of >0.30 mm was used.

The study included 50 patients. Saphenous insufficiency was an exclusion criterion. Reticular veins were removed first by phlebectomy; thereafter the telangiectasias were treated with foam sclerotherapy. On the same leg, several areas were treated using a 26-gauge needle (*n* = 341 areas); other areas (*n* = 356) were treated with a 30-gauge needle. A digital photographic assessment was performed comparing photos taken immediately before the treatment and again after 3 months. A score was calculated (0–10, the latter indicating complete disappearance). For the areas treated with the 26-gauge needle, the score before treatment (2.8/10) increased to 8/10 at 3 months; as for the 30-gauge areas, the score after treatment reached only 5.5/10 (prior treatment score in this group was 3.1/10). Therefore the efficacy of foam was higher when it was injected with a 26-gauge needle.

These results could explain why foam did not reached a higher efficacy than solution in the study of Kern et al,[23] which used a 30-gauge ½-inch needle. But, in the study of Benoit, where the size of the needle was >0.30 mm (27-gauge, ½-inch), chromated glycerin still gave better results than polidocanol 0.5% foam.[25] On the other hand, injecting telangiectasias with a 26-gauge (0.45 mm diameter) needle is certainly appropriate in the treatment of larger telangiectasias, but not for smaller ones (<0.4 mm), as the needle would be larger than the vein.

These foam studies evaluated the results after a single sclerotherapy session, except for the study by Benigni, where assessment was performed after five sessions. Therefore their results cannot be extrapolated to the final visual result, as generally several sessions are needed for complete visual disappearance of the telangiectasias. Furthermore, early results and efficacy of foam can be masked by the side-effects such as microthrombi, which reduce visual aesthetic results. As microthrombi disappear with time, as does most of the pigmentation, it is possible that even if foam does not give a significantly higher score than the solution after one session, it could do so at the end of the treatment, or could permit reduction of the number of sessions.

Prospect of long-term results

Long-term results of foam sclerotherapy are not known. Perhaps the rate of recurrence and recanalization of telangiectasias is less with foam than with solution, as in the treatment of saphenous veins.[36] All these questions remain open, and further comparative trials are needed to answer them.

The rate of recurrence 5 years after liquid sclerotherapy is high.[37] A retrospective study reported new telangiectasias occurring 5 years after treatment in 77% of 52 patients. Of these, 56% had recurrence in the same area and 67% in another area of the leg. In 46% of the patients, telangiectasias occurred both in the treated area and in additional areas. But in 48% of the cases, recurrence was very limited and needed little or no treatment. This high rate of recurrence could be explained by the low concentration of the sclerosing agents used in this study, as chromated glycerin was diluted to half strength and polidocanol liquid concentration started with 0.20% concentration. but was increased up to 0.50% if there were no results with lower concentrations.

Comparative trials: sclerotherapy versus laser

Comparative studies between laser and sclerotherapy are scarce; they include small numbers of patients and therefore do not reach enough statistical power to provide definitive conclusions. Two studies compare liquid conventional sclerotherapy with 1064 nm Nd:YAG laser.[38,39] There are no studies comparing foam with laser.

Lupton et al.[38] performed a clinical comparison study after a first and a second treatment session. Twenty randomized patients presenting with telangiectasias (0.1–1.5 mm diameter) were included in the study. One leg was treated with 0.25% liquid sodium tetradecyl sulfate as the other was treated with a long-pulsed 1064 nm Nd:YAG laser. Photographic assessment was performed 1 month after the first session, and again 1 and 3 months after a second session, by two masked independent assessors using a scale from 0 to 3, where 3 meant a greater than 75% improvement. In this study, telangiectasias responded better to sclerotherapy than to laser as well after the first session as 3 months after the second session. The average clinical improvement scores were 1.7 (sclerotherapy) and 1.1 (laser) 1 month after the first treatment; 2.8 (sclerotherapy) and 1.8 (laser) 1 month after the second treatment; and 2.6 (sclerotherapy) and 1.7 (laser) at the 3-month control. The pain scores were similar in both groups and the laser treatment was not less painful than sclerotherapy. The incidence of side-effects was minimal and equivocal in both treatments groups.

Levy et al[39] published a pilot study comparing four sites of 14 patients presenting with leg telangiectasias ranging from 0.5 to 2 mm in diameter. Only telangiectasias resistant to previous sclerotherapy were included in this study. Resistance was defined as no improvement after at least two sclerotherapy sessions with two sclerosing agents, 6 months before inclusion. The first site was treated with one session of liquid sclerotherapy (polidocanol 0.5%), then 3 weeks later with one session of long-pulsed 1064 nm Nd:YAG laser with contact cooling; the second site was treated with laser 3 weeks later, then with one session of sclerotherapy; the third site was treated with one session of laser; the fourth site was treated with one session of sclerotherapy. The patients were followed up to 3 months after the last treatment. Assessment was performed on digital photographs by blinded observers (scale 1–4, with 4 meaning clearance of more than 75%). The results showed no statistical difference comparing the different treatment groups (sclerotherapy, laser alone, or in combination). However, the sequence sclerotherapy seemed to be give the best results. Side-effects were minimal and comparable.

With regard to these trials, sclerotherapy, in our opinion, should still be the first choice of treatment for telangiectasias. There is no evidence that laser does any better than sclerotherapy, and results could even be worse. Laser is much more expensive for patients, and less cost-effective for them. Last, but not least, unlike laser, sclerotherapy not only treats telangiectasias, but also their feeding reticular veins in the same session; this is probably essential to enhance results and lower short-term recurrence. For these different reasons, laser should be proposed only as a second choice for selected patients with telangiectasias who do not respond to sclerotherapy or who present residual matting.

Complications

These can be divided into early and late complications.

Early complications:

- allergic reactions
- transient visual disorders
- systemic disorders (vasovagal fainting, malaise or nausea)
- intra-arterial injection/vasospasm.

Late complications:

- microthrombus and pigmentations
- telangiectactic matting
- cutaneous ulcerations
- superficial or deep vein thrombosis.

There are no known specific complications linked to the use of foam itself. But the rate of complications can differ between conventional liquid sclerotherapy and foam sclerotherapy of telangiectasias.

Allergic reactions

These are of course related to the sclerosing agent and not to the foam. As only polidocanol foam is actually used in the treatment of telangiectasias, we will limit the discussion to this agent. Allergic reactions against polidocanol are very rare, with an estimated incidence of 0.01%.[2] Most of the time, they present as minor localized or general urticaria. Localized urticaria, which occurs immediately after injection and disappears generally 30 minutes after the treatment,[1,2] should be differentiated from an allergic reaction. It is probably the result of endothelial irritation and/or release of histamine from perivascular mast cells. Bronchospasm or angioedema are exceptional. The company Kreussler GmbH[2] reported one fatal anaphylactic shock. Therefore, resuscitation facilities must be on hand in all practices where sclerotherapy is conducted. Patients must of course be informed about the potential allergic risks of sclerotherapy.

Urticaria is treated with an oral antihistamine medication. Systemic reactions should be treated with subcutaneous or intravenous epinephrine (adrenaline), intravenous antihistamine and steroids.

Transient visual disorders

Transient visual disorders (TVDs) are described with all sclerosing agents, but are more frequent with foam. They generally present as visual scintillation, blurred vision or even amaurosis fugax lasting less than 2 hours.[1,2,22,23,40,41] Visual disturbances can be associated with headache, nausea and vasovagal fainting. Some cases could be classified as ophthalmic migraine.[42,43] Prevalence is low, <0.1%.[22,40] TVDs are more often observed after treatment of reticular veins and telangiectasias than after foam sclerotherapy of saphenous veins. One hypothesis could be that the sessions last longer than the injection in a saphenous vein; Monfreux's method, where foam is less homogeneous and contains larger bubbles, was used more frequently for telangiectasias.

TVDs may recur in subsequent sclerotherapy sessions. A mechanism for the formation of TVDs is still unclear: gaseous emboli have been suggested. However, prevalence of patent foramen ovale is about 20% in the general population.[44] Cardiologists inject 10 mL of a mixture of saline and air into the veins of the arms for echographic diagnosis of patent foramen ovale and very seldom report TVDs. Therefore, if this is the mechanism, prevalence of TVDs should be much greater than has been observed. On the other hand, TVDs also occur after injection of liquid sclerosing agents.[40,41,43] Stroke after sclerotherapy of telangiectasias has never been reported. A case of *migraine ophtalmique* with reversible scotomas after liquid sclerotherapy of telangiectasias with polidocanol 1% was reported.[43] Visual impairment developed five minutes after a fourth session of sclerotherapy of telangiectasias. Only 2 mL of polidocanol were injected during the session. This 23-year-old woman complained of dizziness, right hemianopia, and bilateral prickling on her hands and feet. Ophthalmic examination performed 90 minutes after sclerotherapy revealed homonymous hemianopia. Neurologic examination at 150 minutes was normal. Headache started at the time the visual fields normalized. Two hours later, the headache resolved. A patent foramen ovale was ruled out. The pathophysiologic mechanism was thought to be ophthalmic migraine secondary to cerebral vasospasm, following the localized vasospasm at the injection site provoked by polidocanol. In a personal observation, a TVD occurred in a young woman after injection of chromated glycerin. It presented as a small amputation of the lateral visual fields. This symptom was isolated and not associated with headache in this woman without a history of migraines. It resolved spontaneously after 30 minutes. Clinical neurologic examination was normal. It was the first sclerotherapy session and the patient was very anxious about the treatment. Clinically, she presented some hyperventilation. This benign, mild disorder did not recur during the next session with the same agent.

Even though the phenomenon is clinically worrisome, it is, above all, necessary to reassure the patient that it is purely transitory.

Systemic disorders

Vasovagal fainting (10/12 173 sessions[40]) as well as nausea (1/12 173 sessions[40]) is rarely observed with foam as compared with solution. Pain control, observation of the patient's reaction to treatment and performing sclerotherapy as the patient is lying down is a good prevention for vasovagal reaction.

Intra-arterial injection/vasospasm

Because telangiectasias are located in the derma, their sclerotherapy is not associated with a risk of intra-arterial injection when performed by trained physicians. Intra-arterial injection is one of the mechanisms of cutaneous necrosis and ulceration, which complicate sclerotherapy of telangiectasias. Even if it is an early complication, its classical clinical presentation is an ulceration generally observed 1 week after the session.

Intra-arterial injection has to be distinguished from vasospasm, which can present as a porcelain-white cutaneous reaction immediately after injection.[2] It can progress to a hemorrhagic bulla and to an ulcer.

Microthrombi and pigmentation

Microthrombi and pigmentation are among the most frequent adverse reactions after sclerotherapy of telangiectasias. Their incidence varies from 6.7% to 31% with polidocanol and up to 80% with sodium tetradecyl sulfate.[2] Pigmentations are mainly explained by inflammation-induced melanogenesis stimulation, erythrocyte extravasation, thrombus degradation and subsequent intradermal deposits of hemosiderin.[1,2] The rate of inflammation is related to the power, high concentrations[35] and large volumes of the sclerosing agents injected. For these reasons, microthrombi and pigmentations are more often observed after foam use.[20,22] Clinically, pigmentations are preceded most of the time by microthrombi. Early removal of microthrombi through small stab incisions significantly reduces pigmentation.[32] The presence of a microthrombus is therefore an important factor for postsclerotherapy pigmentation. In a multicenter randomized trial, Scultetus et al performed microthrombectomy 1–3 weeks after a sclerotherapy session. Three blinded experts evaluated photographs. The rate of microthrombi was very high after injection of liquid sodium tetradecyl sulfate (0.25% in the telangiectasias, 0.5% in reticular veins). In this group, 99 patients (101 total) developed microthrombi. This study shows that it is very efficient to perform a microthrombectomy in telangiectasias, as it significantly reduces pigmentation. This effect could not be demonstrated for reticular veins, but in this group thrombectomy was associated with significant pain relief.

Telangiectactic matting

Telangiectactic matting (TM) is defined as new appearance of fine red telangiectasias after treatment of telangiectasias and varicose veins. It can be observed as a nonaesthetic adverse reaction after sclerotherapy as well as after surgery. Commonly, TM appears 3–6 weeks after treatment. It frequently resolves spontaneously between 3 and 12 months later. Only 20% may persist indefinitely.[2] Its incidence in the Australian polidocanol study (16 804 limbs treated) was very low (0.04%).[45] In the study by Kern et al,[23] it was observed in 2% of patients treated with liquid 0.25% polidocanol and in 6% of the patients treated with foam. TM is probably explained by neoangiogenesis, which is proportional to the increase in regional venous pressure, the degree of inflammation and the magnitude of the thrombus.[1,5] For these reasons, TM might be more frequent with foam. The risk of TM may be limited by injecting:

- only territories in which the proximal reflux has been excluded
- small volumes
- low pressure injection – injection should not be performed with syringes of capacity smaller than 3 mL
- small areas – one injection should not clear a surface greater than 1–2 cm^2
- a minimal concentration.

Risk factors for the development of TM could be obesity, estrogen/progestagen hormonal intake, family history of telangiectasias, and old telangiectasias (mean 17 years old).[46]

Treatment of TM can be difficult. In our experience, we recommend waiting and trying to treat the remaining telangiectasias only after 6 months to 1 year, with minimal volumes and concentration of sclerosing agent, using a weak agent (e.g., chromated glycerin, even diluted). In case of lack of response, laser may be a useful alternative.

Cutaneous necrosis

Cutaneous necrosis is a rare complication of sclerotherapy of telangiectasias (<0.01%[40]). The risk is mainly related to the sclerosing agent, its concentration, extravasation, intra-arterial injection or the diffusion of the sclerosing agent through an arteriovenous anastomosis.[1,2,5] Polidocanol foam is used at low concentrations in this indication (0.5% or less). Moreover, its concentration in foam is much less, as the solution/air ratio is 1/4. Polidocanol at these concentrations does not provoke necrosis even when it is accidentally injected into the skin. Therefore, the risk related to paravasal injection or extravasation from the injured vessel is minimal.

Accidental intra-arteriolar injection is very rare. Sometimes ulcerations cannot be explained either by the agent or by its concentration, or the injection technique. In these cases, diffusion of the sclerosing agent through an arteriovenous anastomosis must be suspected. Histologic studies showed that 1 of 26 telangiectasias can be associated with an arteriolar–venous anastamosis and microshunt.[2]

Superficial and deep vein thrombosis

Symptomatic superficial venous thrombosis is a rare complication (< 0.01%[40]). It has to be differentiated from reticular vein thrombi, which can be painful on palpation but do not present clinical inflammation (erythema and intense pain). Most of the time, superficial venous thrombosis is limited when it presents as a complication of telangiectactic sclerotherapy. This complication may be prevented by postsclerotherapy compression. Thrombectomy can have a positive effect on pain. It can be associated with local or oral nonsteroidal anti-inflammatory drugs.

Deep vein thrombosis is exceptional after sclerotherapy of telangiectasias. This risk can be enhanced by unknown thrombophilia, oral contraceptive use, diminished immobilization or incorrect application of compressions bandages (e.g., limited to the thigh).

Complication rate with foam

Henriet[22] reported the following complications after 70 000 foam injections in his three years' experience:

- 9 transitory visual troubles
- 1 episode of vomiting
- 7 episodes of migraine in migraine-known patients
- frequent microthrombi that necessitated complementary micropuncture, especially at the beginning of the experience, probably due to large volumes injected in the same area (>0.5 mL foam)
- pigmentations
- 1 ulceration.

Minor complications with foam were twice as frequent as with liquid (microthrombi, pigmentations and matting) in the pilot study by Benigni et al.[20] Because of this increasing number of side-effects, they proposed the use in the future of lower foam concentrations (0.2% polidocanol).[21]

In the trial by Kern et al, side-effects seemed to be more frequent in patients treated with foam (Table 13.1) when compared with liquid polidocanol and chromated glycerin: the rate of microthrombi was comparable between the three groups. Pigmentation seem to be more frequent with polidocanol than with chromated glycerin. Matting was more frequent in the foam group. Transient visual defects were noticed only in the foam group. However, the number of side-effects was too limited to permit any statistical analysis and conclusions.[23] With foam, matting was more frequent and benign transient visual disturbances were noticed. In Benoit's comparative trial, more side-effects were noticed with polidocanol foam, which at 0.5% concentration provoked three microthrombi and one ulceration at the injection site, whereas neither was experienced with chromated glycerin.[25] One case of matting in both thighs with chromated glycerin as with polidocanol foam happened in a patient aged 57 years hormonal replacement treatment. Matting in this case seemed to be related more to one of the known risk factors[46] than to the sclerosing agent.

Ferrara[24] noticed more micothrombi (39 cases), pigmentation (9 cases) and matting (8 cases) in the area treated with the 26-gauge needle compared with the 30-gauge needle (27 cases of microthrombi, 5 of pigmentation and 4 of matting). This confirms the impression that the more powerful the foam, the more side-effects are noticed. This demonstrates the limiting factor of sclerotherapy treatment of telangiectasias. A future challenge will be to find a powerful agent producing only slight side-effects.

Conclusions

Foam is an efficient agent to treat telangiectasias, but does not seem to be more effective with regard to vessel disappearance rate than liquid sclerotherapy. This is true for short-term results after one session. Final results after several sessions or long-term results are not known.

Foam seems to provoke more aesthetic complications such as pigmentation and matting. This of course negatively influences visual results. But foam has the advantage of reducing the risk of cutaneous necrosis, as its concentration is lower than that of sclerosing solution. On the other hand, benign transient visual troubles are more frequent. Foam permits saving sclerosing agent volume and, from this point of view, money. But it takes more time to prepare foam than liquid. Foam is stable for only a few minutes; therefore it has to be produced continuously during the treatment session. For these various reasons, after initial enthusiasm for foam sclerotherapy of telangiectasias, most phlebologists are actually going back to foam as a second-choice method, which is used only in cases resistant to standard liquid sclerotherapy.

References

1. Ramelet A-A, Kern P, Perrin M. Varicose veins and telangiectasias. Paris: Elsevier SAS, 2004.
2. Goldman MP, Bergan JJ, Guex J-J. Sclerotherapy: Treatment of Varicose and Telangiectactic Leg Veins, 4th edn. Philadelphia: Mosby Elsevier, 2007.
3. Eklof B, Rutherford RB, Bergan JJ, et al, for the American Venous Forum International Ad Hoc Committee for Revision of the CEAP Classification. Revision of the CEAP classification for chronic venous disorders: consensus statement. J Vasc Surg 2004; 40: 1248–52.
4. Uhl JF, Cornu-Thenard A, Carpentier PH, et al. Clinical and hemodynamic significance of corona phlebectatica in chronic venous disorders. J Vasc Surg 2005; 42: 1163–8.
5. Ramelet A-A, Perrin M, Kern P, Bounameaux H. Phlébologie, 5th edn. Paris: Elsevier Masson SAS, 2006.
6. Kröger K, Ose C, Rudofsky G, et al. Symptoms in individuals with small cutaneous veins. Vasc Med 2002; 7: 13–17.
7. Ruckley CV, Evans CJ, Allan PL, et al. Chronic venous insufficiency: clinical and duplex correlations. The Edinburgh Vein Study of venous disorders in the general population. J Vasc Surg 2002; 36: 520–5.
8. Langer RD, Ho E, Denenberg JO, et al. Relationships between symptoms and venous disease: the San Diego Population Study. Arch Intern Med 2005; 165: 1420–4.
9. Criqui MH, Jamosmos M, Fronek A, et al. Chronic venous disease in an ethnically diverse population: the San Diego Population Study. Am J Epidemiol 2003; 158: 448–56.
10. Engelhorn CA, Engelhorn AL, Cassou MF, Salles-Cunha S. Patterns of saphenous venous reflux in women presenting with lower extremity telangiectasias. Dermatol Surg 2007; 33: 282–8.
11. Kern P, Ramelet A-A, Wütschert R, Hayoz D. Compression after sclerotherapy for telangiectasias and reticular leg veins: a randomized controlled study. J Vasc Surg 2007; 45: 1212–16.
12. Kim JR, Kent PJ. Clinical examination of varicose veins – a validation study. Ann R Coll Surg Engl 2001; 83: 171–5.
13. Campbell WB, Niblet PG, Ridler BMF, et al. Handheld Doppler as a screening test in primary varicose veins. Br J Surg 1997; 84: 1541–3.
14. Kent PJ, Weston MJ. Duplex scanning may be used selectively in patients with primary varicose veins. Ann R Coll Surg Engl 1998; 80: 388–93.
15. Mercer KG, Scott DJA, Berridge DC. Preoperative duplex imaging is required before all operations for primary varicose veins. Br J Surg 1998; 85: 1495–7.
16. Wills V, Moylan D, Chambers J. The use of routine duplex scanning in the assessment of varicose veins. Aust NZ J Surg 1998; 68: 41–4.
17. Daher A, Jones V, da Silva AF. The role of popliteal vein incompetence in the diagnosis of saphenous-popliteal reflux using continuous wave Doppler. Eur J Vasc Endovasc Surg 2001; 21: 350–2.
18. Darke SG, Vetrivel S, Foy MA, et al. A comparison of duplex scanning and continuous wave Doppler in the assessment of primary and uncomplicated varicose veins. Eur J Vasc Endovasc Surg 1997; 14: 457–61.
19. Rautio T, Perälä J, Biancari F, et al. Accuracy of handheld Doppler in planning the operation for primary varicose veins. Eur J Vasc Endovasc Surg 2002; 24: 450–5.
20. Benigni JP, Sadoun S, Thirion V, et al. Télangiectasies et varices réticulaires. Traitement par la mousse d'Aethoxisclérol à 0.25%. Présentation d'une étude pilote. Phlebologie 1999; 52: 283–90.
21. Sadoun S, Benigni JP. Bonnes pratiques cliniques et mousse de sclérosant: propositions pour une étude randomisée contrôlée, prospective, multicentrique, comparative, en aveugle, sur le traitement sclérosant par la mousse d'Aetoxysclérol à 0.20%. Phlebologie 1999; 52: 291–7.
22. Henriet JP. Expérience durant 3 années de la mousse de polidocanol dans le traitement des varices réticulaires et des varicosités. Phlebologie 1999; 52: 277–82.
23. Kern P, Ramelet A-A, Wutschert R, et al. Single-blind randomized study comparing chromated glycerin, polidocanol solution and polidocanol foam for treatment of telangiectactic leg veins. Dermatol Surg 2004; 30: 367–72.
24. Ferrara F, Bernbach HR. Efficacité de la sclérothérapie à la mousse en fonction de l'aiguille utilisée. Phlebologie 2005; 58: 229–31.
25. Benoit R. Sclérothérapie des télangiectasies: quel est le meilleur agent sclérosant? Société Européenne de Phlébectomie, 33e réunion, Lisbonne, 2005.
26. Monfreux A. Traitement sclérosant des troncs saphéniens et leurs collatérales de gros calibre par la méthde mus. Phlebologie 1997; 50: 351–3.
27. Tessari L. Nouvelle technique d'obtention de la scléromousse. Phlebologie 2000; 53: 129.

28. Wollmann JC. Schaum – zwischen Vergangenheit und Zukunft. Vasomed 2002; 16: 34–5.
29. Partsch H, Baccaglini U, Stemmer R. Questionnaire regarding the practice of sclerotherapy. Phlebology 1997; 12: 43–55.
30. Goldman MP. How to utilize compression after sclerotherapy. Dermatol Surg 2002; 28: 860–2.
31. Weiss RA, Sadick NS, Goldman MP, Weiss MA. Postsclerotherapy compression: controlled comparative study of duration of compression and its effects on clinical outcome. Dermatol Surg 1999; 25: 105–8.
32. Scultetus AH, Villavicencio JL, Kao TC, et al. Microthrombectomy reduces postsclerotherapy pigmentation: multicenter randomized trial. J Vasc Surg 2003; 38: 896–903.
33. Breu F-X, Guggenbichler S. 2nd European Consensus Meeting on Foam Sclerotherapy. Tegernsee, Germany, 2006. Vasa 2008; 37(Suppl 71): 1–30.
34. Henriet JP. Un an de pratique quotidienne de la sclérothérapie (veines réticulaires et télangiectasies) par mousse de polidocanol: faisabilité, résultats, complications. Phlebologie 1997; 50: 355–60.
35. Norris MJ, Carlin MC, Ratz JL. Treatment of essential telangiectasias: effects of increasing concentrations of polidocanol. J Am Acad Dermatol 1989; 20: 643–9.
36. Hamel-Desnos C, Desnos P, Wollmann JC, et al. Evaluation of the efficacy of polidocanol in the form of foam compared with liquid form in sclerotherapy of the greater saphenous vein: initial results. Dermatol Surg 2003; 29: 1170–5.
37. Lucchi M, Bilancini S, Tucci S. Sclerotherapy for telangiectasias of the leg: results of a 5-year follow-up. Phlebology 1996; 11: 73–5.
38. Lupton JR, Alster TS, Romero P. Clinical comparison of sclerotherapy versus long-pulsed Nd:YAG laser treatment for lower extremity telangiectases. Dermatol Surg 2002; 28: 694–7.
39. Levy JL, Elbahr C, Jouve E, Mordon S. Comparison and sequential study of long pulsed Nd:YAG 1064 nm laser and sclerotherapy in leg telangiectasias treatment. Laser Surg Med 2004; 34: 273–6.
40. Guex JJ, Allaert FA, Gillet JL, Chleir F. Immediate and midterm complications of sclerotherapy: report of a prospective multicenter registry of 12 173 sclerotherapy sessions. Dermatol Surg 2005; 31: 1–6.
41. Tournay R. La sclérose des varices. Paris: Expansion Scientifique Française, 1985.
42. Ratinahirana H, Benigni JP, Bousser MG. Injection of polidocanol foam (PF) in varicose veins as a trigger for attacks of migraine with visual aura. Cephalalgia 2003; 23: 850–1.
43. Künzleberger B, Pieck C, Altmeyer P, Stücker M. Migraine ophtalmique with reversible scotomas after sclerotherapy with liquid 1% polidocanol. Dermatol Surg 2006; 32: 1410–3.
44. Rodriguez CJ, Homma S. Patent foramen ovale and stroke. Curr Treat Options Cardiovasc Med 2003; 5: 233–40.
45. Conrad P, Malouf GM, Stacey MC. The Australian polidocanol (Aethoxysclerol) study. Results at 2 years. Dermatol Surg 1995; 21: 334–6.
46. Davis L, Duffy D. Determination of incidence and risk factors for postsclerotherapy telangiectactic matting of the lower extremity: a retrospective analysis. J Dermatol Surg Oncol 1990; 16: 327–30.

14 Comparison of polidocanol and sodium tetradecyl sulfate in the treatment of varicose and telangiectatic leg veins

Mitchel P Goldman

Introduction

Sclerotherapy is a well tolerated and highly efficacious treatment for varicose and telangiectatic leg veins. Sclerosing solutions act by inducing endothelial damage (endosclerosis) that leads eventually to endofibrosis of the treated vessels. Effective sclerotherapy results when the endothelial damage and associated vascular necrosis is sufficient to destroy the entire vessel wall.[1]

Two of the most widely used sclerotherapy solutions worldwide are sodium tetradecyl sulfate (STS) and polidocanol (POL). These solutions both act as a detergent effecting endothelial destruction through protein-thief denaturization as described below. The relative efficacy of STS and POL has previously been compared, both experimentally in the rabbit ear vein model and clinically in liquid form.[2,3]

Comparative studies of a variety of sclerosing solutions and concentrations performed in the rabbit ear vein model have demonstrated an approximately twofold enhanced efficacy with STS compared with POL. Specifically, 0.25% and 0.5% STS liquid have a similar destructive effect on endothelia as do 0.5% and 1.0% POL, respectively.[2]

A clinical comparison of the liquid forms of POL and STS was performed in 129 patients.[3] Each patient's leg veins that did not have incompetence from the saphenofemoral junction (SFJ) were divided into three categories by size (<1 mm, 1–3 mm, 3–6 mm in diameter). Each leg was randomly treated with 0.25%, 0.5%, or 1.5% of STS, or 0.5%, 1.0% or 3% of POL respective of size. An independent, three-panel, blindly randomized photographic examination was obtained at pretreatment and 4 and 16 weeks thereafter. All patients had an average of 70% improvement and were 70–72% satisfied in all vein categories treated with either solution. There was no significant difference in adverse effects between each group, except for a decrease in ulcerations and swelling in the POL group.

An open clinical trial comparing STS with POL was conducted by 120 physicians in Australia.[4] The results at 2 years showed that 55 of 65 physicians found that POL had a better efficacy than STS, with two claiming decreased efficacy, and 8 seeing no difference. When compared with hypertonic saline (HS), 49 of 58 claimed better efficacy, with 1 physician reporting decreased efficacy and 8 physicians finding no difference. Pain of injection with POL was less than with STS in the experiences of 54 of 65 physicians, with pain being less than HS as reported by 56 of 58 physicians. Finally, the physicians' perceptions of complications were that POL had fewer overall complications (pigmentation, ulceration, phlebitis and telangiectatic matting) according to 58 of 65 physicians as compared with STS, and according to 43 of 58 physicians as compared with HS.

The use of a gas (including room air) to turn the detergent sclerosing solutions into a foam has become popular over the last ten years. Hamel-Desnos and Wollmann have demonstrated both clinical[5,6] and microscopic[7] superior efficacy of foam versus liquid. In vitro studies have been conducted on single layers of endothelial cells in contact during 1.5 s with various concentrations of foam and liquid POL. Histologic examination demonstrates identical cell destruction with 0.5% foam and 3%

liquid. As indicated by Hamel-Desnos et al, better efficacy had been supposed to be related to a longer time of contact; however, they observed that the effect happened in a very short time; therefore there should be missing explanatory links. From a macroscopic point of view, foam seems to work because of the delayed dilution and closer contact between nondiluted sclerosing agent and endothelium; some microscopic phenomena will perhaps be found explaining more precisely what happens.

Before evaluating the relative efficacy of STS and POL foam, one should become more knowledgeable in the specific properties of each of these sclerosing solutions.

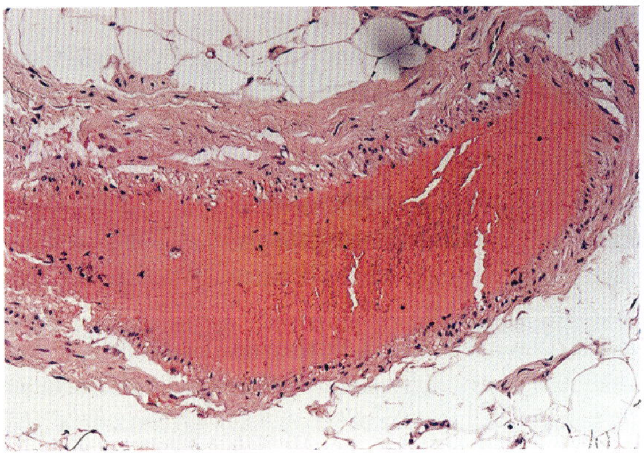

(a)

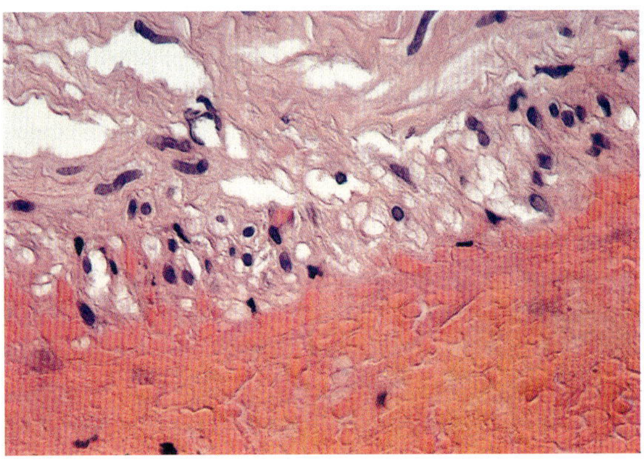

(b)

Figure 14.1 (a) Histologic examination of vein 48 hours after injection with polidocanol 0.5% ×40. (b) Endothelial cell vacuolization with thrombosis is present. ×100 (hematoxylin–eosin). (Reproduced with permission from: Sclerotherapy: Treatment of Varicose and Telangiectatic Leg Veins, 4th edn. Goldman MP, Bergan JB, Guex JJ, eds. Elsevier Mosby, London, 2007)

Sodium tetradecyl sulfate

STS is a synthetic, surface-active substance first described by Reiner in 1946.[8] It has been widely used since the 1950s and many authors have described its safety and efficacy.[1,9–13] It is a long-chain fatty acid salt of an alkali metal with the properties of soap. It is composed of sodium 1-isobutyl-4-ethyloctyl sulfate plus benzyl alcohol 2% (as an anesthetic agent) and phosphate buffered to pH 7.6. It is a clear solution that is nonviscous, has a low surface tension, and is readily miscible with blood, resulting in a uniform distribution postinjection. The mechanism of action is to disrupt the intracellular cement between the endothelial cells, resulting in desquamation of the cells in plaques. Endothelial destruction results in the exposure of subendothelial collagen fibers. The response to the damage is vein spasm, platelet aggregation and subsequent fibrosis that obliterates the vein (Figure 14.1). Excess STS is rapidly diluted and neutralized in the bloodstream, since it attaches to red blood cells resulting in hemolysis (Figure 14.2).

The version of sodium tetradecyl sulfate previously approved by the Food and Drug Administration (FDA) was manufactured and distributed by Elkins Sinn (a division of Wyeth-Ayerth); however, in the year 2000, production of this product was discontinued. Bioniche Pharma Group Ltd. (Inverin, Co. Galway, Ireland) in 2005 obtained FDA approval for the sale and marketing of STS under the same name "Sotradecol." The formulation involves preparation of a solution of the active

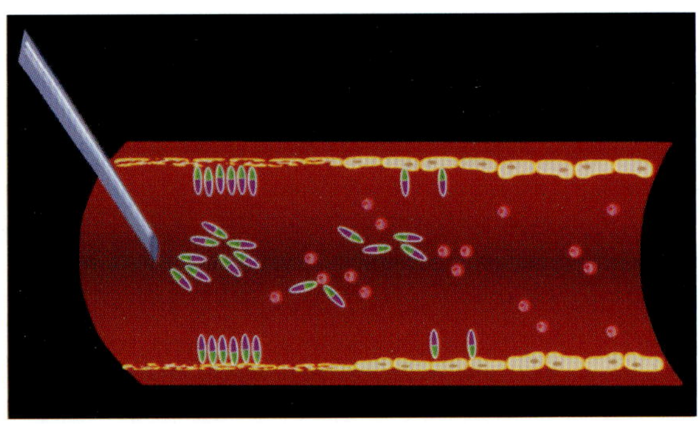

Figure 14.2 Diagramatic representation of the action of a detergent sclerosing solution on the vessel wall, showing formed elements of the blood (Reproduced with permission from: Sclerotherapy: Treatment of Varicose and Telangiectatic Leg Veins, 4th edn. Goldman MP, Bergan JB, Guex JJ, eds. Elsevier Mosby, London, 2007)

ingredient STS and the inactive ingredients benzyl alcohol, dibasic sodium phosphate and water for injection. The Bioniche Active Pharmaceutical Ingredient (API) was tested for the presence of carbitol by gas chromatographic analysis.[1] The test results revealed that no carbitol was detected.

STS can also be obtained from a variety of other sources, most commonly compounding pharmacies, that supply products that have been shown to have a variable concentration, pH and level of contaminants.[14] STS is also available as Trombovein™ (Omega Pharmaceuticals Ltd, Montreal, Canada) and as Fibro-Vein™ (STD Pharmaceutical Products Ltd, Hereford, United Kingdom). Fibro-Vein is available in 2 mL ampules in concentrations of 0.5%, 1%, and 3%, as well as 5 mL vials in 0.2% and 3% concentrations.

STS from Omega Laboratories and STD Pharmaceutical Products is distilled from a compound manufactured as a high-grade detergent used to clean optical surfaces by Nacet (Niagara Falls, NY, United States). The product name is NIAPROOF Anionic Surfactant 4, also known as NAS 4 and NIAPROOF 4. It is manufactured to have between 26% and 28% by weight STS with 20% by weight maximum of diethylene glycol monoethyl ether (carbitol) and 1–2% by weight of sodium chloride. During the manufacture, carbitol is added so that the final product is 3 parts STS to 2 parts carbitol. This 27% parent compound is the same compound provided to each manufacturer of STS for injection. Each manufacturer then purifies the active ingredient, sodium tetradecyl sulfate. Interestingly, analysis performed by an independent laboratory shows that the four major companies that manufacture STS have different levels of impurities, including carbitol. STD contains 0.02% w/v of carbitol; Sotradecol contains 0.6% carbitol, and Trombovar contains 2.6% w/v of carbitol. What effect the carbitol impurity has on efficacy or toxicity is unknown.

Many compounding pharmacies supply STS. Various loopholes in Federal and State regulations allow pharmacies to compound a variety of medications for use in humans. The FDA has no regulatory power over this "branch" of the pharmaceutical industry. Although the compounding pharmacy industry has voluntary standards, no organization exists to test the quality and accuracy of medications that it provides. Our analysis found discrepancies in both the stated concentration and the actual concentration of STS as labeled on the bottle from all three compounding pharmacies. The concentration of the sclerosing solution should be matched to the size and type of vein treated to produce the minimal sclerosing effect.

The reason for the difference in concentration may be related to the variability of the percentage of the bulk STS industrial solution. In temperatures below 15°C, the product fractionates so that the concentration of STS is greater than 27% at the bottom of the drum and below 27% at the top of the drum. An analysis of this 27% STS solution by the Professional Compounding Centers of America (Houston, TX) (PCCA) performed in July 2003 found that the 27% STS contained 27.94% of STS. No analysis of the carbitol component or any other component in the industrial solution was performed. The presence of impurities in any intravenous injection is worrisome.

The presence of both molecules in an injectable product will increase the risk of unwanted side-effects relating to sensitivity and anaphylaxis. I believe that it is not a coincidence that Fibro-Vein has displayed a very low incidence of such side-effects and that this is due to very low levels of carbitol that have been present in Fibro-Vein for the last 25 years.

STS 0.1–0.3% in solution form is commonly used for the treatment of telangiectatic leg veins less than 1 mm in diameter; 0.5–1% in solution form is useful in treating uncomplicated leg veins 1–3 mm in diameter. The use of STS as a foam has expanded its versatility, with 0.25–1.0% in foam formulation (created from a 1:4 ratio of solution to air) being popular for the treatment of larger reticular and varicose veins, usually 3–6 mm in diameter.[15] Treatment with 3% STS foam is popular for reflux in the great saphenous vein, with veins of over 10 mm in diameter being treated successfully.[16]

Polidocanol

This sclerosing solution is composed of a mixture of hydroxypolyethoxydodecane dissolved in distilled water to which 96% ethanol is added to a concentration of 5% to ensure emulsification of POL micelles (which provides a clear solution), and to decrease foaming during the production process. The other ingredients are disodium hydrogen orthophosphate dihydrate and potassium dihydrogen orthophosphate.

POL belongs to the class of detergent sclerosing solutions that are nonionic compounds. It consists of an apolar hydrophobic part, dodecanol, and a polar hydrophilic part, a polyethylene oxide chain, which is esterified. In solution, POL is associated as macromolecules through electrostatic hydrogen bonding between the hydrogen ion of the –OH group in one molecule, and the free electron pair of an O_2 dimer of a second molecule. This bonding results in the formation of a network. The sclerotherapeutic activity results from this double hydrophobic and hydrophilic action, and thus POL is a "detergent."

POL is available as Sclerovein (Resinag, Switzerland) in 30 mL multiuse vials in concentrations of 0.5%, 1%, 2%, 3% and 5%. POL is also available as Aethoxysklerol (Kreussler Pharma, Wiesbaden, Germany) in 2 mL ampules in concentrations of 0.25%, 0.5%, 1%, 2%, 3% and 4%, as well as multiuse 30 mL vials in 0.5% and 1% concentrations.

A randomized study determined that a solution of 0.5% concentration might be ideal for sclerosis of telangiectatic leg veins.[8] POL 1% is recommended for veins that are 1–2 mm in diameter, POL 2% for reticular and varicose veins that are 2–4 mm in diameter, and POL 3% for larger veins that are 4–8 mm in diameter.[1] The use of POL as a foam has expanded its versatility and increased its usage worldwide.

Comparative studies on the quality of foam

The most commonly used system to produce foam today is the DSS (double-syringe system) technique. Here, two syringes are connected by a two- or three-way stopcock, with the sclerosing solution in one syringe and air in the second syringe drawn back and forth by pumping movements.

The longer the sclerosant/air mixture remains as a foam in vivo, the higher the likelihood that the foam will travel into other, nontargeted veins. Foam half-life, the time for a volume of foam to be reduced to half its original volume, is one measure of foam stability. Prolongation of half-life is directly related to increasing the stability of the bubbles that comprise the foam. Bubble stability is dependent on several factors, including the specific sclerosant and concentration used to create the foam, the air-to-sclerosant ratio, the average diameter of the bubbles within the foam, and any additional ingredients used in its preparation. Of interest is the hypothesis that silicone present in disposable equipment such as syringes, infusion tubes and connectors can act as a lubricant and reduce foam stability. It has been postulated that this effect is caused by the destruction by silicone of the foam lamellae.

We first compared the half-life of foam using various connectors and the DSS technique.[17] With the presumption that each connector would vary from one another in their silicone content, it was hypothesized that half-lives would vary depending on the connector used, with the longest half-life attributed to the connector with the lowest relative amount of silicone.

The following standardized technique was employed throughout the study, to determine exact foam half-lives for six different connectors using STS and POL.

Foam creation. A sterile 5 mL syringe with 4 mL of predrawn air was attached to one end of a Stainless Steel 2-Way connector. A sterile 3 mL syringe was then used to draw up 1.0 mL of STS or POL 0.50% sclerosant and connected to the other end of the Stainless Steel 2-Way connector. Using the DSS technique, the 5 mL syringe was pushed to empty the 4 mL of air as much as possible through the connector to the 3 mL syringe with the sclerosant. This action was counted as "one" pump. Immediately thereafter, the air/sclerosant mixture in the 3 mL syringe was emptied through the connector to the 4 mL syringe. This action was counted as "two" pumps. Subsequently, the to-and-fro cycle was repeated for a total of "10" pumps. At completion of the 10 pumps, a homogenous white foam was created and filled the 5 mL syringe.

The 5 mL syringe filled with foam was then disconnected from the Stainless Steel 2-Way connector and placed exactly vertically, with the rubber stopcock of the syringe on the bottom. The timer was started. Over the course of time, as the foam degenerated back into its constituents, the sclerosing solution was found to gradually re-form at the bottom of the syringe. When the bottom of the solution's meniscus attained a volume of exactly 0.5 mL (half the original sclerosing volume of 1.0 mL) as measured by the graduations on the side of the syringe, the timer was stopped and the time was recorded in seconds.

This process was repeated for the remaining five disposable connectors, using POL 0.50% and STS 0.50%. Two sets of recordings were obtained and averaged for each connector used. Results are summarized in Tables 14.1 and 14.2. After two sets of recordings for each connector used in each of the two arms of the study, it was found that the time required for foam to destabilize was approximately the same for the specific sclerosant and

Table 14.1 Times for 0.5 mL of sodium tetradecyl sulfate to settle from a foam mixture containing 1.0 mL of sodium tetradecyl sulfate 0.50%

Connector name	Time 1 (s)	Time 2 (s)	Average time (s)
Stainless Steel 2-Way	88	90	**89**
B/Braun 2-Way	88	91	**89.5**
Kendall 3-Way	89	94	**91.5**
Discofix 3-Way	86	91	**88.5**
Vycon 3-Way	95	93	**94**
Connecta Plus 3-Way	90	94	**92**
Average time		**91**	

Table 14.2 Times for 0.5 mL of polidocanol to settle from a foam mixture containing 1.0 mL of polidocanol 0.50%

Connector name	Time 1 (s)	Time 2 (s)	Average time (s)
Stainless Steel 2-Way	50	52	**51**
B/Braun 2-Way	48	50	**49.5**
Kendall 3-Way	53	50	**51.5**
Discofix 3-Way	52	47	**49.5**
Vycon 3-Way	51	54	**52.5**
Connecta Plus 3-Way	50	54	**52**
Average time		**51**	

concentration used, and not the type of connector used. For STS 0.50%, the average time recorded was 90.75 s (range: 88.5–94.0), and for POL 0.50%, the average time recorded was 51.00 s (range: 49.5–52.5).

The Stainless Steel 2-Way connector was used as a control as it does not contain silicone, and yet the difference in foam dissolution times with this connector compared to others was not statistically significant. Likewise, the Connecta Plus 3-Way connector, which has the largest surface area and likely the highest amount of silicone as compared with the other connectors, also had time variations that were not statistically significant.

Bubble stability, and hence foam half-life, is not diminished by the type of connector used in the DSS technique described in this study. It is possible that the amount of silicone in the disposable connectors was negligible. Alternatively, the cohesive forces of silicone molecules to the disposable connectors may have been stronger than the adhesive forces between the foam bubbles and the silicone. Finally, the amount of silicone in the 3 mL and 5 mL syringes could be the most important factor.

Perhaps the most important discovery in this study is the difference in stability between the two tested sclerosing agents: STS was twice as stable as a foam than POL. Whether this has any measurable effect on either efficacy or adverse effects between the two sclerosing solutions awaits further study.

Comparative clinical study of STS and POL foam

While there have been previously reported comparisons between liquid STS and POL, only one study has been published to date comparing the safety and efficacy of STS and POL in foam form. Rao et al[18] performed a direct comparison between STS (Fibrovein, STD

Pharmaceuticals, Hereford, United Kingdom) and POL (Aethoxysklerol, Kreussler Pharma, Wiesbaden, Germany) in 20 patients with varicose, reticular, and/or telangiectatic leg veins without incompetence at the saphenofemoral or saphenopopliteal junctions. Each patient's leg veins were evaluated for extent, quality and size, and placed into one of the following three study categories: (1) veins less than 1 mm in diameter, 2) veins 1–3 mm in diameter and (3) veins 3–6 mm in diameter. Patients were then randomized to have the veins of either the right leg or left leg treated with STS, and the contralateral leg veins treated with POL. Selection of concentration and formulation (solution or foam) of sclerosing agent was based on the protocol outlined in Table 14.3. The treating physician was blinded as to the agent being injected.

The foam used consisted of 1 mL of sclerosing solution and 4 mL of air, mixed using the DSS technique. All patients were required to wear class II graduated compression stockings (30–40 mmHg) around the clock for 7 days following treatment. After having the first leg treated, patients returned 1 week later for treatment of the contralateral leg. Patients were seen every 4 weeks thereafter for follow-up.

High-quality digital photographs were taken prior to treatment and at 12 weeks post-treatment. At the end of study, four independent physicians, who were blinded to the sclerosing agents administered, assessed these images for overall clearance of vessels based on vessel size.

STS and POL were found to be equally effective in causing the clearance of veins in all size categories, as per independent, blinded physician evaluations (Table 14.4). Adverse events were expected and in proportion to the size and extent of treated leg veins. As detailed in Table 14.5, the incidence of adverse events of treatment were comparable between the two sclerosing agents used, with ecchymosis and hyperpigmentation being the most common. Of note, no skin necrosis was observed in any person treated with either agent. All patients tolerated STS and POL very well and were pleased with their treatments (Table 14.6). Both agents demonstrated equally high subject tolerability and satisfaction. It is worth noting that the results of this study correlate with previous trials comparing these sclerosing agents.[3–5]

Table 14.3 Randomization protocol

Veins <1 mm
STS 0.25% solution or POL 0.5% solution
Veins 1–3 mm
STS 0.5% solution or POL 1% solution
Veins 3–6 mm
STS 0.5% foam or POL 1% foam

Conclusion

Both STS and POL have been found to be equally efficacious when used either in liquid or foam form to treat varicose and telangiectatic leg veins. Since STS has approximately twice the destructive effects of POL, one cannot use these solutions interchangeably. STS should be used at one-half the concentration of POL, in either

Table 14.4 Clearance scores at 12 weeks as determined by four physician evaluators[a]

Evaluator	Veins <1 mm		Veins 1–3 mm		Veins 3–6 mm	
	STS	**POL**	**STS**	**POL**	**STS**	**POL**
1	4	4	4	4	3	3
2	4	4	4	4	4	4
3	5	5	5	4	4	4
4	4	5	5	5	4	4
Average	**4.25**	**4.5**	**4.5**	**4.25**	**3.75**	**3.75**

[a] Disappearance scoring scale (1–5): 1 = worse than before treatment, 2 = no change, 3 = minimal disappearance (50%), 4 = moderate disappearance (75%), 5 = complete disappearance (100%).
STS, sodium tetradecyl sulfate; POL, polidocanol.

Table 14.5 Adverse events by treatment group (N = 20)

Adverse event	STS	POL
Ecchymosis	18	17
Hyperpigmentation	10	9
Coagulum formation	7	8
Local urticaria	5	4
Telangiectatic matting	2	2
Skin necrosis	0	0
Allergic reaction	0	0

STS, sodium tetradecyl sulfate; POL, polidocanol.

Table 14.6 Average subject tolerability and satisfaction at 12 weeks post-treatment (N = 20)

	STS	POL
Tolerability[a]	0.40	0.35
Satisfaction[b]	4.34	4.30

[a] Tolerability scale (0–3): 0 = no discomfort, 1 = mild discomfort, 2 = moderate discomfort, 3 = severe discomfort.
[b] Satisfaction scale (1–5): 1 = worse than before treatment, 2 = no change, 3 = minimal disappearance, 4 = moderate disappearance, 5 = complete disappearance.
STS, sodium tetradecyl sulfate; POL, polidocanol.

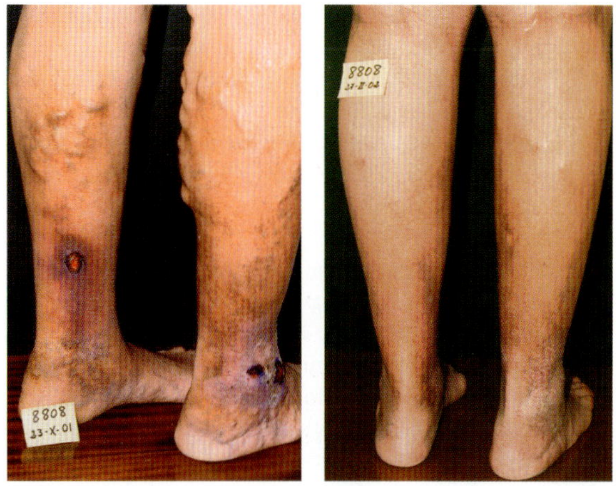

(a) (b)

Figure 14.3 (a) A 64-year-old woman with bilateral leg ulcers present for 1 and 2 years (right and left, respectively). She had had varicose veins for the past 20 years. Duplex examination revealed bilateral great saphenous vein incompetence from the groin to the ankle and an incompetent perforating vein near the left ulcer. (b) Four months after treatment with 1% polidocanol foam injected in two sessions 2 weeks apart and one further injection 4 weeks later, the varicose veins are reduced and the ulcers healed (Courtesy of DDI Wright and JC Cabrera. Reproduced with permission from: Sclerotherapy: Treatment of Varicose and Telangiectatic Leg Veins, 4th edn. Goldman MP, Bergan JB, Guex JJ, eds. Elsevier Mosby, London, 2007)

the liquid or the foam form. In addition, we have demonstrated that using a sclerosing solution in its foamed form with room air approximately doubles the sclerosing "power" or effect of the solution. Therefore, we recommend the following as a guide to using either STS or POL as a foam in treating varicose veins (Figure 14.3):

- STS 0.25% foam and/or POL 0.5% foam are to treat vessels between 1 and 3 mm in diameter.
- STS 0.5% foam and/or POL 1.0% are to treat vessels between 3 and 6 mm in diameter.
- STS 1% and/or POL 2% are to treat vessels between 6 and 9 mm in diameter.
- STS 3% and/or POL 5% are to treat incompetent great saphenous veins greater than 9 mm in diameter.
- The use of a ***liquid*** sclerosing solution is to treat vessels less than 1 mm in diameter.

References

1. Goldman MP, Bergan JJ, Guex JJ. Sclerotherapy: Treatment of Varicose and Telangiectatic Leg Veins. 4th edn. London: Elsevier Mosby, 2007.
2. Goldman MP, Kaplan RP, Oki LN, et al. Sclerosing agents used in the treatment of telangiectasia: comparison of the clinical and histologic effects of intravascular polidocanol, sodium tetradecyl sulfate, and hypertonic saline in the dorsal rabbit ear vein. Arch Dermatol 1987; 123: 1196–201.
3. Goldman MP. Treatment of varicose and telangiectatic leg veins. Double-blind prospective comparative trial between Aethoxyskerol and Sotradecol. Dermatol Surg 2002; 28; 52–5.
4. Conrad P, Malouf GM, Stacy MC. The Australian polidocanol (Aethoxysklerol) study: results at two years. Dermatol Surg 1995; 21: 334–6.
5. Hamel-Desnos C, Desnos P, Wollmann JC, et al. Evaluation of the efficacy of polidocanol in the form of foam compared with liquid form in sclerotherapy of

the greater saphenous vein: initial results. Dermatol Surg 2003; 29: 1170–5.
6. Wollmann JC. Schaum – zwischen Vergangenheit und Zukunft. Vasomed 2002; 16: 34–5.
7. Hamel-Desnos C, Allaert FA, Benigni JP, et al. Etude 3/1. Mousse de Polidocanol 3% versus 1% dans la grande veine saphène. Premiers résultats. Phlebologie 2005; 58(2): 165–73.
8. Reiner L. The activity of anionic surface active compounds in producing vascular obliteration. Proc Soc Exp Biol Med 1946; 62: 49.
9. Nabatoff RA. Recent trends in the diagnosis and treatment of varicose veins. Int Abstr Surg 1950; 90: 521.
10. Tretbar LL. Spider angiomata: treatment with sclerosant injections. J Kansas Med Soc 1978; 79: 198.
11. Shields JL, Jansen GT. Therapy for superficial telangiectasias of the lower extremities. J Dermatol Surg Oncol 1982; 8: 857–60.
12. Carlin MC, Ratz JL. Treatment of telangiectasia: comparison of sclerosing agents. J Dermatol Surg Oncol 1987; 13: 1181–4.
13. Kahle B, Leng K. Efficacy of sclerotherapy in varicose veins – prospective, blinded, placebo-controlled study. Dermatol Surg 2004; 30: 723–8.
14. Goldman MP. Sodium tetradecyl sulfate for sclerotherapy treatment of veins: Is compounding pharmacy solution safe? Dermatol Surg 2004; 30: 1454–6.
15. Barrett J, Allen B, Ockelford A, Goldman MP. Microfoam ultrasound-guided sclerotherapy for varicose veins in a subgroup with diameter at the junction of >10 mm compared with a subgroup <10 mm. Dermatol Surg 2004; 30: 1386–90.
16. Lucchi M, Bilancini S, Tucci S. Sclerosis with foam of the great saphenous vein – short term results. Phlebologie 2003; 4: 389–94.
17. Rao J, Goldman MP. Stability of foam in sclerotherapy. Difference between sodium tetradecyl sulfate and polidocanol and the type of connector used in the double syringe system (DSS) technique. Dermatol Surg 2005; 31: 19–22.
18. Rao J, Wildemore JK, Goldman MP. Double-blind prospective comparative trial between foamed and liquid Aethoxysklerol and Fibrovein in the treatment of varicose and telangiectatic leg veins. Dermatol Surg 2005; 31: 631–5.

15 Lesser importance of the saphenous vein in varicose vein treatment

Paul Pittaluga and Sylvain Chastanet

Introduction

For many decades, the so-called radical therapeutic approach to varicose disease has attempted to eliminate saphenous reflux using surgical treatment, combining crossectomy and stripping of the saphenous vein (SV).[1,2] This treatment fits in with the traditional pathophysiologic description of varicose disease, which is considered to develop from the junctions between the deep venous system and the SVs. According to this theory, the appearance of reflux at the terminal valve of the SV is the key point in the progression of saphenous insufficiency, leading to the appearance of varicose veins in the tributaries throughout the SV from proximal to distal.[3,4]

The description of a new hemodynamic theory of varicose disease treatment by Franceschi at the end of the 1980s[5] has not won many people over, even 25 years later, although some practitioners are convinced that the CHIVA cure (French acronym for *Cure Hémodynamique de l'Insuffisance Veineuse Ambulatoire*) is well founded.

Experience with less invasive approaches to surgical treatment using thermal laser energy or radiofrequency energy in the late 20th century led to the appearance of new methods and techniques using an endovascular route, just as in arterial surgery.[6,7] At the same time, sclerotherapy was revolutionized by the use of foam sclerosants, which were considerably more effective in larger veins,[8,10] and which therefore provided serious competition to traditional surgical and endovenous techniques.

These technical developments took place without calling into question the principle behind surgical treatment, namely, the systematic ablation of the refluxing SV, which is supposed to be responsible for the appearance of varices in its tributaries. However, to make the procedures less invasive, crossectomy no longer accompanied thermal ablation or sclerotherapy of the SV. This "detail" caused the utility of crossectomy, which was inseparable from traditional surgical treatment, to be called into question. The absence of routine elimination of ostial reflux led to the importance of the descending hemodynamic theory of varicose disease, with progression from the SV being doubted.[11] This was supported by work based on an increased hemodynamic understanding, thanks to the development of ultrasound technology.[12–16] Some observations supported the idea that varicose disease developed from distally to proximally.[11–18] A minimally-invasive surgical approach appeared, based on treatment of the superficial varicose reservoir (SVR) by means of phlebectomy and preservation of the SV, even if the SV presented preoperative reflux.[11,19] Supporters of this conservative approach cited the physiological role played by the SV, as well as the hemodynamic and clinical efficacy in the medium term of a rigorous, isolated resection of the SVR.[17]

If this theory turns out to be well founded, the challenge for foam echosclerotherapy will be to show itself capable of treating the varicose reservoir, whilst still preserving the SV as precisely and reliably as ambulatory phlebectomy.

The objectives of this chapter are to summarize briefly current theories and knowledge of the pathophysiology of varicose disease, to explain as objectively as possible the role occupied by SV treatment in various varicose vein treatment techniques, and to consider the advantages of SV ablation based on published results.

Pathophysiologic data

Varicose vein etiology and pathogenesis

The "hemodynamic hypothesis" is based on the idea of upstream SV insufficiency being caused by insufficiency of the terminal valves or the valves in the perforating femoral veins. This theory has been widely accepted for a long time, but it is now being called into question by the well-substantiated arguments put forward by supporters of the "parietal hypothesis." These arguments concern an initial alteration in the venous wall that leads to venous dilation, which in turn causes incompetence of the valves as their leaflets no longer meet properly.[18,20–22]

Insufficiency of the superficial venous network

It is accepted that incompetence of the valves in the superficial veins is responsible for reflux in the superficial venous network in an orthostatic (standing) position. In practice, this reflux can only appear when the pressure in the deep veins is greater than the pressure in the superficial veins, which (aside from when there is deep venous insufficiency) is only possible when the muscles in the calves dilate. In this way, at rest or when the muscles contract, the superficial veins present an anterograde flow.

Furthermore, numerous ultrasound hemodynamic observations have shown that superficial venous reflux does not necessarily develop from the knee distally, and that often refluxing segments are isolated to the SV or the nonsaphenous network.[12–16,18] Conceptions of the refluxing SVR's effect on the scale and extension of reflux in the SV have recently been updated.[11,18]

These observations also run contrary to the hemodynamic hypothesis.

Clinical consequences of reflux

The increase in pressure in the superficial venous system is largely behind the cascade phenomena that cause the problems at a macroscopic level, particularly at a microcirculatory level, which lead to the clinical manifestations of chronic venous insufficiency.[18,23–25]

Once again, it seems that the role of the SVR is crucial, as it plays a major role in the scale of the reflux and in the existence of high pressure in the superficial venous network.

Role of the saphenous vein in various treatments for varicose disease

Traditional surgery or "radical" treatment

Principles. As described at the beginning of the 20th century,[1,2] traditional surgery is based on the hemodynamic hypothesis, which states that the main cause of reflux is the SV extending from the saphenous junction (SJ) distally, in accordance with the theory of retrograde reflux progression. The appearance of varices in the tributaries is the consequence of chronic venous hypertension in the superficial venous network derived from saphenous reflux. Saphenous reflux progresses by retrograde valvular insufficiency from the ostial valve to the malleolar region, promoted by standing[3,4] (Figure 15.1).

Hemodynamic exploration initially involved only a

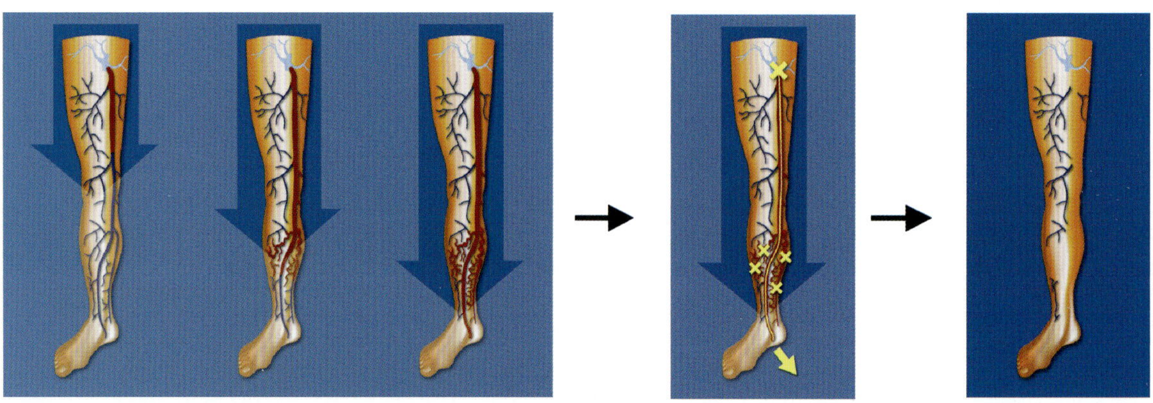

Figure 15.1 Theory of retrograde evolution of the superficial venous insufficiency and treatment by traditional surgical procedure with crossectomy + stripping + phlebectomy

clinical examination using the Valsalva maneuver and a Trendelenburg test; and was not intended to check for the existence of saphenous reflux, but rather to find out whether the great saphenous vein (GSV) and/or the small saphenous vein (SSV) were affected.[26] Phlebography was sometimes recommended before surgery.[27] Doppler and then echo-Doppler examinations improved hemodynamic understanding, but they remained superfluous in many practices until recently. Such was the rigidity of the thinking about treatment.

Ablation of the SV is central to traditional surgical treatment, since it involves the rigorous elimination of all the refluxing veins and all the reflux points. In its original description, complete surgical treatment combined ablation of the SJ and all its tributaries (extended crossectomy), ablation of refluxing perforating veins, and SV resection. It was made simple and quick by techniques of stripping by telescoping or invagination.[28] Debates on the necessity of performing a long stripping right down to the malleolus, or a short stripping to below the knee, are based on the risk of recurrence for those in favor of long stripping, and on the risk of injuring the saphenous nerve for those in favor of short stripping. Treatment of the SVR is obviously advised for the most serious varices, but it is not the treatment's central element.

- *The key element of traditional surgery is the ablation of the SV, which may cause involution of the residual varices due to the suppression of superficial venous hypertension by the stripping, potentially facilitated by postoperative sclerotherapy.*[29]

Results. Comparative studies relating to traditional surgical treatment compare either isolated crossectomy with crossectomy associated with stripping,[30,31] or isolated sclerotherapy with complete surgical treatment.[31–33] They tend to show better results for aggressive and extensive surgical treatment of the refluxing veins and the sources of the reflux.

However, studies of the long-term results report an extremely variable varicose clinical recurrence rate of 6–66%,[34–40] depending on the authors, the era, the surgical technique, the length of the follow-up period and the monitoring methods (Table 15.1). But none of them includes the preoperative SVR volume and the criteria that led to the treatment decision. Be that as it may, none of the studies report a sufficiently low recurrence rate to justify using the adjective "radical" when referring to surgical treatment, although this term adjective has persisted.

Postsurgery varicose recurrence is traditionally attributed to several factors including poor surgical technique, anatomical and tactical errors, the natural progression of the disease, pregnancy, and lifestyle and health factors.[38–41] Poor surgical technique leads to the persistence of reflux sources,[34,35] most frequently due to an incomplete or overly distal crossectomy, or even because of the persistence of perforating veins, and this is usually attributed to substandard surgical training.[42] Neovascularization around the SJ appears as a new cause of postsurgery recurrence, and is even the most frequently cited cause in recent publications.[43,44] Logically, as extended crossectomy became widespread, the frequency of residual SJ reflux fell whilst the frequency of

Table 15.1 Frequency of varicose vein recurrence after traditional surgical treatment by crossectomy and saphenous vein stripping

First author	Date	*N*	Follow-up (years)	Recurrence (%)	Assessment
Rivlin[34]	1975	1708	5–10	6	Clinical
Royle[35]	1986	367	5	18	Clinical
Fischer[36]	2001	125	34	48	Clinical
				60	Ultrasound
van Rij[37]	2003	137	5	47.1	Clinical
				93	Ultrasound
				66	Air plethysmography
Kostas[38]	2004	113	5	25	Clinical
Winterborn[39]	2004	133	11	62	Clinical
Fischer[40]	2006	1261[a]	6.6 (mean)	19.2	Ultrasound

[a]Multicentric study.

neovascularization as the main source of postsurgery recurrence increased.

Although traditional surgical techniques were standardized with the advent of surgeons' specialization and the standardization of their training, the postsurgery recurrence rate remained stable, even though there were wide disparities between published results. The most reliable figure is probably the proportion represented by recurrence surgery within practitioners' overall varicose vein surgery workload, which is around 20% and has been stable for many years.[39,41]

- *An analysis of the results in the literature therefore enables us to state that rigorous ablation of the SV does not prevent varicose recurrence; in fact, the contrary might be true. Creton even raises the possibility that extensive ablation of the SVs could increase the rate of postsurgery recurrence.*[45]

The CHIVA cure

Principles. Franceschi vizualized a different therapeutic approach for treatment of varicose veins, based on a new hemodynamic theory.[5] The therapeutic principle is the redistribution of the superficial venous reflux to the deep veins using a system of shunts, with a combination of staggered ligatures using the perforating veins and thanks to very precise preoperative echo mapping and a hemodynamic study. In the initial description, ablation of the varices was not strictly necessary, as they should drain into the deep venous system and therefore subside.[5] At a later date, certain authors recommended ablation of the varices in association with the CHIVA cure, due to the risk of patient dissatisfaction.[46] Even more recently, authors have developed this point even further, creating "CHIVA 2," which reverses the initial description and where the ablation of the varicose collaterals is the treatment's first port of call, followed by a crossectomy if reflux persists in the SV.[47] This description of "CHIVA 2" seems to undermine the very principle behind the CHIVA cure.

- *In fact, in the initial description of the CHIVA cure, the SV does undergo first-line therapy with the performance of staged ligatures.*

Results. The results published vary widely, depending on the author. Supporters of the CHIVA cure have published studies, including some with very good techniques and excellent results,[47,48] whereas others note high recurrence rates.[49] As poor results are often not published, it is difficult to assess the CHIVA cure objectively. The controversial nature of the CHIVA cure, as well as its conceptual complexity and difficult execution, could be the cause of the poor results sometimes reported, and could explain why few teams still practice the technique. (These teams are almost exclusively situated in Europe, although very few of them are based in France.)

- *CHIVA cure supporters promote the preservation of the SV, essentially so that it is available for use as an arterial bypass at a later date.*

Endovenous laser treatment (EVLT)

Principles. As for arterial surgery, it was tempting to vizualize an endovascular treatment for varicose disease via the SV. Lasers were perfectly adapted to this idea, since by using a small fiberoptic cable (600 μm), it is possible to deliver a larger amount of thermal energy and occlude the SV. The fiberoptic cable is introduced percutaneously, in the same way as for any endovascular procedure (introducer sheath and guide wire), allowing an aggressive surgical stripping procedure to be avoided.

The laser's (810 nm, 940 nm, 980 nm, 1064 nm, 1320 nm) effect on the vein wall is not yet clearly understood, but the idea is to heat the vein wall so that intimal lesions are created, leading to a retraction of the parietal collagen and edema of the wall, which in turn causes the vein to be obliterated and then to undergo fibrosis.

From a practical point of view, the catheter is introduced above the knee or the malleolus for the GSV, and at the malleolus for the SSV. In general, the sural GSV (i.e., in the calf) and the distal third of the SSV are not treated, due to the risk of injuring the internal or external saphenous nerve.

The procedure starts downstream of the ostial valve, and generally preserves the first abdominal collateral of the SJ.[50] The SJ is therefore not treated, which represents a fundamental difference compared with traditional surgery.

Two types of procedure are used:

1. A sequential procedure during which the laser is pulsed for a set time. The fiber is then retracted a few millimeters and the laser is pulsed again.

2. A continuous procedure where the laser is continuously turned on as the fiber is retracted at a regulated speed.

Authors agree that the efficacy of the procedure is dependent on the quantity of energy[51] and on the laser fluence, for which the diameter of the SV has to be taken into account.[52]

Some authors treat varices during the laser procedure,[53] whereas others treat them separately.[50]

- *As for traditional surgery, ablation of the SV (distal to the first abdominal collateral) is therefore the central element of the endovenous laser procedure, treatment of the SVR being a corollary.*

Results. Authors initially reported that EVLT is feasible and of low risk, and also that it gave excellent immediate results.[6] Some short- and medium-term results have now been published[51,52,54,55] (Table 15.2). The SV recanalization rate seems to be heavily dependent on the energy used during the procedure. Proebstle suggests a threshold energy of 6.3 J/cm per millimeter diameter of the vein treated, enabling the SV obliteration rate after 1 year to be increased from 82.7% to 97%.[52]

Reflux disappearance at the SJ, with drainage of the abdominopelvic collaterals toward the deep veins, is certainly the most remarkable observation, since it challenges the utility of crossectomy.

Although the SV occlusion rate is the key element in all the publications, the clinical results, and in particular the varicose recurrence rate during follow-up, are very poorly documented.

The problem when analyzing the results is, first of all, the quality of the publications, which include a large amount of imprecise data (e.g., numbers lost to follow-up and clinical recurrence), and second, the wide technical variations (e.g., laser manufacturer, type of wavelength, continuous or sequential pulse mode, and whether or not the SV was bloodless or full), making comparisons impossible.

A comparative study of EVLT and traditional surgery (crossectomy + stripping) reports less ecchymosis and edema, as well as greater patient satisfaction, for EVLT and the same hemodynamic results as for traditional surgery.[56] However, these comparative studies do not make precise records of the scale of the preoperative SVR or its mode of treatment.

- *Therefore, an analysis of the literature does not tell us what influence the obliteration of the SV using an endovenous laser has on clinical results and, in particular, on the varicose recurrence rate.*

Radiofrequency (RF) treatment

Principles. Like EVLT, the physical principle of RF treatment is to deliver endovenous thermal energy with a view to occluding the SV. We know more about the effects of RF treatment than we do about EVLT: thermal energy is applied using an RF wave (50 Hz) from a diathermal electrode, along the same lines as an

Table 15.2 Results after treatment of superficial venous insufficiency by endovenous laser

First author	Date	Initial *N*	Follow-up	Follow-up *N*	Saphenous occlusion (%)	Recurrence
Min[54]	2003	499	2 years	121 (24.2%)	93.4	Unknown
Timperman[51]	2004	111	29.5 weeks (mean)	107 (93.4%)	77.5	Unknown
Proebstle[52]	2006	263	1 years	188 (71.5%)	95.7	Unknown
Agus[55]	2006	1076[a]	3 years	Unknown	97	6% (leading to an adjuntive procedure)

[a]Multicentric study.

electrosurgical unit. The electrode comes in a tulip shape with peripheral anodes and a central cathode. The opening of this "tulip," after retraction of the external sheath, enables the anodes to be applied directly to the vein wall and deliver heat when they come into direct contact with the wall. This heat denatures the collagen fibers and causes the wall to retract, which in turn leads to the obliteration of the SV. There must be no blood when performing RF treatment, because if the electrode comes into contact with blood, a thrombus can be formed, and this reduces the procedure's efficacy.[7]

The RF introducer is slightly larger than for laser treatment (5 or 7 F), but the procedure goes ahead in the same way as any endovascular procedure. The catheter can be introduced percutaneously at the knee or above the knee, but it is inadvisable to treat the GSV below the knee due to the risk of thermal diffusion (1.5 mm). For the same reason, it is inadvisable to treat the SSV using RF therapy. After an initial period when surgical crossectomy was combined with RF treatment,[7] and then a period when the SJ was obliterated endovascularly,[7,57] the SJ is now not treated: the procedure starts after the first abdominal collateral.[58]

In contrast to EVLT, there is only one treatment kit available, marketed as CLOSURE® (VNUS Medical Technologies, Inc., San Jose, California, United States). The procedure is therefore perfectly standardized. Also in contrast to EVLT, it is not recommended to treat an SV that is larger than 15 mm although practitioners are pushing back the boundaries of this limit, and larger diameters have already been treated.[58]

As with EVLT, varicose veins can be treated during the same procedure, or separately. Some authors favor treatment limited to the saphenous trunk, leading to spontaneous regression of the varices in 28–65% of cases after obliteration of the SV, without any procedure being performed on the varicose reservoir, with, however, a short follow-up period (6–9 months).[59,60]

- *As for EVLT, ablation of the SV (after the first abdominal collateral) is the main priority of this procedure, before ablation of the SVR.*

Results. In contrast to EVLT, RF treatment is completely standardized, making it easier to compare the published studies and their results. Right from the outset, several multicenter prospective studies were started, with a much more robust methodology than that used for studies published on EVLT.[7,57] We now have access to studies with follow-up periods of 3–5 years[58,61,62] (Table 15.3). The results of the studies are similar, with an excellent SV occlusion rate after 3 or 5 years (80–85%) and excellent symptom results (70–94% improvement), but with a non-negligible varicose recurrence rate (20–30%).[58,61,62] The progression of the untreated SJ in the medium term shows that, as with EVLT, there is a physiologic flow toward the deep vein in over 90% of cases, supporting the theory that crossectomy is of limited use.[63] However, all of these studies include a limited number of lower extremities reviewed after 2, 3 or 5 years (20–33%).

Occlusion failure indicators are essentially the fiber being removed too quickly and a high body mass index.[57,61] In some studies, incomplete obliteration of the SV is a risk factor for varicose recurrence,[61] although this is not necessarily correlated with the symptom results.[62]

Table 15.3 Results after treatment of superficial venous insufficiency by radiofrequency

First author	Date	Initial *N*	Follow-up (years)	Follow-up *N*	Saphenous occlusion (%)	Recurrence (%)
Merchant[58]	2005	1222[a]	5	406 (29.5%)	87.2	27.4
Nicolini[61]	2005	330[a]	3	68 (20.6%)	88	12.8
Creton[62]	2006	330[a]	5	103 (31.2%)	82	27

[a]Multicentric study.

Most authors note an absence of neovascularization, which is one of the advantages of endovenous treatment,[7,58,61–63] but some publications have mentioned inguinal neovascularization[64] or perivenous neovascularization[65] after endovenous treatment.

Several studies have compared traditional surgery (crossectomy + stripping) and RF treatment. Lurie[66] concluded that RF treatment gives the best results in terms of patients being able to resume their daily activities and quality of life, with identical clinical and hemodynamic results after 2 years. Rautio[67] concluded that RF treatment is better overall, but Perälä[68] concluded that RF treatment leads to greater recurrence after 3 years. Once again, these comparative studies do not take account of the scale of the preoperative SVR or its mode of treatment.

We are therefore not able to draw any conclusions on the influence that SV elimination has on the quality of the clinical results, but it is very striking that the varicose recurrence rate is always higher than the SV repermeation rate. This is particularly true for the 5-year results, with a recurrence rate around 30%, whereas the SV repermeation rate is only around 15%.[58,62] This very clearly shows, as with traditional surgery, that eliminating the SV does not prevent varicose vein recurrence.

Sclerotherapy

Principles. Liquid sclerotherapy has been practiced for nearly a century, but has been revolutionized in recent years by the appearance of foam echosclerotherapy.[8] This foam is obtained by mixing the sclerosant with air or carbon dioxide. Foam sclerosants have many advantages compared with liquid sclerosants, as, among other things, they enable larger veins to be treated and offer excellent ultrasonic visualization due to the fact that ultrasound picks up the foam particularly well.

Although foam echosclerotherapy enables large varicose collaterals to be treated, its main application has been its treatment of the SV, where it is much more effective than liquid sclerotherapy, since the foam does not mix with blood, limiting its dilution and enabling it to fill up the port by pushing back the blood. Various techniques are described, with open or closed access.[69,70] Another slightly different technique involves using a long catheter that is inserted up the SV and then withdrawn as the foam is injected[71]; this is a real endovenous treatment along the same lines as endovenous EVLT and radiofrequency treatment. In general, the treatment stops at the first abdominal collateral, and the SJ is not treated. Foam echosclerotherapy is known as "chemical ablation" of the SV, as the philosophy behind the procedure is similar to thermal ablation by means of RF or laser. Therefore, for foam echosclerotherapy, as for traditional surgery and thermal endovenous techniques, the elimination of the refluxing SV is the essential step in the treatment strategy for varicose veins with saphenous reflux.

- *We should note that, in contrast to EVLT and RF treatment, foam echosclerotherapy offers the possibility of extensive treatment of the SV and the SVR using the same procedure. On the other hand, no publications currently describe a tested and reproducible technique to treat the SVR without eliminating the SV.*

Results. The results published on foam echosclerotherapy are encouraging in the short term, with 85% efficacy

Table 15.4 Results after treatment of superficial venous insufficiency by foam echosclerotherapy

First author	Date	Initial *N*	No. of injections	Injected volume (mean) (mL)	Follow-up	Follow-up *N*	Saphenous occlusion (%)	Recurrence (%)
Hamel-Desnos[9]	2003	45	1	2.5	1 year	45 (100%)	80	Unknown
Barrett JM[72]	2004	112	2.19 (mean)	8.7	22.5 months (mean)	112 (100%)	76.8	5
Smith PC[73]	2006	1411	1 (26.6%) 2 (44.5%) 3 (25.6%) >3 (3.3%)	10	11 months (mean)	504 (35.7%)	86.1	5.2

for elimination of the treated vein. This can reach 95% if three subsequent injection sessions are utilized[9,72,73] (Table 15.4).

All of the studies use the elimination of the SV as the efficacy criterion, without assessing the scale of the SVR before the procedure or the exact methods for its treatment.

- *Furthermore, we do not have any foam echosclerotherapy data with a long enough follow-up period to be able to assess the recurrence rate in connection with the SV elimination rate.*

Mini-invasive surgical approaches

Principles. The appearance of endovenous techniques has called the utility of crossectomy into doubt. The realization that ostial reflux was reversible after endovenous procedures[58,61–63] led practitioners to wonder if truncal reflux could be reversed after treatment of the SVR. Some authors had reported that SV reflux was reversible by means of simple phlebectomies,[74,75] that deep venous reflux could disappear after treating saphenous reflux[76–78] and that the diameter of the SV could be reduced after ablating the refluxing collateral.[79] A new pathophysiologic concept has been mentioned recently: varicose disease could come about at the level of the reticulum, stemming from the subfascial veins, which are the most superficial and the most exposed, and whose walls are the thinnest.[11,18] The subfascial veins could be the first to dilate through decompensation of their parietal strength. Progression could initially remain subfascial, creating a dilated and refluxing venous network. When this refluxing network becomes large enough, it could create an aspiratory effect in the intrafascial SV, leading to decompensation of the vein wall, moving forward to reach the saphenofemoral or popliteal junction. The SV is the superficial vein with the thickest and most muscular wall. Furthermore, the enveloping subcutaneous fascia in which it resides protects it. It would therefore be the last vein to experience decompensation as varicose disease progresses. Numerous publications challenge the theory of descending progression, citing the possibility of local or multifocal early distal evolution, sometimes ascending or anterograde, based on precise and detailed echo-Doppler explorations.[12–16] The fact that the ostial valve is frequently competent (>50%) when there is truncal reflux has been clearly proven.[80–82] We recently reported on an anatomoclinical study based on 2275 echo-Doppler results, showing a correlation between the extent of the reflux in the SV and age, with the reflux appearing to progress in an antegrade manner from the superficial collaterals to the SV and then to the SJ.[16]

This pathophysiologic theory has two consequences. If there were no saphenous reflux, early treatment of varicose veins would be useful in order to prevent reflux spreading to the SVs. If there were saphenous reflux, and up until a certain stage of the disease, first-line therapy should include ablation of the SVR and not elimination of the saphenous reflux, which is potentially reversible (Figure 15.2).

Saphenous stripping would only be indicated in cases where saphenous reflux seems to be irreversible. This approach therefore involves selective management of

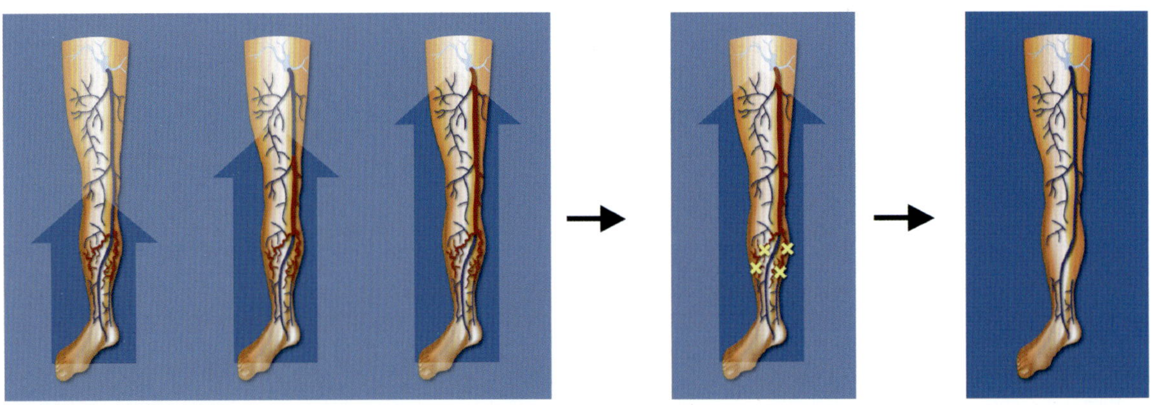

Figure 15.2 Theory of anterograde evolution of the superficial venous insufficiency and treatment by the ASVAL (Ambulatory Selective Varices Ablation under Local anesthesia) surgical procedure, leading to disappearance of the saphenous reflux

superficial venous reflux, depending on the clinical and hemodynamic context found in each case. This rejection of traditional surgery, systematically including crossectomy and stripping, is known as the ASVAL method (Ambulatory Selective Varices Ablation under Local anesthesia) – only the SVR is treated by phlebectomy, and the refluxing SV is preserved.[11,19]

The ASVAL method differs from the CHIVA cure, which preserves the SV without really questioning its role in the appearance of varices. In fact, the principle behind the CHIVA cure is to redistribute the superficial venous flow from the superficial veins to the deep veins, using a system of shunts in the saphenous and perforating veins.[5]

Results. Since the publication of the preliminary results of the ASVAL method (303 lower limbs with a mean follow-up period of 7–8 months),[11] the initial cohort has been followed up regularly, and the medium-term results were recently published.[17] The hemodynamic results are remarkably stable after 1, 2 and 3 years of follow-up, with a major improvement in saphenous hemodynamics in 90% of cases: reflux is less than 0.5 s in 70% of cases; and in 20% of cases reflux is reduced by over 50% in duration compared with the preoperative values. The clinical results are also stable after 3 years of follow-up, with improvement or disappearance of symptoms in 80–90% of cases, and a cosmetic improvement in 90% of cases. The varicose recurrence rate after 3 years (15.7%) is close to the figures obtained after RF treatment or traditional stripping (Table 15.5), and the number of complementary procedures performed is low (2.3%).

As the recurrence rate for the ASVAL method in the short and medium term is not higher than for techniques that involve removal of the SV, we can legitimately ask ourselves whether a conservative approach is not justified as a first-line therapy when there is only partial SV reflux and when the SV is only moderately dilated. The main argument in favor of this conservative approach is the physiologic role that the SV could play in superficial drainage, and to a lesser extent its availability as revascularization material.

In the literature, there are reports of the harmful effect that resection of the SV has on the long-term progression of SV insufficiency.[45] The conservative approach of the ASVAL method needs to be validated in the longer term, with prospective studies and more precise data so that criteria for preserving the SV can be established. In fact, the pathophysiology is not dependent on a single cause, as during the study of the 2275 preoperative echo-Doppler results, we found SV reflux without varicose veins in 7.2% of cases.[16] It could be early saphenous incompetence with a high prevalence of trophic problems (20% at stage C_4–C_6), even though there is no deep venous pathology. Elimination of the SV seems completely justified in this case.

For three years now, when removal of the SV is necessary, we have used a technique involving stripping but no crossectomy, which in our experience gives results that are equivalent to the results obtained from endovenous techniques. Pittaluga and colleagues recently reported – at the American Venous Forum 19th Annual Congress, San Diego, CA, on 14 February 2007 – on a retrospective study of 112 lower limbs followed-up for a mean period of 24.4 months.[83] The SJ guaranteed physiological drainage of its collaterals toward the femoral vein in 98.2% of cases; we noted neovascularization in only 0.9% of cases, and there was a recurrence rate of 6.3%.

- *The medium-term results of isolated ablation of the SVR with preservation of the preoperative refluxing SV (ASVAL) are encouraging enough to lead us to believe that ablation of the SV is perhaps a secondary measure in the treatment of varicose veins.*

Table 15.5 Comparison of results after treatment of superficial venous insufficiency by ASVAL, radiofrequency and traditional surgery

	ASVAL[17]	Radiofrequency[58,61,62]	Surgery[33,43]
Follow-up (years)	3	3	2–3
Persistence of significant reflux (%)	10.7	12–18	10–15
Improvement of symptoms (%)	83.1	70–85	65–80
Recurrence (%)	15.7	10–20	10–25

Discussion

Saphenous junction treatment

The results that we have published after SV stripping with preservation of the SJ[83] are at least comparable, or even superior, to the data published after 2 years of follow-up after endovenous treatment using RF treatment or EVLT, where reflux absence in the SJ varied between 80% and 97%.[52,54,58,61–63] In view of these results, we can ask ourselves whether carrying out a surgical stripping in association with extensive phlebectomies improves the hemodynamics of the preserved SJ, given the fact that the SV cannot become permeable again and, perhaps especially, given the ablation of the varicose reservoir. The hemodynamic benefits of ablation of the varicose reservoir are mentioned in the literature.[11,19]

Despite an inguinal approach, the rate of inguinal neovascularization after 2 years was very low (1.8% at 2 years) in our series of SV stripping with preservation of the SJ.[83] This figure is not higher than the figures recorded after endovenous treatment, where the neovascularization rate varied from 0% to 2.8%,[58,61–63] and it is much lower than traditional surgical series including extended crossectomy, with rates of 20–53%.[37,41,43] It seems that preserving the superficial abdominal and perineal venous drainage by not dissecting the SJ and by not disconnecting the collaterals enables neovascularization to be avoided. Using a limited inguinal approach without dissecting the SJ does not therefore seem to cause more neovascularization, since it preserves the drainage of the SJ collaterals into the femoral vein.[19,83]

The clinical recurrence rate observed after SV stripping with preservation of the SJ[83] was 6.3%, which can be compared with series of stripping associated with traditional extended crossectomy, where the figures varied from 10% to 25% after 2 years.[33,43] This recurrence rate after SV stripping with preservation of the SJ is also better than that observed after endovenous treatment with an identical follow-up period, where there was a 12–15% clinical recurrence rate.[58,61–63] It is difficult to compare the different series, because the extent of the preoperative varices and the extent of the SVR resection are never mentioned. Moreover, after SV stripping with preservation of the SJ, clinical recurrence was independent of SJ reflux in 6 cases out of 7,[83] just as the ablation of the SV did not prevent recurrence in the series of endovenous treatments.[58,61–63] These observations support the theory that varicose disease develops from the superficial distal venous network, which is increasingly mentioned in the literature,[12–16] contrary to the traditional description whereby varicose disease develops downward from the junctions between deep and superficial venous networks.[3,4]

However, a serious postoperative complication was observed after SV stripping with preservation of the SJ, with SJ thrombosis complicated by an extension to the femoral vein and by a pulmonary embolism, fortunately without after-effect.[83] Saphenofemoral junction (SFJ) thrombosis extending to the femoral vein has been reported in the literature after endovenous treatment.[57,58,66,84] This potentially serious complication risk should probably be taken into account when preserving the SFJ by means of targeted prevention, for example, by using low-molecular-weight heparin treatment or a traditional enlarged crossectomy in cases of thrombophilia, history of thrombosis or very dilated junctions (>20 mm). An early postoperative echo-Doppler examination (e.g., after 24–48 hours) could also be recommended in order to detect thromboembolic complications.[84]

Saphenous vein treatment

Before the description of the ASVAL method, authors reported that simple phlebotomies could change the hemodynamics and the diameter of the SV.[74,75,79] The short-term results after ASVAL that we reported previously[11] show that the percentage of patients experiencing no saphenous reflux remains at 70%, and if we add patients with moderate reflux (<50% than the initial reflux), the saphenous hemodynamic improvement is considerable in nearly 90% of cases, consistently at 6 months, 1 year, 2 years and 3 years.[17] Despite SV preservation, these hemodynamic results are close to the results obtained using endovenous techniques with thermal ablation of the SV, in which 85% of patients experience no saphenous reflux after 3 years.[58,61,62] Studies assessing hemodynamic results after stripping, at 2 and 3 years of follow-up, do not show better results.[33,43]

From a clinical point of view, our results show the same stability, since functional improvement remains above 80% for the cohort followed-up for 3 years, whilst the cosmetic benefit is close to 90%.[17] Following up our original ASVAL cohort for a longer period of time has allowed us to note the appearance of varicose recurrences, which essentially occurred in the second year; the recurrence level at 3 years was 15.7%.[17] We have used a broad definition for recurrence, including the REVAS criteria,[85] that is, recurrent varices after surgery, regardless of where they are located. This figure is also close to that obtained with endovenous techniques: authors report between 10% and 20% recurrence after 3 years, whilst saphenous occlusion rates are nearly 90%.[58,61,62] It is interesting to note that in our research recurrence was only accompanied by saphenous reflux in 7 of the 19 cases, and that the reflux was only major in 1 case. Furthermore, the limbs with recurrent varices had a preoperative varicose surface area that was significantly larger than that of the limbs that had no further problems.[17] This points toward the natural progression of varicose disease, which develops differently depending on the individual, and supports the theory of development from the reticulum, which is increasingly gaining ground.[12–16] Consequently, it is logical to envisage following up patients treated for varicose veins in the long term, adapting procedures and techniques to each individual case, and abandoning systematic treatments.[86–89]

A new deal

There is no longer any place for systematic elimination of the SJ and the SV: numerous studies show that extensive ostial-trunk reflux is involved in only a minority of cases.[12–16,80,81] Regardless of the technique chosen, the procedure should be adapted to each individual case and should involve the least aggressive option.

Therefore, it seems that first-line therapy should always consider the option of preserving the SV, depending on the clinical examination (signs and symptoms, antecedents, and professional considerations), the echo-Doppler data (dilation of the SV and seat of the reflux) and the patient's reason for consulting (cosmetic, functional, preventative or trophic problems). Isolated treatment of the SVR with preservation of the SV at stage C_2 of the CEAP classification will probably, therefore, often be the most appropriate course of action. Ablation of the SV using traditional surgery, EVLT and RF treatment could then be limited to the advanced stages of varicose disease.

In terms of isolated treatment of the SVR, ambulatory phlebectomy seems to be the most appropriate technique, but foam echosclerotherapy is also possible,[90] provided that it blocks the sclerosant from entering the SV – which is not an easy thing to do.

Conclusion

The notion of traditional surgical treatment for varicose veins, combining crossectomy and stripping, being seen as the "gold standard" seems to have had its day. Several important steps forward have revolutionized varicose vein treatment: the appearance of thermal endovenous techniques that are less aggressive but effective in the medium term, and the development of foam sclerosants that have enabled sclerotherapy to compete with other varicose vein treatments in the shorter term. The appearance of these new techniques has called into question the utility of crossectomy, and therefore opened the way for another pathophysiologic theory of varicose veins that questions whether the SV is initially responsible for disease development. It has therefore seemed logical to envisage a conservative approach to the SV with rigorous treatment of the SVR by means of ambulatory phlebectomy, or even foam echosclerotherapy. Aside from advanced stages of the disease, the results of this conservative strategy seem to be equivalent in the medium term to the results of techniques that involve ablation of the SV, which are more aggressive for the physiology of the superficial venous network. It could well be that ablation of the SV for the treatment of varicose veins should only be suggested at advanced stages of varicose disease or if isolated treatment of the SVR has failed. Longer-term studies need to be completed in order to clarify all of the issues involved in the treatment of the SV in varicose disease.

References

1. Mayo CH. Treatment of varicose vein. Surg Gyn Obst Br J Surg 1906; 2: 385–8.
2. Babcock WW. A new operation for the extirpation of varicose veins of the leg. New York Med J 1907; 86: 153–6.
3. Trendelenburg F. Ueber die Unterbindung der Vena Saphena magna bei Unterschenkel Varicen. Beitr Klin Chir 1890–91; 7: 195–210.
4. Ludbrook J, Beale G. Femoral venous valves in relation to varicose veins. Lancet 1962; i: 79–81.
5. Franceschi C. Théorie et pratique de la cure conservatrice hémodynamique de l'insuffisance veineuse en ambulatoire. Percy sous Thil: Editions de l'Armaçon, 1988.
6. Navarro L, Min RJ, Bone C. Endovenous laser: a new minimally invasive method of treatment for varicose

veins – preliminary observations using an 810 nm diode laser. Dermatol Surg 2001; 27: 117–22.
7. Chandler JG, Pichot O, Sessa C, et al. Treatment of primary insufficiency by endovenous saphenous vein obliteration. Vasc Surg 2000; 38: 201–14.
8. Cabrera Garrido JR, Cabrera Garcia Olmedo JR, Garcia Olmedo D. Nuevo metodode esclerois en las varices trunculares. Pathol Vasculares 1993; 1: 55–72.
9. Hamel-Desnos C, Desnos P, Wollman JC, et al. Evaluation of the efficacy of polidocanol in the form of foam compared with liquid form in sclerotherapy of the greater saphenous vein: initial results. Dermatol Surg 2003; 29: 1170–5.
10. Guex JJ. Foam sclerotherapy: an overview of use for primary venous insufficiency. Semin Vasc Surg 2005; 18: 25–9.
11. Pittaluga P, Réa B, Barbe R, Guex JJ. ASVAL method: principles and preliminary results. In: Becquemin JP, Alimi YS, Watelet J, eds. Updates and Controversies in Vascular Surgery. Torino: Minerva Medica, 2005: 182–9.
12. Labropoulos N, Giannoukas AD, Delis K, et al. Where does venous reflux start? J Vasc Surg 1997; 26: 736–42.
13. Labropoulos N, Leon L, Kwon S, et al. Study of the venous reflux progression. J Vasc Surg 2005; 41: 291–5.
14. Cooper DG, Hillman-Cooper CS, Barker SG, Hollingsworth SJ. Primary varicose veins: the sapheno-femoral junction, distribution of varicosities and patterns of incompetence. Eur J Vasc Endovasc Surg 2003; 25: 53–9.
15. Engelhorn CA, Engelhorn AL, Cassou MF, Salles-Cunha SX. Patterns of saphenous reflux in women with primary varicose veins. J Vasc Surg 2005; 41: 645–51.
16. Pittaluga P, Chastanet S, Réa B, et al. Classification of saphenous refluxes: implications for treatment. Phlebology 2008; 23: 2–9.
17. Pittaluga P, Chastanet S, Réa B, et al. Saphenous vein preservation: is it the new gold standard? In: Becquemin JP, Alimi YS, eds. Updates and Controversies in Vascular Surgery. Torino: Minerva Medica, 2007: 391–9.
18. Perrin M. Insuffisance veineuse superficielle: notion fondamentales. Techniques chirurgicales – Chirurgie vasculaire [43-161-A]. Paris: Elsever Masson, 2007.
19. Perrin M. Chirurgie à ciel ouvert de l'insuffisance veineuse superficielle. Principes. Techniques. Résultats. Techniques chirurgicales – Chirurgie vasculaire [43-161-B]. Paris: Elsever Masson, 2007.
20. Rose SA, Ahmed A. Some thoughts on the etiology of varicose vein. J Cardiovasc Surg (Torino) 1986; 27: 534–43.
21. Clarke GH, Vasdekis SN, Hobbs JT, Nicolaides AN. Venous wall function in the pathogenesis of varicose veins. Surgery 1992; 111: 402–8.
22. Travers JP, Brookes CE, Evans J, et al. Assessment of wall structure and composition of varicose veins with reference to collagen, elastin and smooth muscle content. Eur J Vasc Endovasc Surg 1996; 11: 230–7.
23. Leu AJ, Leu HJ, Franzeck UK, Bollinger A. Microvascular changes in chronic venous insufficiency: a review. Cardiovasc Surg 1995; 3: 237–45.
24. Bollinger A, Leu AJ, Hoffmann U, Franzeck UK. Microvascular changes in venous disease: an update. Angiology 1997; 48: 27–32.
25. Jünger M, Steins A, Hahn M, Häfner HM. Microcirculatory dysfunction in chronic venous insufficiency (CVI). Microcirculation 2000; 7: 3–12.
26. Zelikovski A, Zamir B, Hadar H, Urca I. Sapheno-femoral valve insufficiency in varicose veins of the lower limb. Angiology 1981; 32: 807–11.
27. Perrin M. L'apport de la phlébographie dans le traitement chirurgical de l'insuffisance veineuse chronique des membres inférieurs. Phlebologie 1988; 41: 115–34.
28. Creton DE. Eveinage traditionnel: techniques, complications, résultats. In: Kieffer E, Bahnini A, eds. Chirurgie des Veines des Membres Inférieurs. Paris: AERCV, 1990: 125–44.
29. Perrin M. Chirurgie des varices des membres inférieurs. Encyclopédie Med Chir Paris. Techniques chirurgicales – Chirurgie vasculaire, [43-161-A]. Paris: Elsevier, 1995.
30. Dwerryhouse S, Davies B, Harradine K, Earnshaw JJ. Stripping the long saphenous vein reduces the rate of reoperation for recurrent varicose veins: five-year results of a randomized trial. J Vasc Surg 1999; 29: 589–92.
31. Miyazaki K, Nishibe T, Sata F, et al. Long-term results of treatments for varicose veins due to greater saphenous vein insufficiency. Int Angiol 2005; 24: 282–6.
32. Hobbs JT. Surgery and sclerotherapy in the treatment of varicose veins. A random trial. Arch Surg 1974; 109: 793–6.
33. Rutgers PH, Kitslaar PJ. Randomized trial of stripping versus high ligation combined with sclerotherapy in the treatment of the incompetent greater saphenous vein. Am J Surg 1994; 168: 311–15.
34. Rivlin S. The surgical cure of primary varicose veins. Br J Surg 1975; 62: 913–17.
35. Royle JP. Recurrent varicose vein. World J Surg 1986; 10: 944–53.
36. Fischer R, Linde N, Duff C, et al. Late recurrent saphenofemoral junction reflux after ligation and stripping of the greater saphenous vein. J Vasc Surg 2001; 34: 236–40.

37. Van Rij AM, Jiang P, Solomon C, et al. Recurrence after varicose vein surgery: a prospective long-term clinical study with duplex ultrasound scanning and air plethysmography. J Vasc Surg 2003; 38: 935–43.
38. Kostas T, Ioannou CV, Touloupakis E, Daskalaki E, et al. Recurrent varicose veins after surgery: a new appraisal of a common and complex problem in vascular surgery. Eur J Vasc Endovasc Surg 2004; 2: 275–82.
39. Winterborn RJ, Foy C, Earnshaw JJ. Causes of varicose vein recurrence: late results of a randomized controlled trial of stripping the long saphenous vein. J Vasc Surg 2004; 40: 634–9.
40. Fischer R, Chandler JG, Stenger D, et al. Patient characteristics and physician-determined variables affecting saphenofemoral reflux recurrence after ligation and stripping of the great saphenous vein. J Vasc Surg 2006; 43: 81–7.
41. Perrin MR, Labropoulos N, Leon LR Jr. Presentation of the patient with recurrent varices after surgery (REVAS). J Vasc Surg 2006; 43: 327–34.
42. Negus D. Recurrent varicose veins: a national problem. Br J Surg 1993; 80: 823–4.
43. Jones L, Braithwaite BD, Selwyn D, et al. Neovascularisation is the principal cause of varicose vein recurrence: result of a randomised trial of stripping the long saphenous vein. Eur J Vasc Endovasc Surg 1996; 12: 442–5.
44. De Maeseneer MG, Vandenbroeck CP, Van Schil PE. Silicone patch saphenoplasty to prevent repeat recurrence after surgery to treat recurrent saphenofemoral incompetence: long-term follow-up study. J Vasc Surg 2004; 40: 98–105.
45. Creton D. A nondraining saphenous system is a factor of poor prognosis for long-term results in surgery of great saphenous vein recurrences. Dermatol Surg 2004; 30: 744–9.
46. Bahnini A, Bailly M, Chiche L, Franceschi C. Cure conservatrice hémodynamique de l'insuffisance veineuse en ambulatoire: technique, résultats. In: Kieffer E, Bahnini A, eds. Chirurgie des Veines des Membres Inférieurs. Paris: AERCV, 1990: 167–81.
47. Escribano JM, Juan J, Bofill R, et al. Durability of reflux-elimination by a minimal invasive CHIVA procedure on patients with varicose veins. A 3-year prospective case study. Eur J Vasc Endovasc Surg 2003; 25: 159–63.
48. Zamboni P, Escribano JM. Regarding "Reflux elimination without any ablation or disconnection of the saphenous vein. A haemodynamic model for venous surgery" and "Durability of reflux-elimination by a minimal invasive CHIVA procedure on patients with varicose veins. A 3-year prospective case study." Eur J Vasc Endovasc Surg 2004; 28: 567.
49. Franco G. Ambulatory and hemodynamic treatment of varicose veins (CHIVA cure). Revolution or regression? J Mal Vasc 1992; 17: 301–7.
50. Guex JJ, Min RJ, Pittaluga P. Traitement de l'insuffisance veineuse de la grande saphène par photo coagulation laser endoveineux: technique et indication. Phlebologie 2002; 55: 239–43.
51. Timperman PE, Sichlau M, Ryu RK. Greater energy delivery improves treatment success of endovenous laser treatment of incompetent saphenous veins. J Vasc Interv Radiol 2004; 15: 1061–3.
52. Proebstle TM, Moehler T, Herdemann S. Reduced recanalization rates of the great saphenous vein after endovenous laser treatment with increased energy dosing: definition of a threshold for the endovenous fluence equivalent. J Vasc Surg 2006; 44: 834–9.
53. Mekako A, Hatfield J, Bryce J, et al. Combined endovenous laser therapy and ambulatory phlebectomy: refinement of a new technique. Eur J Vasc Endovasc Surg 2006; 32: 725–9.
54. Min RJ, Khilnani N, Zimmet SE. Endovenous laser treatment of saphenous vein reflux: long-term results. J Vasc Interv Radiol 2003; 14: 991–6.
55. Agus GB, Mancini S, Magi G; IEWG. The first 1000 cases of Italian Endovenous-laser Working Group (IEWG). Rationale, and long-term outcomes for the 1999–2003 period. Int Angiol 2006; 25: 209–15.
56. De Medeiros CA, Luccas GC. Comparison of endovenous treatment with an 810 nm laser versus conventional stripping of the great saphenous vein in patients with primary varicose veins. Dermatol Surg 2005; 31: 1685–94.
57. Manfrini S, Gasbarro V, Danielsson G, et al. Endovenous management of saphenous vein reflux. Endovenous Reflux Management Study Group. J Vasc Surg 2000; 32: 330–42.
58. Merchant RF, Pichot O. Long-term outcomes of endovenous radiofrequency obliteration of saphenous reflux as a treatment for superficial venous insufficiency. J Vasc Surg 2005; 42: 502–9.
59. Monahan DL. Can phlebectomy be deferred in the treatment of varicose veins? J Vasc Surg 2005; 42: 1145–9.
60. Welch HJ. Endovenous ablation of the great saphenous vein may avert phlebectomy for branch varicose veins. J Vasc Surg 2006; 44: 601–5.
61. Nicolini P, and the Closure Group. Treatment of primary varicose veins by endovenous obliteration with the VNUS closure system: results of a prospective multicentre study. Eur J Vasc Endovasc Surg 2005; 29: 433–9.
62. Creton D, et le Groupe Closure. Oblitération tronculaire saphène par le procédé radiofréquence closure:

résultats à 5 ans de l'etude prospective multicentrique. Phlebologie 2006; 59: 67–72.
63. Pichot O, Kabnick LS, Creton D, et al. Duplex ultrasound scan findings two years after great saphenous vein radiofrequency endovenous obliteration. J Vasc Surg 2004; 39: 189–95.
64. Salles-Cunha SX, Comerota AJ, Tzilinis A, et al. Ultrasound findings after radiofrequency ablation of the great saphenous vein: descriptive analysis. J Vasc Surg 2004; 40: 1166–73.
65. Labropoulos N, Bhatti A, Leon L, et al. Neovascularization after great saphenous vein ablation. Eur J Vasc Endovasc Surg 2006; 31: 219–22.
66. Lurie F, Creton D, Eklof B, et al. Prospective randomised study of endovenous radiofrequency obliteration (closure) versus ligation and vein stripping (EVOLVeS): two-year follow-up. Eur J Vasc Endovasc Surg 2005; 29: 67–73.
67. Rautio T, Ohinmaa A, Perala J, et al. Endovenous obliteration versus conventional stripping operation in the treatment of primary varicose veins: a randomized controlled trial with comparison of the costs. J Vasc Surg 2002; 35: 958–65.
68. Perälä J, Rautio T, Biancari F, et al. Radiofrequency endovenous obliteration versus stripping of the long saphenous vein in the management of primary varicose veins: 3-year outcome of a randomized study. Ann Vasc Surg 2005; 19: 669–72.
69. Guex JJ. Foam sclerotherapy: an overview of use for primary venous insufficiency. Semin Vasc Surg 2005; 18: 25–9.
70. Guex JJ, Hamel-Desnos C. Quelle technique pour la sclérose des varices? Sang Thrombose Vaisseaux 2006; 18: 441–5.
71. Milleret R. Garandeau C, Brel D, Allaert FA. Sclérose des grandes saphènes à la mousse délivrée par un cathéter écho-guidé sur veine vide "Alpha-Technique." Phlebologie 2004; 57: 15–20.
72. Barrett JM, Allen B, Ockelford A, Goldman MP. Microfoam ultrasound-guided sclerotherapy of varicose veins in 100 legs. Dermatol Surg 2004; 30: 6–12.
73. Smith PC. Chronic venous disease treated by ultrasound guided foam sclerotherapy. Eur J Vasc Endovasc Surg 2006; 32: 577–83.
74. Vidal-Michel JP, Bourrel Y, Emsallem J, Bonerandi JJ. Respect chirurgical des crosses saphènes internes modérement incontinentes par "effet siphon" chez les patients variqueux. Phlebologie 1993; 1: 143–7.
75. Zamboni P, Cisno C, Marchetti F, et al. Reflux elimination without any ablation or disconnection of the saphenous vein. a haemodynamic model for venous surgery. Eur J Vasc Endovasc Surg 2001; 21: 361–9.
76. Walsh JC, Bergan JJ, Beeman S, Comer TP. Femoral venous reflux abolished by greater saphenous vein stripping. Ann Vasc Surg 1994; 8: 566–70.
77. Sales CM, Bilof ML, Petrillo KA, Luka NL. Correction of lower extremity deep venous incompetence by ablation of superficial venous reflux. Ann Vasc Surg 1996; 10: 186–9.
78. Puggioni A, Lurie F, Kistner RL, Eklof B. How often is deep venous reflux eliminated after saphenous vein ablation? J Vasc Surg 2003; 38: 517–21.
79. Creton D. Diamater Reduction of the proximal long saphenous vein after ablation of a distal incompetent tributary. Dermatol Surg 1999; 25: 394–7.
80. Abu-Own A, Scurr JH, Coleridge Smith PD. Saphenous vein reflux without incompetence at the saphenofemoral junction. Br J Surg 1994; 81: 1452–4.
81. Pichot O, Sessa C, Bosson JL. Duplex imaging analysis of the long saphenous vein reflux: basis for strategy of endovenous obliteration treatment. Int Angiol 2002; 21: 333–6.
82. Wong JK, Duncan JL, Nichols DM. Whole-leg duplex mapping for varicose veins: observations on patterns of reflux in recurrent and primary legs, with clinical correlation. Eur J Vasc Endovasc Surg 2003; 25: 267–75.
83. Pittaluga P, Chastanet S, Guex JJ. Great saphenous vein stripping with preservation of the sapheno–femoral confluence: hemodynamic and clinical results. J Vasc Surg 2008; 47: 1300–5.
84. Puggioni A, Kalra M, Carmo M, et al. Endovenous laser therapy and radiofrequency ablation of the great saphenous vein: analysis of early efficacy and complications. J Vasc Surg 2005; 42: 488–93.
85. Perrin M, Guex JJ, Ruckley CV, et al., and the REVAS group. Recurrent varices after surgery (REVAS): a consensus document. Cardiovasc Surg 2000; 8: 233–45.
86. Schanzer H, Skladany M. Varicose vein surgery with preservation of the saphenous vein: a comparison between high ligation–avulsion versus saphenofemoral banding valvuloplasty–avulsion. J Vasc Surg 1994; 20: 684–7.
87. De Ross KP, Nieman FH, Neumann HA. Ambulatory phlebectomy versus compression sclerotherapy: results of a randomized controlled trial. Dermatol Surg 2003; 29: 221–6.
88. Pittaluga P, Marionneau N, Creton D, et al. Traitement chirurgical des varices des membres inférieurs: approche moderne. Phlebologie 2004; 3: 149–56.
89. Creton D. Faire moins pour faire mieux. Phlebologie 2006; 59: 67–72.
90. Guex JJ. Clinical methods for sclerotherapy of varicose veins. In: Goldman MP, Bergan JJ, Guex JJ, eds. Sclerotherapy: Treatment of Varicose and Telengiectatic Leg Veins, 4th edn. Philadelphia: Mosby Elsevier, 2007: 284.

16 Efficacy of polidocanol foam compared with polidocanol liquid in sclerotherapy of venous insufficiency

Takashi Yamaki

Introduction

Polidocanol (hydroxypolytetradodecane) was originally developed as a local anesthetic, and is now the most frequently used detergent sclerosing solution in Europe. In Japan, it is the only sclerosant that has been approved by the Japanese Ministry of Health, Labor and Welfare, in 2006. It is also commonly used in the United States; however, it is not yet approved by the Food and Drug Administration (FDA) as a pharmaceutical product. Following the introduction of sclerosing foam, many phlebologists are now in favor of the use of polidocanol foam instead of polidocanol liquid. However, few studies have focused on the efficacy of polidocanol foam compared with polidocanol liquid in the sclerotherapy of venous insufficiency.

Historically, Orbach first described the macrobubble foam preparation with sclerosing solution in 1950.[1] Using his technique, however, only 20% of the sclerosant was transformed into foam, with relatively large bubbles of irregular shape, and side-effects caused by this method led to its abandonment.[2] Therefore, foam sclerotherapy did not become popular until the mid-1990s after the introduction of new methods of formulating sclerosing solutions.[3–9] There have been several different methods reported to produce foam forms. In 1997, Cabrera and associates started the production of complex foam with carbon dioxide and an unknown tension-active agent.[4] Monfreux described a technique that generated a simple foam with air in glass syringe.[5] Henriet reported his experience using Monfreux's technique for minor varices.[6,7] Mingo-Garcia developed a special device for producing a foam form with compressed air.[8] In 2000, Tessari reported a new method for the production of foam using two syringes connected with a three-way stopcock, and it has been widely accepted as producing a stable foam.[10]

Producing polidocanol foam

Three methods are recommended for preparation of stable foam according to the European consensus meeting on foam sclerotherapy.[11] Of these, sclerosing foam is easily produced by Tessari's method using two syringes and a three-way stopcock. Basically, 1% or 3% polidocanol is used. A syringe of 5 mL capacity is filled with 0.5 mL of polidocanol solution, and 2.5 mL of air are aspirated with another syringe of 5 mL. The two syringes are attached to a three-way stopcock, and the stable sclerosing foam is obtained by mixing the contents through multiple passages between the two syringes.

Patient selection

Generally, patients who have primary valvular insufficiency with reflux in the superficial and perforating veins are good candidates for foam sclerotherapy. In principle, all vein calibers with primary valvular insufficiency and recurrent varicose veins are suitable for foam sclerotherapy.[11] The larger the diameter of the vein, the more viscous the foam should be to obtain better results, and a lower diameter threshold exists for using viscous foams. In contrast, an upper diameter threshold is recognized with liquid foam, although no lower caliber limit exists with viscous foams.[11] Favorable results are also obtained in patients with symptomatic venous malformations.[12–14]

Compression sclerotherapy is best performed on an ambulatory basis. Therefore, sclerotherapy should not be performed on patients who need long-distance travel or who are bedridden. Patients with known allergic reaction to sclerosant and previous history of deep vein thrombosis and/or pulmonary embolism should not be treated with sclerotherapy. Patients who have known thrombophilia, a family history of thromboembolism, or severe arterial insufficiency of the limbs (stage 3 or 4) are also excluded from treatment with sclerosing solutions. Systemic disease and hyperthyroidism are absolute contraindications for sclerotherapy.[15]

Diagnostics before sclerotherapy

Proper evaluation of the patients is key to obtaining successful results. Diagnostic examination includes medical history, clinical examination and Doppler ultrasonography. Nowadays, duplex scanning is considered an important front-line test in patients with primary valvular insufficiency. Duplex scanning can detect the distribution of venous reflux as well as the extent of reflux. Over 90% of patients with primary valvular insufficiency have superficial venous insufficiency with or without deep and perforating vein incompetence.[16] Even in patients with combined superficial and deep vein insufficiency, ablation of reflux in the superficial venous system may lead to abolishment of deep vein reflux. Therefore, foam sclerotherapy is a good treatment option for these patients.

Additionally, functional testing can detect improvement of venous function. Recent studies have shown that air plethysmography (APG) can provide quantitative measurements of venous reflux, and the amount of reflux is closely related to disease severity.[17,18] Combination with noninvasive diagnostic testing is also useful in the follow-up of patients after sclerotherapy.

Duplex-guided sclerotherapy

Theoretically, duplex-guided sclerotherapy should give improved results when treating a refluxing great saphenous vein (GSV). Using duplex guidance, safe injections are carried out by an experienced sclerotherapist.[19,20] Bishop and associates reported a GSV obliteration rate of only 6% when treating the refluxing GSV without duplex guidance.[21] In contrast, Kanter and associates demonstrated recanalization rates of 24.1% at 1 year and 35.7% at 2 years with duplex-guided sclerotherapy, which appears to be superior to that achieved by conventional sclerotherapy.[22] At present, a wide range of different practices are being performed in sclerotherapy. At the consensus conference on sclerotherapy held in Padua in 1994–95, duplex-guided sclerotherapy was recommended for lesser saphenous varicose veins, anterior saphenous varicose veins, recurrent varicose veins, perforators and obese patients.[23] No agreement had been reached regarding the need for duplex-guided sclerotherapy, or the advantages of this treatment, for GSV incompetence.[22] At the European consensus meeting on foam sclerotherapy held in Tegernsee in 2003, however, duplex guidance was recommended for GSV incompetence, because foam is easily identified by duplex scanning, and the initial effects are visible in real time.[11]

Comparative study between duplex-guided foam sclerotherapy and liquid sclerotherapy

To confirm the safety and efficacy of duplex-guided polidocanol foam sclerotherapy (DGFS), and to compare the preliminary results of hemodynamic changes between DGFS and duplex-guided polidocanol liquid sclerotherapy (DGLS), we conducted a comparative study in patients with superficial venous insufficiency.[23]

Patients

Between 2001 and 2002, 77 limbs in 77 patients with isolated GSV incompetence were selected for duplex-guided sclerotherapy. The patients comprised 15 males and 62 females, ranging in age from 21 to 84 years (mean 54.6 years). Of these, 37 limbs were treated with DGFS and the remaining 40 limbs were treated with DGLS. All of the patients' lesions were classifiable according to the CEAP classification into no signs of venous disease (C_0), telangiectasias or reticular veins (C_1), varicose veins (C_2), edema (C_3), changes in the skin and subcutaneous tissue ($C_{4a,b}$), or chronic ulcers (C_5 and C_6). Patients with myocardial ischemia, with arterial insufficiency (ankle–brachial index <0.8) or with active thrombophlebitis (i.e., those with active ulcers) were excluded. The follow-up period of the patients was 12 months.

Duplex scanning

A pretreatment examination was performed to detect venous reflux at the saphenofemoral junction (SFJ) and in the GSV. Venous reflux was assessed with the patient in a standing position, by applying distal manual compression followed by sudden release. Venous reflux was considered to be present if the duration of reflux exceeded 0.5 s. Venous obstruction and recanalization were screened by serial post-treatment duplex examination (Figures 16.1–16.3).

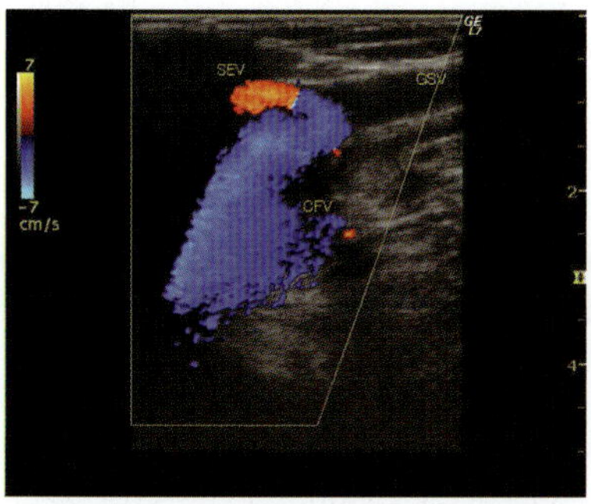

Figure 16.1 Postsclerotherapy duplex scanning showing an occluded great saphenous vein (GSV) with patent superficial epigastric vein (SEV) at the saphenofemoral junction (SFJ). CFV, common femoral vein

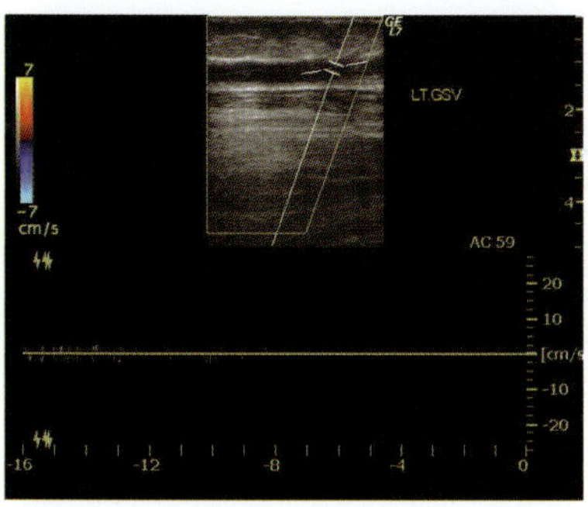

Figure 16.2 Postsclerotherapy duplex scanning showing an occluded great saphenous vein (GSV) in the above-knee segment

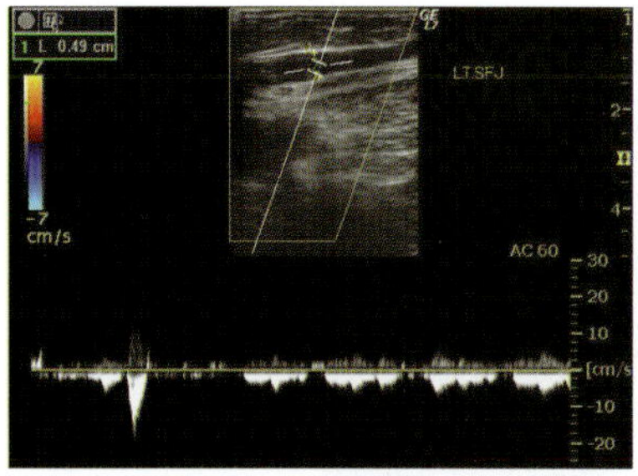

Figure 16.3 Postsclerotherapy duplex scanning showing a partially recanalized great saphenous vein (GSV) with no reflux in the above-knee segment

Air plethysmography

Pretreatment APG measurements were obtained, including the venous filling index (VFI), ejection fraction (EF), and residual venous fraction (RVF). Post-treatment APG analysis was performed 3, 6, 9 and 12 months after the sclerotherapy.

Duplex-guided sclerotherapy

The sclerosing foam was produced by Tessari's method using 1% and 3% polidocanol. Each visible varicose tributary vein draining into the GSV was injected first, with 2 mL of 1% polidocanol foam or 1% polidocanol liquid. Then 0.5 mL of 3% polidocanol foam or 3% polidocanol liquid were injected under duplex guidance, starting 3–4 cm distal to the SFJ, and a second injection was

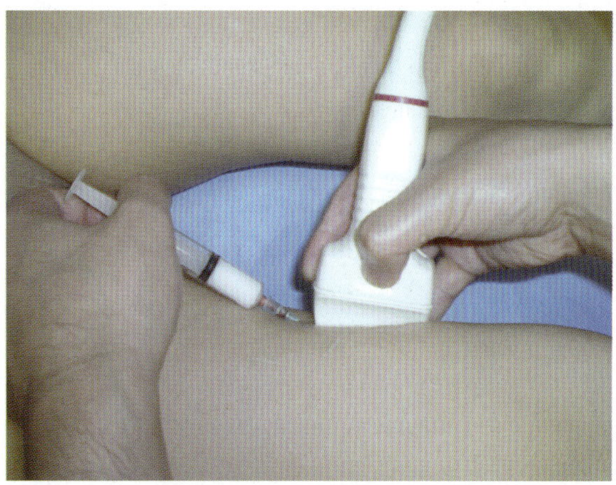

Figure 16.4 Duplex-guided polidocanol foam sclerotherapy of the great saphenous vein

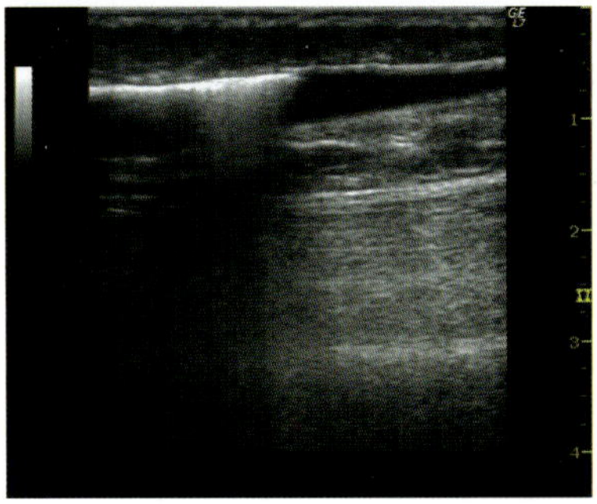

Figure 16.5 Duplex scanning showing the injection of foam

made 5–10 cm distal to the initial point with 0.5 mL of 3% polidocanol foam or 3% polidocanol liquid (Figures 14.4 and 14.5). Immediately after sclerotherapy, compression pads and elastic bandages were applied, and kept on continuously for the first two days. All patients were encouraged to ambulate after the treatment. On postsclerotherapy day 3, elastic bandages and compression pads were removed, and a Class II thigh-high compression stocking was applied.

Statistical analysis

Wilcoxon's nonparametric rank sum test and chi-square analysis or Fisher's exact test were used to evaluate differences between group of patients. Statistical significance was defined as $P < 0.05$.

Results

There were no significant differences in age, male-to-female ratio or clinical presentation between the two groups, and CEAP clinical classes were all matched (Table 16.1).

The incidence of venous reflux at the 12-month follow-up point is shown in Table 16.2. Duplex scanning demonstrated complete occlusion in the GSV for DGFS in 25 limbs (67.6%), which was a significantly higher proportion than for the DGLS (7 limbs, 17.5%, $P < 0.0001$). There was no statistically significant difference in the proportion of partial recanalization without reflux ($P = 0.580$). Similarly, there was no significant difference in the proportion of partial recanalization with reflux between the two groups ($P = 0.171$). Complete recanalization with reflux was detected in 5 patients (13.5%) in the DGFS group, and 22 patients (55%) in the DGLS group, which was statistically significant ($P = 0.0001$). Recurrent varicose veins were found in 3 patient (8.1%) in the DGFS group, and 10 patients (25%) in the DGLS group. This was statistically significant ($P = 0.048$; Figure 16.6A, B).

Table 16.3 demonstrates the pre-and post-treatment APG examinations. The pretreatment APG examinations showed reflux in both groups (4.34 ± 2.22 mL/s and 4.39 ± 2.53 mL/s, respectively). In the DGFS group, VFI values remained normal during the subsequent follow-up examinations, whereas in the DGLS group, VFI began to increase, and there was a significant difference at 6 months between the DGFS and the DGLS groups

Table 16.1 Baseline characteristics of the study patients (derived from Yamaki et al[24]). There were no statistical differences in age, gender, and CEAP clinical manifestations between the two groups

	Foam (*n* = 37)	Liquid (*n* = 40)	*P*-value
Age (years) ± SD	54.3 ± 13.9	54.8 ± 14.7	0.617[a]
Female sex	30 (81.1%)	32 (80%)	0.905[b]
CEAP clinical class[c]			
C_2	27 (73.0%)	31 (77.5%)	0.645[b]
C_3	2 (5.4%)	4 (10%)	0.577[b]
$C_{4a,b}$	5 (13.5%)	3 (7.5%)	0.388[b]
C_5	3 (8.1%)	2 (5%)	0.580[b]

Foam = duplex-guided polidocanol foam sclerotherapy; Liquid = duplex-guided polidocanol liquid sclerotherapy.
[a]Wilcoxon's nonparametric rank sum test.
[b]Pearson's χ^2 test or Fisher's exact test.
[c]CEAP clinical classification: C_0, no visible or palpable signs of venous disease; C_1, telangiectases, reticular veins; C_2, varicose veins; C_3, edema without skin changes; C_4, changes in the skin and subcutaneous tissue; C_5, healed ulcer; C_6, active ulcer.

Table 16.2 Incidence of occlusion, recanalization and recurrence rate after treatment (derived from Yamaki et al[24]). There was a statistically higher proportion of occlusion in duplex-guided polidocanol-foam sclerotherapy, and there was a statistically higher proportion of reflux in duplex-guided polidocanol liquid sclerotherapy. Recurrence was statistically predominant in duplex-guided polidocanol liquid sclerotherapy

Great saphenous vein	Foam (n = 37)	Liquid (n = 40)	P-value
Occluded	25 (67.6%)	7 (17.5%)	< 0.0001
Partial recanalization with no reflux	3 (8.1%)	2 (5%)	0.580
Partial recanalization with reflux	4 (10.8%)	9 (22.5%)	0.171
Complete recanalization with reflux	5 (13.5%)	22 (55%)	0.0001
Recurrence	3 (8.1%)	10 (25%)	0.048

Foam = duplex-guided polidocanol-foam sclerotherapy; Liquid = duplex-guided polidocanol-liquid sclerotherapy.

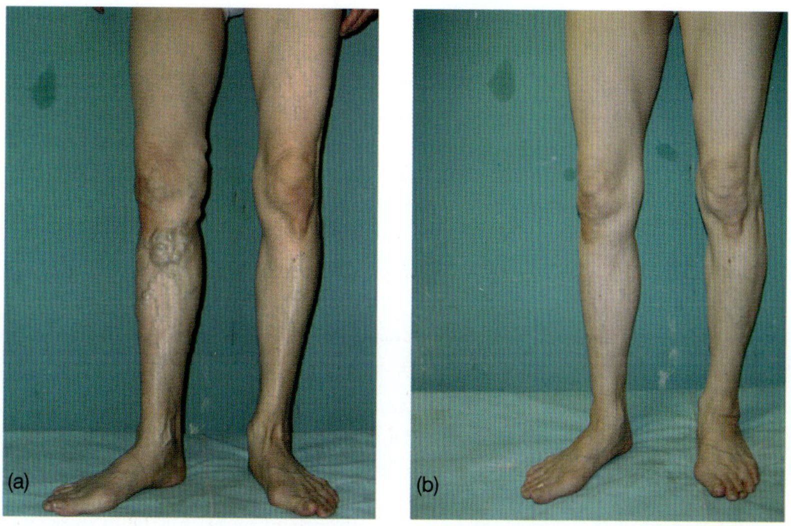

Figure 16.6 (a) Patient showing great saphenous vein incompetence with elongated tortuous varicose veins. (b) No recurrent varicose veins, 12 months after one session of duplex-guided polidocanol foam sclerotherapy

Table 16.3 Comparison of hemodynamic variables before and after treatment (derived from Yamaki et al[24]). Values are expressed as mean ± SD. VFI began to increase in duplex-guided polidocanol-liquid sclerotherapy, and there was a significant difference at 6 months between the two groups. At 9 months, there was a significant difference in RVF between the two groups, and the RVF value continued to improve in duplex-guided polidocanol foam sclerotherapy

	Pretreatment	3 months	6 months	9 months	12 months
Venous filling index (VFI) (mL/s):					
Foam	4.3 ± 2.2	1.4 ± 0.4	1.1 ± 0.4[a]	1.2 ± 0.6[b]	1.2 ± 0.8[c]
Liquid	4.4 ± 2.5	2.3 ± 1.6	2.2 ± 0.6	2.2 ± 0.6	2.3 ± 0.7
Ejection fraction (EF) (%):					
Foam	51.0 ± 22.9	55.8 ± 14.6	54.4 ± 20.7	51.2 ± 16.8	52.0 ± 13.5
Liquid	47.7 ± 18.5	58.1 ± 16.6	54.2 ± 40.7	51.9 ± 39.4	50.7 ± 40.4
Residual venous fraction (RVF) (%):					
Foam	39.6 ± 19.9	28.6 ± 9.2	26.9 ± 22.8	21.2 ± 22.5[c]	22.7 ± 26.1[c]
Liquid	36.7 ± 19.8	35.8 ± 16.5	37.0 ± 14.6	35.6 ± 22.8	39.5 ± 16.8

Foam = duplex-guided polidocanol foam sclerotherapy; Liquid = duplex-guided polidocanol liquid sclerotherapy.
[a]Foam vs liquid, $P < 0.0005$. [b]Foam vs liquid, $P < 0.0003$. [c]Foam vs liquid, $P < 0.033$.

($P < 0.0005$). There was no significant difference in EF value between pre- and post-treatment examinations in either group. At 9 months, there was a significant difference in RVF between the two groups, and the RVF value continued to improve in the DGFS group ($P = 0.033$). No adverse events were found using either foam or liquid sclerosing solutions in this series.

Conclusions

After the introduction of the foam form of sclerosing solution, foam sclerotherapy rapidly gained popularity. However, few studies have compared the safety and efficacy between polidocanol foam and polidocanol liquid. This comparative study confirmed that polidocanol foam has extensive advantages over polidocanol liquid. A variety of venous disorders can be treated with foam sclerotherapy with a low rate of adverse events.

References

1. Orbach EJ. Contribution to the therapy of the varicose complex. J Int Coll Surg 1950; 13: 765–71.
2. Henriet JP. History of foam In: Foam Sclerotherapy: State of the Art. Editions Phlébologique Françaises. Paris: 2002.
3. Tessari L, Cavezzi A, Frullini A. Preliminary experience with a new sclerosing foam in the treatment of varicose veins. Dermatol Surg 2001; 27: 58–60.
4. Cabrera Garrido JR, Cabrera Garcia-Olmedo JR, Garcia-Olmedo Dominguez MA. Elargissement des limites de la sclérothérapie: nouveaux produits sclérosants. Phlebologie 1997; 50: 181–8.
5. Monfreux A. Traitement˙ sclérosant des troncs saphènies et leurs collatérals de gros caliber par le method MUS. Phlebologie 1997; 50: 351–3.
6. Henriet JP. Un an de pratique quotidienne de la sclérothérapie par mousse de polidocanol (veines réticulaires et télangiectasies): faisabilité, resultants, complications. Phlebologie 1997; 50: 351–3.
7. Henriet JP. Expérience durant trois années de la mousee de polidocanol dans le traitement des varices réticulaires et des varicosités. Phlebologie 1999; 52: 277–82.
8. Mingo-Garcia J. Esclerosis venosa con espuma: Foam Medical System. Rev Esp Med Cir Cosmet 1999; 7: 29–31.
9. Benigni JP, Sadoun S, Thirion V, et al. Télangiectasies et varices réticulaires. Traitement par la mousee d'Aetoxisclérol à 0.25%. Présentation d'une etude pilote. Phlebologie 1999; 52: 29–31.
10. Tessari L. Nouvelle technique d'obtention de la scleromousee. Phlebologie 2000; 53: 129.
11. Breu FX, Guggenbichler S. European consensus meeting on foam sclerotherapy, 4–6 April, 2003, Tegernsee, Germany. Dermatol Surg 2004; 30: 709–17.
12. Yamaki T, Nozaki M, Sasaki K. Color duplex-guided sclerotherapy for the treatment of venous malformations. Dermatol Surg 2000; 26: 323–8.
13. Yamaki T, Nozaki M, Fujiwara O, Yoshida E. Duplex-guided foam sclerotherapy for the treatment of the symptomatic venous malformations of the face. Dermatol Surg 2002; 28: 619–22.
14. Bergan JJ, Pascarella L, Mekenas L. Venous disorders: treatment with sclerosant foam. J Cardiovasc Surg 2006; 47: 9–18.
15. Rabe E, Pannier-Fischer F, Gerlach H, et al. Guidelines for Sclerotherapy of Varicose Veins (ICD 10: I83.0, I83.1, I83.2, and I83.9). Dermatol Surg 2004; 30: 687–93.
16. Yamaki T, Nozaki M, Fujiwara O, Yoshida E. Comparative evaluation of duplex-derived parameters in patients with chronic venous insufficiency: correlation with clinical manifestations. J Am Coll Surg 2002; 195: 822–30.
17. Yamaki T, Nozaki M, Sasaki K. Quantitative assessment of superficial venous insufficiency using duplex ultrasound and air plethysmography. Dermatol Surg 2000; 26: 644–8.
18. Yamaki T, Nozaki M, Sakurai H, et al. Quantification of venous reflux parameters using duplex scanning and air plethysmograpy. Phlebology 2007; 22: 20–8.
19. Schadeck M. Ultrasound guided sclerotherapy In: Schadeck M, ed. Duplex and Phlebology. Napoli: Gnocchi, 1994: 115–28.
20. Zummo M, Forrestal M. Sclerotherapy of the long saphenous vein: a prospective duplex controlled comparative study. Phlebology 1994; Suppl. 1: 571–3.
21. Bishop CCR, Fronek HS, Fronek A, et al. Real-time color duplex scanning after sclerotherapy of the greater saphenous vein. J Vasc Surg 1991; 14: 505–10.
22. Kanter A, Thibault P. Saphenofemoral incompetence treated by ultrasound-guided sclerotherapy. Dermatol Surg 1996; 22: 648–52.
23. Baccaglini U, Spreafico G, Castoro C, Sorrentino P. Consensus conference on varicose veins of lower extremity. Phlebology 1997; 12: 2–16.
24. Yamaki T, Nozaki M, Iwasaka S. Comparative study of duplex-guided foam sclerotherapy and duplex-guided liquid sclerotherapy for the treatment of superficial venous insufficiency. Dermatol Surg 2004; 30: 718–22.

17 Studies on safety of foam sclerotherapy

Nick Morrison

Introduction

Whilst many studies in the literature mention the safety of foam sclerotherapy anecdotally,[1–11] and some studies examine specific complications of foam,[12–14] reports that critically examine the overall safety of foam for sclerosis of abnormal leg veins remain scant.[15–17]

In order to shed more light on the subject of the physiological effects of foamed sclerosants, we have conducted a series of clinical trials and exercises designed firstly to examine the safety profile of foamed sclerosants, and then to look at specific effects of foam sclerotherapy.

Study 1

Objective. This was a prospective clinical trial, enrolling patients with truncal or nontruncal superficial venous insufficiency, treated with ultrasound-guided injection of 1% polidocanol air-based foam, analyzing rates of toxicity and complications in the perioperative period, and establishing an adverse effect profile.

Materials and methods. Forty-nine patients with truncal or nontruncal venous insufficiency, all of whom had had previous ablation of the proximal great saphenous vein, were treated with 1% polidocanol foam, injected under ultrasound guidance into the distal great or small saphenous veins and/or their tributaries. Polidocanol foam was produced by the Tessari method, using room air and 1% Sclerovein®, mixed in a 4-to-1 ratio. Injected volumes ranged from 8 to 52 mL (mean: 26 mL). Nurse-conducted patient interviews and monitoring of blood pressure, pulse rate, respiratory rate, electrocardiogram and pulse oximetry were carried out preoperatively, at 15-minute intervals during treatment, immediately postoperatively, and 30 and 60 minutes after completion of treatment (longer if symptoms occurred). Patients were then interviewed 2, 6 and 24 hours post-treatment. Adverse effects were monitored for 24 hours or until resolution, and included changes in blood pressure, pulse rate, electrocardiogram or partial oxygen pressure (Po_2), chest discomfort, dry cough, dizziness, visual disturbances and nausea.

Results. Statistically significant decreases in heart rate occurred ($P < 0.001$), less than 5 bpm, which were not physiologically significant. Blood pressure, respiratory rate, electrocardiogram, and Po_2 did not change significantly during or for 60 minutes after the injection session ($P > 0.05$). The most commonly occurring adverse effects were dry cough, chest discomfort and visual disturbances, although only with dry cough was there a positive correlation with increasing volume of injectate. Chest discomfort was seen in 8.2% of patients (4/49). Visual disturbances were experienced by 8.2% (4/49). Other adverse effects included dizziness reported in 12% and nausea in 4%. Adverse effects rarely lasted more than one to four hours. No deep vein thromboses (DVTs) were detected by follow-up duplex scan performed in response to symptoms.

Conclusions. Ultrasound-guided injection of polidocanol foam, in large volumes, appears to be associated with few, if any, significant complications, although some short-lived adverse effects do occur. Concerning these adverse effects, only dry cough appeared to have a direct correlation with the volume of foam injected.

Study 2

As interest grew in replacing the air used to produce foam with a more soluble and diffusible gas,[4–6,9] a second clinical trial was conducted to test the theory that, because of its presumably more rapid dissolution carbon dioxide (CO_2)-based foam would produce fewer adverse effects than air-based foam.

Objective. This was a prospective clinical trial, involving patients with previous truncal or nontruncal superficial venous insufficiency, treated with ultrasound-guided injection of 1% polidocanol CO_2-based foam, analyzing rates of toxicity and complications in the perioperative period, and establishing an adverse effect profile.

Materials and methods. This study was a follow up to Study 1, and was performed in precisely the same manner on 128 patients who also had previously undergone saphenous vein ablation procedures. In this study, pure CO_2 instead of air was used to produce the foamed sclerosant and the range of injected foam was 6–45 mL (mean: 26 mL).

Results. As in Study 1, no physiologically significant changes were seen whilst monitoring blood pressure, electrocardiogram, heart rate, respiratory rate, or Po_2. Dry cough, chest tightness, and dizziness occurred in 1.6% (2/128), 3.9% (5/128) and 3.1% (4/128) respectively, statistically significantly less often than with air-based foam ($P = 0.02$). Visual disturbances and nausea were seen to trend lower to an incidence of 3.1% (4/128) and 2% (3/128), respectively, compared with the air-based foam group ($P = 0.15$) (Table 17.1).

Conclusions. Adverse effects decreased statistically significantly (or trended downward) if CO_2 rather than air was employed to produce the sclerosing foam.

Table 17.1 Comparison of side-effects of patients treated with CO_2-based foam and air-based foam

Symptom	Air	CO_2	χ^2
Chest tightness	9 (18%)	4 (3.1%)	$P < 0.001$
Dry cough	8 (16%)	2 (1.6%)	$P < 0.001$
Dizziness	6 (12%)	4 (3.1%)	$P = 0.019$
Metallic/medicinal taste	0 (0%)	2 (1.6%)	$P = 0.39$
Nausea	2 (4%)	3 (2%)	$P = 0.53$
Circumoral paresthesia	0 (0%)	1 (0.8%)	$P = 0.53$

Study 3

Another specific safety concern regarding complications of foam sclerotherapy is the incidence of DVT.[2,6,8,17–19] In our center, we noticed a seemingly high incidence of thrombosis in duplicated femoral vein segments following ultrasound-guided foam sclerotherapy. This study was conducted to see if the presence of a duplicated femoral vein represents a risk factor for thrombosis.

Objective. Because the incidence of duplicated femoral vein segment had been reported as high as 25%,[20] and the incidence of deep vein DVT following ultrasound-guided foam sclerotherapy is generally reported to be <1%,[8,17–19] the aim was to determine if the presence of a duplicated femoral vein segment is a risk factor for development of DVT following ultrasound-guided foam sclerotherapy.

Materials and methods. Forty-three patients with duplex ultrasound-documented true duplicated segments of femoral veins were treated with ultrasound-guided foam sclerotherapy for superficial venous insufficiency, using a foam volume range of 1.5–9 mL. Polidocanol or sodium tetradecyl sulfate (STS) at 1–3% foamed with air or CO_2 gas was injected into truncal and nontruncal superficial veins of the lower extremity. Standard postsclerotherapy treatment included immediate and continued ambulation and compression with 30–40 mmHg hose for 3 weeks. Detailed duplex examination of the treated leg was conducted within 48 hours, including evaluation of the common femoral vein, femoral vein, profunda femoral vein, popliteal vein, posterior tibial veins, anterior tibial veins, peroneal veins and gastrocnemius veins. If thrombosis of any vein was identified, follow-up duplex examination was continued until resolution or stabilization of the thrombosis was confirmed. If no thrombosis was identified, the patient was re-examined at 1 week and 6 weeks.

Results. Five of 43 patients (8.6%) were found to have complete thrombosis of the duplicated femoral vein segment. (Figure 17.1) In four of the five patients with thrombosis, 3% STS air-based foam was used; in the

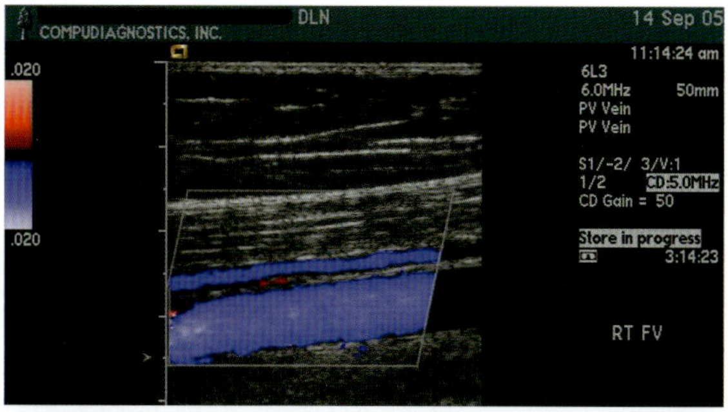

(a)

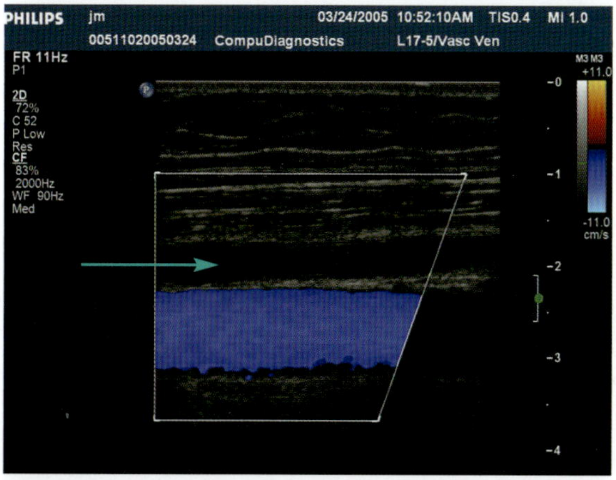

(b)

Figure 17.1 (a) color Doppler showing antegrade flow in a duplicated femoral vein segment. (b) Color Doppler after foam sclerotherapy showing a thrombosed duplicated femoral vein segment (green arrow). (Courtesy of Compudiagnostics—D Neuhardt)

remaining patient, 3% polidocanol CO_2-based foam was used. No other DVTs were identified.

Conclusion. The presence of a duplicated femoral vein segment in patients undergoing ultrasound-guided foam sclerotherapy appears to be a risk factor for DVT in the duplicated segment.

Because of uncertainty regarding the extent to which foam travels from the target vein and the belief expressed in scientific assemblies that the dispersal of foam, once injected, could be controlled and specifically prevented from entering the deep venous system, a series of exercises were designed and conducted to follow the course of foam injected into peripheral superficial leg veins.

Exercise 1

Objective. The aim of the exercise was to follow the course of foam from a peripheral vein injection site to the deep venous system and heart.

Materials and methods. Twenty-one patients undergoing ultrasound-guided foam sclerotherapy using 1% foamed sclerosant were injected with 1–2 mL of foamed sclerosant into a 1–2 mm peripheral superficial leg vein. The foam was produced by the standard Tessari method,[9] with a 4-to-1 ratio of room air to 1% liquid polidocanol. All patients had a preoperative transthoracic echocardiogram, which was negative for right-to-left shunts. All patients had simultaneous transthoracic echocardiography with ultrasound-guided injection of foam (Figure 17.2).

Results. Bubbles could be identified by ultrasound in the injected peripheral vein, perforator vein, deep venous system, inferior vena cava and the right heart 10–30 seconds after every injection. Furthermore, bubbles could still be seen in the right heart more than 2 minutes after each injection.

Conclusion. Small volumes of foamed sclerosants injected into peripheral venous leg tributaries are quickly and persistently identified within the perforators, deep venous system, inferior vena cava, and heart, even several minutes following the initial injection. Dispersal of foam microbubbles is rapid and extensive.

Exercise 2

Some patients undergoing ultrasound-guided foam sclerotherapy complain of neurologic or visual symptoms during or shortly after a sclerotherapy session. Because bubbles had been found to pass quickly to the right heart, the next exercise was designed to determine if a right-to-left shunt could be identified by means of the appearance of bubbles in the left heart.

Objective. Is it possible to reliably identify right-to-left shunting during ultrasound-guided foam sclerotherapy using simultaneous transthoracic echocardiography?

Materials and methods. Twenty-one patients with symptoms of visual disturbances, headache, or altered mentation following ultrasound-guided foam sclerotherapy were studied with additional ultrasound-guided foam sclerotherapy simultaneously with transthoracic

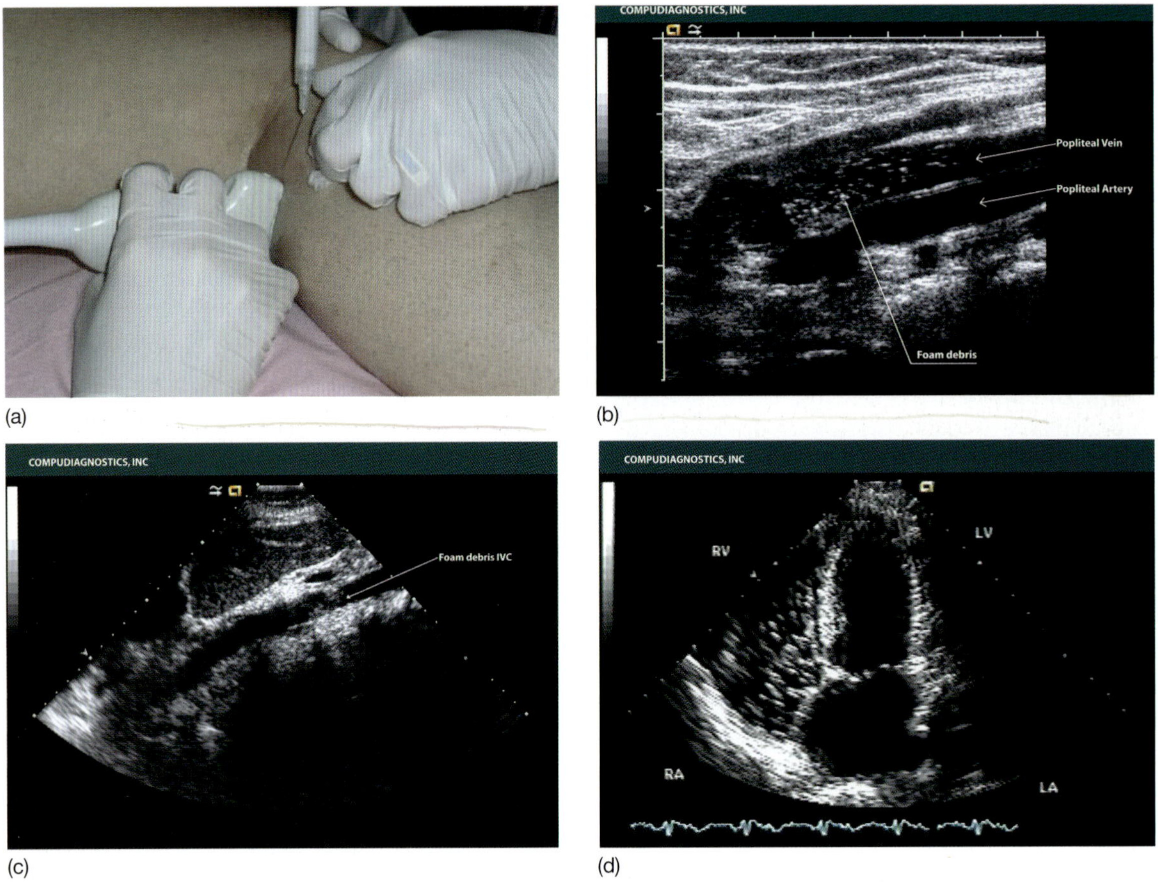

Figure 17.2 (a) Under ultrasound guidance, a 1 mm peripheral leg vein is injected with foam. (b) Popliteal vein with foam debris (arrow). (c) Abdominal inferior vena cava (IVC) with foam debris. (d) Foam debris opacifies the right atrium (RA) and right ventricle (RV). (Courtesy of Compudiagnostics—D Neuhardt)

echocardiography. For the latter study, the patients were positioned in a reversed Trendelenberg and modified left lateral decubitus position, during and after injection of 1–3 mL of foam into a peripheral leg vein. Pressure gradients were then established by asking patients to perform a Valsalva maneuver or to cough.

Results. No right-to-left shunts could be demonstrated on preoperative transthoracic echocardiography and none were seen immediately following ultrasound-guided foam injection into a peripheral leg vein, even though bubbles were readily identified in the right heart. However, following the establishment of pressure gradients with Valsalva maneuver or cough, right-to-left shunting in 7 of 21 patients (30%) was demonstrated with bubbles visible in the left heart (Figure 17.3). This ratio approximates that in the normal population expected to have patent foramen ovale.[21]

Conclusion. It is possible to reliably identify right-to-left shunts in patients undergoing peripheral leg vein ultrasound-guided foam sclerotherapy with the use of transthoracic echocardiography and the creation of a pressure gradient.

Exercise 3

Because bubbles could readily be identified in the left heart in patients with right-to-left shunts, the question arose as to whether bubble emboli could be identified by trancranial Doppler monitoring of the middle cerebral arteries in patients with proven right-to-left shunts.

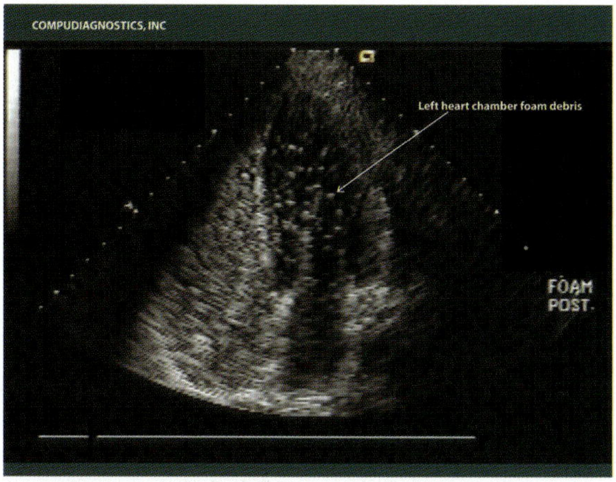

Figure 17.3 Arrow points to foam debris within the left heart. (Courtesy of Compudiagnostics—D Neuhardt)

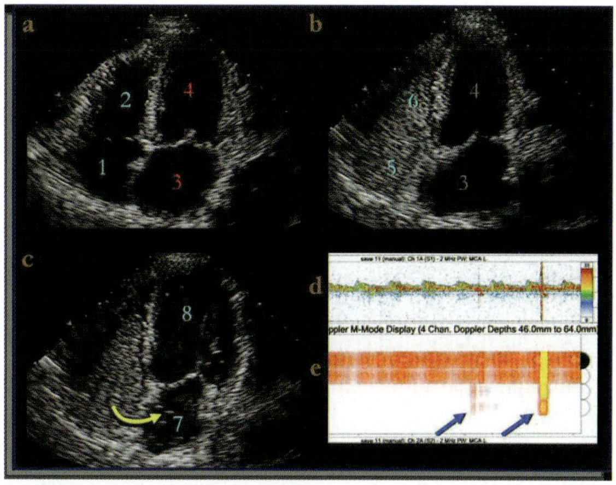

Figure 17.4 (a) Four-chamber view of the heart on transthoracic echocardiography. (b) Bubbles filling right atrium and ventricle following injection of foam sclerosant into a peripheral leg vein. (c) Bubbles (yellow arrow) progressing from right atrium through a patent foramen ovale into the left atrium. (d, e) Transcranial Doppler images depicting high-intensity transient signals (HITS) (blue arrows) in the middle cerebral artery following foam injection into a peripheral leg vein (Courtesy of Compudiagnostics—D Neuhardt)

Objective. The aim of this exercise was to examine the middle cerebral artery for emboli during and following ultrasound-guided foam sclerotherapy by means of transcranial Doppler via the temporal window in patients with known right-to-left shunts undergoing ultrasound-guided foam sclerotherapy.

Materials and methods. Seven patients were found to have right-to-left shunts during simultaneous ultrasound-guided foam sclerotherapy of peripheral superficial veins of the lower extremity and transthoracic echocardiography. These patients were re-examined, adding bilateral transcranial Doppler monitoring of their middle cerebral arteries. Volumes of 1–3 mL of foam were injected into a peripheral leg vein 1–2 mm in diameter under ultrasound guidance, with the patient in a modified, left lateral supine position (in order to permit simultaneous ultrasound-guided foam sclerotherapy, transthoracic echocardiography and transcranial Doppler monitoring), followed by multiple active calf pumps to mobilize the foam into the central circulation.

Results. Four of seven patients were found to have middle cerebral artery HITS (high-intensity transient signals) during the transcranial Doppler examination, confirmed with a 97% likelihood to be emboli (Figure 17.4).

Conclusions. Emboli can be detected by transcranial Doppler in patients with right-to-left shunts who are undergoing ultrasound-guided foam sclerotherapy.

Exercise 4

Because the exercise described above is cumbersome for patients, technologists and physicians, we attempted to simplify our investigations by designing a protocol wherein only bilateral transcranial Doppler monitoring would be performed during ultrasound-guided foam sclerotherapy on a series of patients in whom the status of any right-to-left shunting was unknown. We have observed that patients frequently will not develop neurologic or visual symptoms until they move upon completion of the foam sclerotherapy session. We examined the timing of the symptoms to test for a temporal correlation to emboli in the middle cerebral arteries.

Objective. The aim of this exercise was to identify the incidence of right-to-left shunt in patients undergoing ultrasound-guided foam sclerotherapy by means of bilateral transcranial monitoring of middle cerebral arteries, and determine whether there exists a temporal correlation between the onset of neurologic or visual symptoms and middle cerebral artery emboli.

Materials and methods. Ongoing investigation of 34 patients undergoing ultrasound-guided foam sclerotherapy of peripheral superficial veins of the lower extremities had continuous bilateral (when feasible) monitoring of the middle cerebral arteries from just prior to foam injection until 20 minutes after the last injection of foam. Foam volumes ranged from 5 to 37 mL injected over the course of 45 minutes. The patients were initially placed in a supine position and remained immobile following injection of foam. No cough or Valsalva maneuver was attempted.

Results (preliminary). Thus far, emboli have been identified in the middle cerebral arteries in 15/34 (44%) of patients following injection of foam ranging from 9 to 37 mL. No emboli were identified in patients injected with less than 9 mL of foam; thus, injection of foam volumes above 9 mL was associated with an increased risk of emboli. There was also a positive correlation between the volume of foam injected and the number of emboli seen. Furthermore, increased emboli were detectable 20 minutes after the last injection, when the patient transferred from a supine to a sitting position. Neurologic and/or visual symptoms were rarely reported, but when these symptoms occurred, it was usually when the patient made this transfer of position.

Conclusions. Transcranial Doppler monitoring of middle cerebral arteries in patients undergoing ultrasound-guided foam sclerotherapy will reliably identify emboli, confirmative of right-to-left shunts. Injection of less than 9 mL of foam was not associated with cerebral emboli, and the higher the volume of foam injected, the more cerebral emboli were identified. Further, increased numbers of middle cerebral artery emboli often occur concurrent with active patient movement and the (rare) onset of neurologic or visual symptoms in these patients. Immobilization of the patient for as long as 20 minutes following small-volume foam injection does not appear to be protective of cerebral bubble emboli or symptoms. Also, interestingly, a higher incidence of apparent right-to-left shunts is demonstrated in this study than might be expected based on historical data in the literature regarding such right-to-left shunts (data to be published).

Study 4

A major question that remains is whether neurologic or visual symptoms can be correlated with bubble emboli in the cerebral circulation. One could postulate that these emboli could lodge in the cerebral microcirculation, causing ischemia, which produces the transient symptoms described by patients. An elegant study was conducted by Eckmann et al,[12] sponsored in part by the manufacturer of a commercial foam preparation, to compare the flow characteristics of commercial foam with those of so-called "homemade" foam, such as is prepared in all vein treatment centers currently using foam sclerotherapy.

Objective. This study aimed to determine the relationship between polidocanol microfoam formulation and arteriolar embolization bubble lodging and clearance in vivo.

Materials and methods. Polidocanol microfoam formulations using different physiologic gas mixtures composed primarily of oxygen and CO_2 were mixed with venous blood and injected into the rat cremaster arterial microcirculation. Bubble dimensions and dynamics were recorded using intravital microscopy. This was, in essence, a comparison of so-called "homemade" foam (air-based polidocanol foam as produced by the majority of phlebologists using the Tessari method) and commercially prepared foam (Varisolve – Provensis, BTG).

Results. Bubble entry frequency, size and dynamics depended on microfoam formulation. Air-based bubbles lodged, obliterating blood flow. Varisolve bubbles entered, but either did not lodge or cleared within seconds. Bubble size and number were different among these microfoams. The commercially prepared foam bubbles were smaller than "homemade" foam bubbles, and did not appear to obstruct micro-arterial flow as did the bubbles from "homemade" foam.

Conclusions. The Varisolve formulations produced smaller embolism bubbles than occurred with air-based microfoam. Rapid clearance of Varisolve bubbles suggests that they are so small that they do not have adequate surface area available for significant binding interactions with arteriolar endothelium. Larger air-based bubbles obstruct arteriolar vessels and block blood flow.

Testing theories

Whilst Eckmann et al did not speculate as to whether neurologic or visual symptoms might be caused by obstruction in the cerebral arterial microcirculation by bubble emboli, several centers have postulated that certain maneuvers might have a protective effect on the cerebral circulation by limiting or preventing bubbles from arriving in the brain. We conducted a series of experiments designed to test the efficacy of these maneuvers in limiting or preventing the dispersal of micro-bubbles.

Theory 1

If the patient is kept in a moderate Trendelenberg position, foam injected into truncular veins of the leg under ultrasound guidance will "rise" to the distal leg rather than progress into the central circulation.

Method. An aliquot of 3 mL of 1% polidocanol air-based foam was injected into the great saphenous vein in the distal thigh under ultrasound guidance in 5 patients (Figure 17.5).

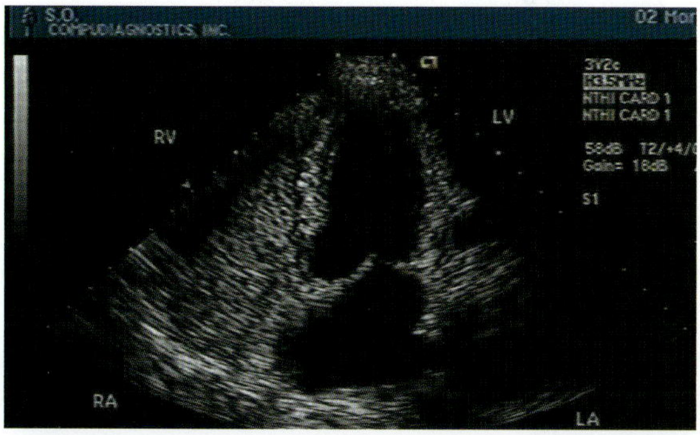

Figure 17.5 Four-chamber transthoracic echocardiogram 3 s following injection. Bubbles are seen to fill the right atrium and ventricle marked RV and RA to side. (Courtesy of Compudiagnostics – D Neuhardt)

Conclusion. The Trendelenberg position does not prevent foam from entering the central circulation.

Theory 2

Keeping patients immobile following ultrasound-guided foam sclerotherapy will prevent bubbles from dispersing into the central circulation.

Method. An aliquot of 2 mL of 1% polidocanol air-based foam was injected into a 1.7 mm peripheral leg vein under ultrasound guidance, with the patient immobile for over 10 minutes, whilst continuously monitoring the heart for bubbles using transthoracic echocardiography (Figure 17.6).

Conclusion. Having the patient remain immobile for a period of time following an ultrasound-guided foam

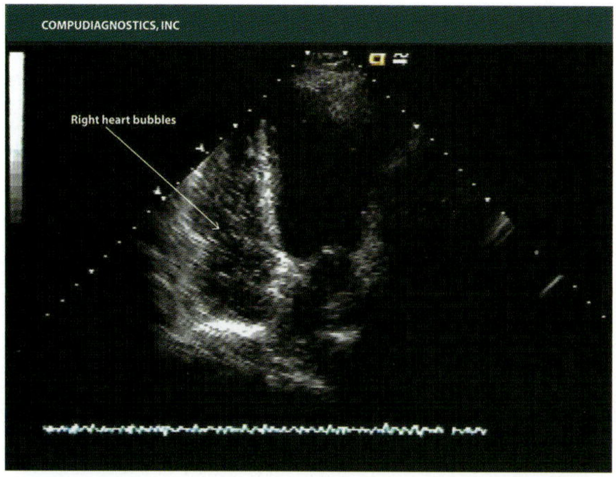

Figure 17.6 Four-chamber transthoracic echocardiogram following ultrasound-guided injection. Arrow points to foam debris within right heart. (Courtesy of Compudiagnostics – D Neuhardt)

injection into a peripheral leg vein will not prevent bubbles from entering the central circulation.

Theory 3

If the patient is kept immobile during ultrasound-guided foam sclerotherapy, bubbles will not pass into the left heart through a right-to-left shunt (Figure 17.7).

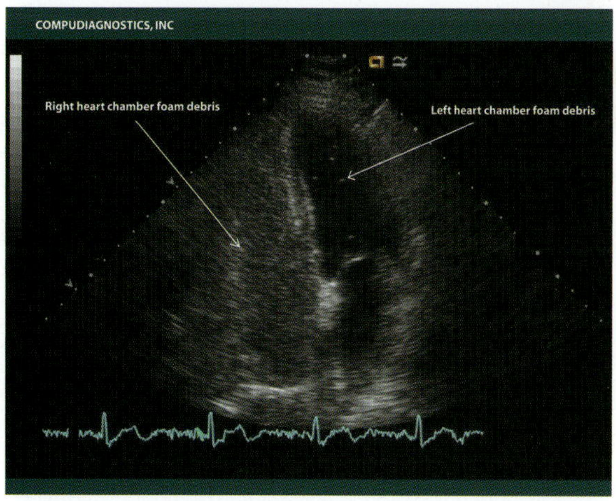

Figure 17.7 Four-chamber transthoracic view of the heart showing the right heart filled with bubbles (arrow), and bubbles in the left ventricle (arrow). (Courtesy of Compudiagnostics – D Neuhardt)

Conclusion. In patients with right-to-left shunts (whether or not the shunts have been diagnosed), keeping the patient immobile following ultrasound-guided foam sclerotherapy does not prevent bubbles from circulating to the left heart.

Theory 4

If the patient remains immobile for several minutes after ultrasound-guided foam sclerotherapy, foam will not embolize to the cerebral circulation (Figure 17.8).

Conclusion. Following injection of a small peripheral leg vein, using small volumes of foamed sclerosant, just as foam is detected in the left heart in patients with right-to-left shunts following ultrasound-guided foam sclerotherapy, emboli can also be detected in the middle cerebral artery whilst the patient remains immobile for as long as 15 minutes.

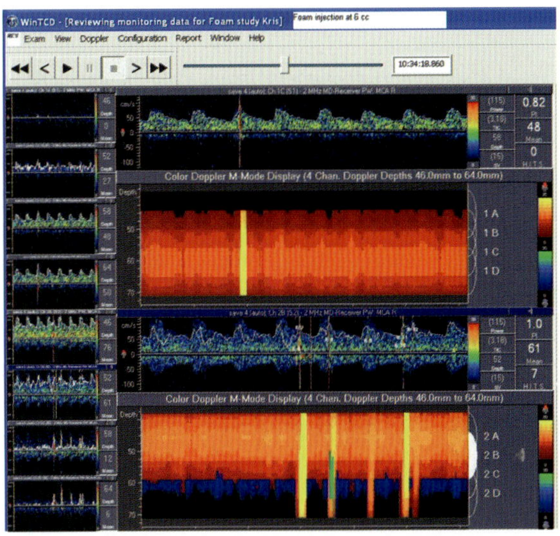

Figure 17.8 Transcranial Doppler (TCD) tracing of middle cerebral artery in a patient 15 minutes after being injected with 3 mL of 1% foamed sclerosant into a 2 mm peripheral leg vein under ultrasound guidance. The patient remained immobile following the injection, and then carefully (to avoid disruption of the TCD monitoring device) sat up. Several emboli can be identified in the middle cerebral artery (lower row 2A–2D) (Courtesy of Compudiagnostics—D Neuhardt)

Theory 5

Using low volumes of foam during ultrasound-guided foam sclerotherapy will prevent cerebral embolization (Figure 17.8).[21]

Conclusion. Cerebral emboli can readily be detected by transcranial Doppler following injection of as little as 3 mL of foam during ultrasound-guided foam sclerotherapy. Limiting the volume of foam injected in any one sclerotherapy session will not prevent cerebral emboli in patients with right-to-left shunts. However, it appears that the use of lower volumes of foam per session may reduce the absolute number of cerebral emboli.

Other studies

Some reports in the literature regarding the safety profile of ultrasound-guided foam sclerotherapy have demonstrated that no adverse neurologic or visual events occurred.[4,15]

There are numerous reports in the literature describing infrequent or rare neurologic or visual disturbances.[2,5,6,9–11,16,17,23,24]

Questions

Whilst some information may be gleaned from these studies, other questions have arisen or remain unanswered:

- Do the bubbles seen in the heart on transthoracic echocardiography during ultrasound-guided foam sclerotherapy contain active sclerosing agent?
- Are the cerebral emboli seen on transcranial Doppler following ultrasound-guided foam sclerotherapy gas bubbles, cellular debris, or other particles with or without active sclerosant agent?
- Does the number of emboli have a positive correlation with the development of symptoms?
- Lastly, since all of the adverse effects in Table 17.2 have been reported following the use of liquid sclerosants,[14] are these symptoms now reported following ultrasound-guided foam sclerotherapy related to the sclerosant itself, cellular debris from vein wall destruction, the foam transmission agent and resultant gas bubbles, or something else entirely?

Table 17.2 Adverse effects of ultrasound-guided foam sclerotherapy

• Dry cough	• Occular migraine
• Migraine	• Visual disturbance
• Chest tightness	• Panic attack
• Circumoral paresthesia	• Respiratory difficulty
• Metallic taste	• Cutaneous necrosis
• Nausea	• Deep vein thrombosis
• Dizziness	• STP
• Hyperpigmentation	

The answers to some of these questions may come as a result of carefully-conducted clinical trials currently ongoing in the United States, specifically looking for adverse effects of cerebral, cardiac and renal origin.

Conclusions

In spite of the fact that it is not possible to control the course and dispersal of foam injected into peripheral or truncal superficial veins, and in light of the thousands of foam sessions performed throughout the world on a daily basis with minimal or rare adverse effects, ultrasound-guided foam sclerotherapy appears to be a reasonably safe method of superficial venous ablation. Limitation of injected foam volume may reduce the risk of cerebral emboli, but may not significantly reduce the risk of the development of symptoms. It may be imprudent to believe that the final chapter on the safety of foam sclerotherapy has been written, and thus caution should be the phlebologist's guide until more information on the physiological effects of foam is forthcoming.

References

1. Barrett JM, Allen B, Ockelford A, Goldman MP. Microfoam ultrasound-guided sclerotherapy of varicose veins in 100 legs. Dermatol Surg 2004; 30: 6–12.
2. Cabrera J, Redondo P, Becerra A, et al. Ultrasound-guided injection of polidocanol microfoam in the management of venous leg ulcers. Arch Dermatol 2004; 140: 667–73.
3. Cavezzi A, Frullini A. The role of sclerosing foam in ultrasound guided sclerotherapy of the saphenous veins and of recurrent varicose veins: Our personal experience. Aust NZ J Phlebol 1999; 3: 49–50.
4. Kakkos SK, Bountouroglou DG, Azzam M, et al. Effectiveness and safety of ultrasound-guided foam sclerotherapy for recurrent varicose veins: immediate results. J Endovasc Ther 2006; 13: 357–64.
5. Kern P, Ramelet AA, Wutschert R, et al. Single-blind, randomized study comparing chromated glycerin, polidocanol solution, and polidocanol foam for treatment of telangiectatic leg veins. Dermatol Surg 2004; 30: 367–72.
6. Myers KA, Jolley D, Clough A, Kirwan J. Outcome of ultrasound-guided sclerotherapy for varicose veins: medium-term results assessed by ultrasound surveillance. Eur J Vas Endovasc Surg 2007; 33: 116–21.
7. Rabe E, Pannier-Fischer F, Gerlach H, Breu FX, et al. Guidelines for sclerotherapy of varicose veins (ICD 10: 183.0, 183.1, 183.2, and 183.9). Dermatol Surg 2004; 30: 687–93.
8. Coleridge Smith P. Chronic venous disease treated by ultrasound guided foam sclerotherapy. Eur J Vasc Endovasc Surg 2006; 32: 577–83.
9. Tessari L, Cavezzi A, Frullini A. Preliminary experience with a new sclerosing foam in the treatment of varicose veins. Dermatol Surg 2001; 27: 58–60.
10. Wright D, Gobin JP, Bradbury AW, et al. Varisolve polidocanol microfoam compared with surgery or sclerotherapy in the management of varicose veins in the presence of trunk vein incompetence: European randomized controlled trial. Phlebology 2006; 21: 180–90.
11. Henriet JP. Expérience durant trois années de la mousse de polidocanol dans le traitement des varices réticulaires et des varicosities. Phlebologie 1999; 52: 277–82.
12. Eckmann DM, Kobayashi S, Li M. Microvascular embolization following polidocanol microfoam sclerosant administration. Dermatol Surg 2005; 31: 636–43.
13. Hoffman K. An unusual complication of facial sclerotherapy. Dermatol Surg 2003; 29: 423–4.
14. Benigni JP, Ratinahirana H, Bousser MG. Polidocanol 400 foam injection and migraine with visual aura [abstract]. ACP 16th Annual Congress; Fort Lauderdale, FL: American College of Phlebology, 2002.
15. Alòs J, Carreño P, López JA, et al. Efficacy and safety of sclerotherapy using polidocanol foam: a controlled clinical trial. Eur J Vas Endovasc Surg 2006; 31: 101–7.
16. Frullini A, Cavezzi A. Sclerosing foam in the treatment of varicose veins and telangiectases: history and analysis of safety and complications. Dermatol Surg 2002; 28: 11–5.
17. Guex JJ, Allaert FA, Gillet JL, Chleir F. Immediate and

midterm complications of sclerotherapy: Report of a prospective multicenter registry of 12 173 sclerotherapy sessions. Dermatol Surg 2005; 31: 123–8.
18. Creton D, Uhl JF. Foam sclerotherapy combined with surgical treatment for recurrent varicose veins: short term results. Eur J Vasc Endovasc Surg 2007; 33: 619–24.
19. Pascarella L, Bergan JJ, Mekenas LV. Severe chronic venous insufficiency treated by foamed sclerotherapy. Ann Vasc Surg 2006; 20: 83–91.
20. Dona E, Fletcher JP, Hughes TM, et al. Ramanathan I. Duplicated popliteal and superficial femoral veins: incidence and potential significance. Aust NZ J Surg 2000; 70: 438–40.
21. Meier B, Lock JE. Contemporary management of patent foramen ovale. Circulation 2003; 107: 5–9.
22. Breu FX, Guggenbichler S. European Consensus Meeting on Foam Sclerotherapy, April 4–6, 2003, Tegernsee, Germany. Dermatol Surg 2004; 30: 709–17.
23. Hamel-Desnos C, Guias B, Jousse S, et al. Foam echosclerotherapy by puncture-direct injection: technique and quantities. J Mal Vasc 2006; 31: 180–9.
24. O'Hare JL, Earnshaw JJ. The use of foam sclerotherapy for varicose veins: a survey of the members of the Vascular Society of Great Britain and Ireland. Eur J Vasc Endovasc Surg 2007; 34: 232–5.

Editorial comment

This chapter was solicited from Dr Morrison because he has extensive, detailed and longstanding experience using ultrasound to detect the passage of foam particles in the circulation from the lower extremities, through the carotid arteries and into the cerebral circulation, as well as through a patent foramen ovale in those patients who have this structural defect. A casual reading of his detailed work would frighten any thoughtful physician and would stop all foam sclerotherapy. However, several facts cause us to rethink the problem after seeing Dr Morrison's chapter.

First is the very small incidence of adverse reactions that have been reported by many who experience foam sclerotherapy. This would suggest that the findings of Dr Morrison, whilst accurate, are not relevant to the clinical production of adverse events.

Second is the complete disappearance of adverse events of all kinds when the foam-treated legs are raised 45° and kept in this position for 5–10 minutes. The objective of such a maneuver is to allow the foam in the lower extremities to revert to its liquid state before circulating throughout the body.

In our experience in La Jolla, this has been accomplished. There have been no ocular signs, chest pain, dry cough, migraine, amblyopia or neurologic deficits of any kind since initiating this practice in January 2006. Thus, well over 500 patients have been treated and the incidence of adverse events has been reduced to zero.

Notwithstanding that this chapter reveals passage of foam particles to every part of the body during all maneuvers designed to prevent foam from leaving the lower extremities, the fact is that all adverse events can be prevented by raising the legs to 45° for 5–10 minutes after introduction of foam. It is apparent that the foam does revert to its liquid state and does not circulate throughout the body.

During this experience with foam sclerotherapy of varicose veins, many patients were treated for telangiectasias without raising the legs. A few of them displayed a dry cough for a short time after treatment, showing that during concurrent experience, foam particles did cause some symptoms when the legs were not raised, but all adverse events were prevented by the maneuver described.

18 Treatment of recurrent varicose veins by sclerosant foam

John Bergan and Van Le Cheng

Introduction

> "... we suggest that ultrasound guided foam sclerotherapy should be the first-line treatment."
> M Perrin and JL Gillet.[1]

Varicose veins recur frequently after primary surgery. The acknowledged rate of recurrence is at least 25%,[2] simply because no mechanical means of varicose vein treatment changes heredity or the propensity for varicose veins to follow the Mendelian laws of inheritance.

Recurrent varicose veins are more prevalent after great saphenous ligation (35%) than after stripping (18%).[3,4] A review of publications on the subject of variceal recurrence from 1954 to 1988 found rates of return of varices following surgery of varicose veins to range from 14% to 80%, with the majority of the papers reporting 30–70% recurrent varices (Table 18.1).

Among patients who have had surgery, the most commonly cited cause is incorrect surgery. Erik Lofgren,[10] the respected and pioneering phlebologic surgeon of the Mayo Clinic, said in 1977: "Early recurrence of varicosities within 2–3 years of the vein stripping operation is interpreted as being caused by incomplete surgery and recurrence beyond 3 years is interpreted as being caused by breakdown of other veins that were clinically normal at the operation." With the broad use of diagnostic ultrasound, that conclusion has been challenged.[11] Allegra, for example, stated, "Varicose veins recurred despite technically correct surgery confirmed on post-operative duplex ultrasonography."

Twenty percent of recurrent varicose veins are believed to be due to neovascularization, and a scattered few are due to abnormal anatomy. Fischer reported three main patterns of neovascularization among patients who had late recurrent saphenofemoral junction reflux after ligation and stripping. Figure 18.1 charts these as single-channel (29%), multichannel (41%) and circumjunctional (29%).

Table 18.1 Varicose vein recurrence rates in limbs treated by conventional surgical techniques

First author	Year	Incidence	Percentage
Van Rij[5]	2003	23/100	23%
Kostas[6]	2004	28/113	25%
Fischer[7]	2001	59/125	47%
Winterborn[8]	2004	83/133	62%
Frings[9]	2004	348/500	70%

Personal experience

Patients were received over 48 months in referral at a single-site private practice office. A history detailing previous treatments and complications was recorded. A focused physical examination was supplemented by a standardized duplex ultrasound examination.[12] A venous map was created for each lower extremity considered for treatment (Figure 18.2).

Patients with recurrent varices, whether of primary or post-thrombotic etiology, in the great or small saphenous vein distribution were included in this study. These were limbs with protuberant, saccular varicose veins and a history of previous intervention by surgery, laser or radiofrequency closure. Exclusions were limbs treated by sclerotherapy without surgery, isolated telangiectasias, limbs that were a part of the Klippel–Trenaunay

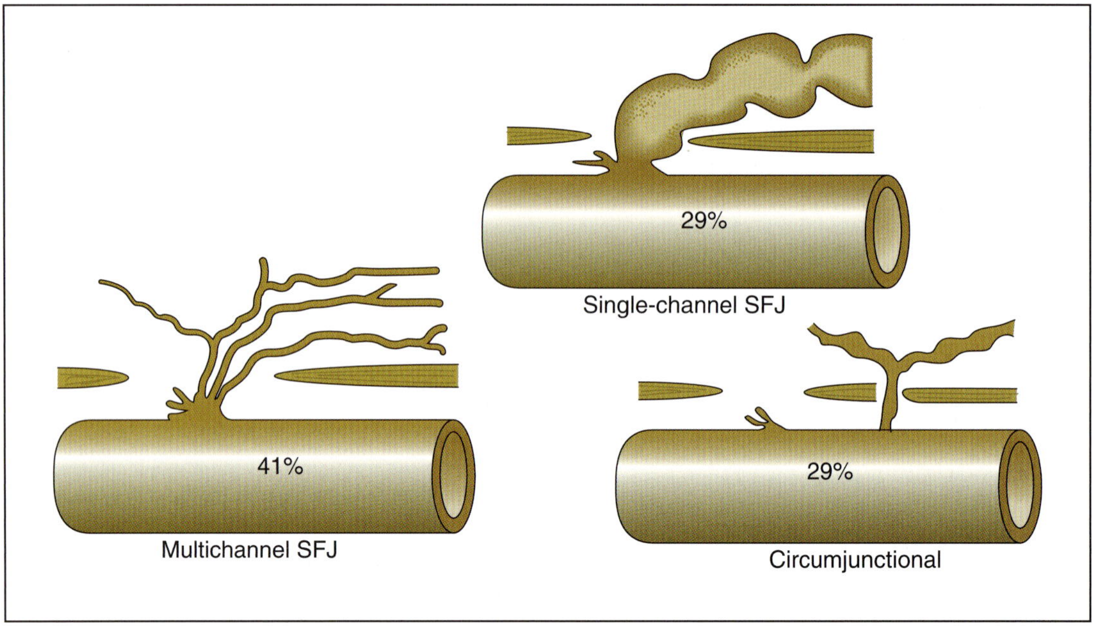

Figure 18.1 Diagrammatic illustration of the three main patterns of neovascularization among patients who had late recurrent saphenofemoral junction reflux after ligation and stripping: single-channel (29%), multichannel (41%) and circumjunctional (29%) (Adapted from Fischer R, Linde N, Duff C, et al. Late recurrent saphenofemoral junction reflux after ligation and stripping of the greater saphenous vein. J Vasc Surg 2001; 34: 236–40)

syndrome, limbs with congenital or acquired arteriovenous malformations, and limbs with venous malformations. Not excluded were legs with venous ulceration, a history of ulceration and/or lipodermatosclerosis (CEAP classification C_4, C_5 and C_6).

Patients and methods

A total of 75 lower extremities from 62 patients had recurrent varicose veins following either great saphenous stripping (35 lower extremities), ligation and phlebectomy (38 lower extremities), or VNUS Closure® (2 lower extremities). There were 49 women (mean age: 52.7 years) and 13 men (mean age: 59.6 years) who had 68 limbs that were symptomatic by CEAP classification C_2, five were C_4, 1 was C_3 and 1 was C_6.

Sclerosant foam was made by the two-syringe Tessari technique with a 1/4 sclerosant-to-air mixture. The sclerosant was polidocanol administered through one or more varices, directed by massage into previously marked varicose veins using ultrasound guidance. For the most part, the great saphenous vein was absent or obliterated, so this was not regularly a target for therapy.

After instillation of foam, the treated limb was held in a 45° elevated position for 10 minutes to fix the foam distally and to allow foam to revert to its liquid state. This was done to avoid adverse events and was successful. The dosage of sclerosant foam ranged from 5 to 17 mL per limb (1% polidocanol in 2 limbs, 3% in 18 limbs and 2% in the remaining 55 limbs). The number of treatments ranged from 1 to 4 (average: 2.1). Class II or III thigh-high support stockings with added focal pressure over large varices were applied immediately after treatment and left in place for 48–72 hours. Afterwards, the stockings were worn only during the day for 2 weeks or for comfort according to patients' wishes. Deep venous thrombosis (DVT) surveillance was done at 7 and 21 days.

Results

Immediately after treatment, all patients returned to normal activity. None were instructed to forced ambulation. Absence of sedation, analgesia and anesthesia

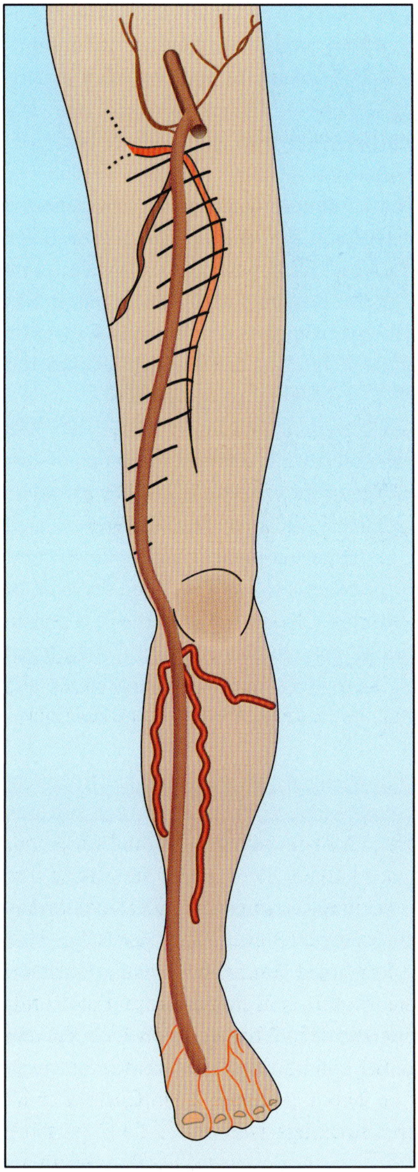

Figure 18.2 Venous map generated from ultrasound data. The great saphenous vein (GSV) that previously had endovenous laser therapy (EVLT) is obliterated, as shown by the hatch-marks. The bold lines represent recurrent varicose veins as seen by transillumination and by ultrasound

allowed unaccompanied patients to drive themselves from the office. No adverse events such as dry cough, ocular signs, chest pain or panic attacks developed. Unlike surgical interventions, no treatment hematomas or wound infections developed.

After treatment, one ulcer remained unhealed. Three limbs remained C_4, but the inflammatory component of lipodermatosclerosis slowly disappeared following direct ultrasound-guided perforating vein injections. The remaining 71 became either C_0 or C_1. (The CEAP score was not designed to provide an evaluation of clinical results in general, but in this study did show elimination of recurrent varicose veins.)

Clinical and an associated duplex examination led to supplemental treatment with foam injection in all but three limbs. These three received only one treatment. In 60 of 75 limbs, the second treatment was the last required. Thus, 84% of limbs with recurrent varicose veins received satisfactory treatment with one or two sessions.

The unhealed ulcer in a diabetic patient remained unhealed despite subsequent placement of an iliac venous stent, performance of a femorotibial arterial bypass and six treatments with foam injections. The ulcer eventually responded to biological dressings. The unimproved C_4 limbs responded to direct perforator vein foam injections, as mentioned above.

No paresthesias were encountered after foam injections. Foot and ankle swelling immediately after treatment was encountered, but this was usually caused by the compression dressings. Narcotics were not required for pain management, but analgesics were taken whenever the compression dressing interfered with sleep. End-results, as assessed by the patients and by the treating physician, were satisfactory for most of the cases. There was elimination of varicose veins and sources of venous reflux in every case. No DVTs or treatment ulcerations were detected.

Discussion

The idea of enhancing the action of liquid sclerosant by mixing it with air was introduced by German clinicians. Flückiger, the most prominent of these, recognized the futility of injecting a liquid sclerosing agent in an orthograde fashion toward the heart, where the agent would flow into vessels of progressively larger diameter and tributaries would not be sclerosed.[13] He then described the essential elements of present-day techniques of foam sclerotherapy: peripherally directed injection, steep leg elevation and manual guidance of the sclerosant. In the absence of ultrasound imaging, he guided the foam by noting subcutaneous crepitus.

Interventions for recurrent varicose veins actually follow the same pattern as primary treatment. That is, sources of reflux such as neovascularization are diagnosed with a venogram (Figure 18.3). These reservoirs of varicose veins that receive such reflux need to be closed, and this can be achieved surgically with a single operation. But such procedures are tedious at best, and dangerous and incomplete at worst. The stump of saphenous vein remaining in the groin must be approached through scar, and great difficulty is encountered when the femoral vessels are encased in scar and neovascularization is present. In such situations, a lateral approach to the femoral vessels is advocated.[14]

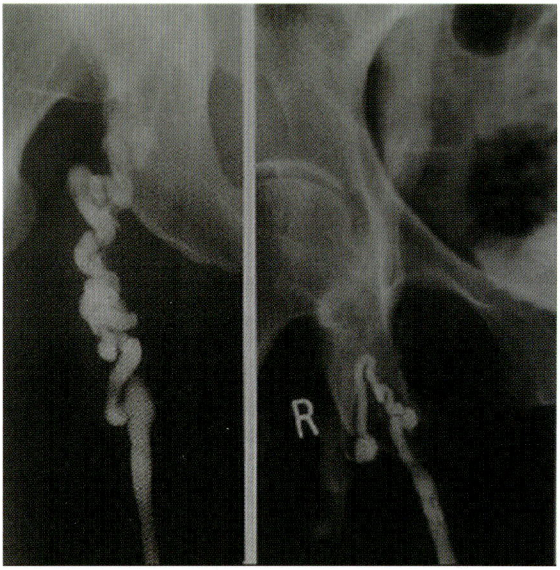

Figure 18.3 Venogram illustrating neovascularization feeding a previously ligated, and still refluxing, great saphenous vein

Actually, there are many patterns of varicose recurrence. Van Rij found neovascular reconnection and persistent abnormal venous function as the major contributors to disease recurrence.[5] The Freiberg group found no junctional recurrence in 68% of their limbs with recurrent varices,[15] and Rutherford et al from the Royal Surrey County Hospital in the United Kingdom focused on perforating veins as a cause of recurrent varices.[16]

Clearly, a technique designed to deal with these several patterns of recurrence must have broad applicability to all patterns of recurrent varices. Foam sclerotherapy does this: the foam can be manipulated into each of the areas of recurrence with little effort.

Finally, the best treatment of recurrent varicose veins should minimize post-treatment discomfort and disability and have a reliably successful outcome. Our experience in treating recurrent varices demonstrates that success has been achieved with no need for sedation, analgesia or anesthesia.

Our experience is almost identical to that reported from the Ealing Hospital in London, where 38 patients with recurrent varicose veins were treated by the same techniques used in the present study.[17] Their report was that in 87% of all legs, complete elimination of varicose veins and all reflux points was achieved. Also, they did not encounter DVT or systemic complications.

The absence of complications in our experience and from the Ealing Hospital are in contrast to reports of surgical treatment of recurrent varicose veins. For example, in a report from Milan, 61 lower extremities were treated surgically.[18] The immediate complications included hemorrhage (1.6%), wound infections (4.9%) and one case of lymphorrhagia. Similarly, from Naples comes a report in which 98 limbs in 82 patients were treated for recurrent varicose veins.[19] There were five wound infections and four lymphorrheas, but no thrombotic or phlebitic complications.

It must be acknowledged that conventional treatment of recurrent varicose veins is no more successful than primary treatment. Eklof reviewed published reports of results of surgical treatment of recurrent varicose veins[4] and found that the long-term results revealed a recurrence rate of approximately 35% for the "re-do" surgery. Thus, it must be concluded that neither standard primary surgical treatment of varicose veins nor secondary surgical treatment of recurrent varicose veins gives acceptable results with minimal complications. Foam sclerotherapy holds promise as being a better treatment for both primary and recurrent varicose veins.

Conclusions

This experience in treating 62 patients having 75 lower extremities with recurrent varicose veins showed that foam sclerotherapy of recurrent varicose veins is successful and causes little morbidity. Treatment with foam sclerotherapy is quick and efficient: no operating room time, no local or general anesthesia, and no time off work or away from normal activities make the technique attractive to the patient and to the physician.

References

1. Perrin M, Gillet JL. Recurrent varices at the groin and popliteal fossa after surgical treatment. J Mal Vasc 2006; 31: 236–46.
2. Royle JP. Recurrent varicose veins. World J Surg 1986; 10: 944–53.
3. Bradbury AW, Stonebridge PA, Ruckley CV, Beggs I. Recurrent varicose veins: correlation between preoperative clinical and hand-held Doppler ultrasonographic examination, and anatomical findings at surgery. Br J Surg 1993; 80: 849–51.
4. Eklof, B, Juhan C. Recurence of varicose veins. In: Eklof B, Gores JE, Thulesius O, Bergqvist D, eds. Controversies in Management of Venous Disorders. London: Butterworths; 1989: 220–33.
5. Van Rij AM, Jiang P, Solomon C, et al. Recurrence after varicose vein surgery: a prospective long-term clinical study with duplex ultrasound scanning and air plethysmography. J Vasc Surg 2003; 38: 935–43.
6. Kostas T, Ioannou CV, Touloupakis E, et al. Recurrent varicose veins after surgery: a new appraisal of a common and complex problem in vascular surgery. Eur J Vasc Endovasc Surg 2004; 27: 275–82.
7. Fischer R, Linde N, Duff C, et al. Late recurrent saphenofemoral junction reflux after ligation and stripping of the greater saphenous vein. J Vasc Surg 2003; 34: 236–40.
8. Winterborn RJ, Foy C, Earnshaw JJ. Causes of varicose vein recurrence: late results of a randomized controlled trial of stripping the long saphenous vein. J Vasc Surg 2004; 40: 634–9.
9. Frings N, Nelle A, Tran P, Fischer R. Krug W. Reduction of neoreflux after correctly performed ligation of the saphenofemoral junction. A randomized trial. Eur J Vasc Endovasc Surg 2004; 28: 246–52.
10. Lofgren, K. Treatment of long saphenous varicosities and their recurrence: a long-term follow-up. In: Bergan JJ, Yao JST, eds. Venous Problems. New York: Yearbook Publishers, 1978: 285–9.
11. Allegra C, Antignani PL, Carlizza A. Recurrent varicose veins following surgical treatment: our experience with five years follow-up. Eur J Vasc Endovasc Surg 2007; 33: 751–6.
12. Mekenas L, Bergan JJ. Venous reflux examination: technique using miniaturized ultrasound scanning. J Vasc Tech 2002; 26: 139–44.
13. Flückiger, P. Nicht-operative Varizenverödung mit Varsylschaum, Schweiz Med Wochenschri 1956, 48: 1368–70.
14. Belardi P, Lucertini G. Advantages of the lateral approach for re-exploration of the sapheno-femoral junction for recurrent varicose veins. Cardiovasc Surg 1994; 2: 772–4.
15. Hartmann K, Klode J, Pfister R, et al. Recurrent varicose veins: sonography-based re-examination of 210 patients 14 years after ligation and saphenous vein stripping. Vasa 2006; 35: 21–6.
16. Rutherford EE, Kianifard B, Cook SJ, et al. Incompetent perforating veins are associated with recurrent varicose veins. Eur J Vasc Endovasc Surg 2001; 21: 458–60.
17. Kakkos SK, Bountouroglou DG, Azzam M, et al. Effectiveness and safety of ultrasound-guided foam sclerotherapy for recurrent varicose veins: immediate results. J Endovasc Ther 2006; 13: 357–64.
18. Viani MP, Poggi RV, Pinto A, et al. Re-exploration of the saphenofemoral junction in the treatment of recurrent varicose veins. Int Surg 1996; 81: 382–4.
19. Canonico S, Campitiello F, Lauletta V, et al. Diagnostic and surgical approaches to recurrent varicose veins of lower limbs. Panminerva Med 1997; 39: 287–90.

19 Vascular malformations

Juan Cabrera, Antonio Martinez de la Cuesta and Alejandro Sierra

Classification and clinical characteristics

Vascular malformations are benign, nontumoral lesions that are present at birth but sometimes not visible until weeks or months later.[1,2] The incidence of vascular malformation is 1.5%, two-thirds of which are of venous predominance,[3] and males and females are equally affected, with no distinction between racial groups. Unlike hemangiomas, vascular malformations do not have a cycle of growth followed by spontaneous regression, but persist and grow slowly throughout the lifespan of patients, sometimes in relation to traumas, infections or hormonal changes. Blood or lymph pressure changes can also produce a rapid or even sudden growth. A characteristic of vascular malformations is that they progressively produce ectasia of vascular structures, increasing the diameter but not the number of vessels, expanding by hypertrophy and not by the hyperplasia observed in hemangiomas.

Vascular malformations are diffuse or localized embryologic development disorders, classically attributed to sporadic mutations. However, recently published evidence has indicated their possible hereditary familial nature. Studies of genetic linkage in familial cases of venous and glomovenous malformations showed the mutation to be localized in different chromosomes: 9p21 and 1p21, respectively. The angiopoietin receptor gene (*TIE2/TEK*)[4,5] is implicated in venous malformations and the glomulin gene in glomovenous malformations. In addition, changes in vascular neurologic modulation have been reported in at least two types of vascular malformation.[6,7] Thus, venular malformations are probably due to a relative or absolute deficiency in the autonomic innervation of the postcapillary venular plexus, and arteriovenous malformations are due to the same deficiency but at the precapillary sphincter level.[8]

More than 25 years ago, in 1982, Mulliken and Glowacki[9] proposed a biological classification of congenital vascular anomalies based on the pathologic characteristics of the predominant epithelium and the natural evolution of the disease. In 1996, a modification of this classification by Mulliken and Young[10,10a] was adopted by the International Society for the Study of Vascular Anomalies (ISSVA) and is now, with minimal changes, considered to be the classic system (Table 19.1). The so-

Table 19.1 Modified ISSVA classification of vascular anomalies (Rome 1996)

Vascular tumors	
Hemangiomas	
Others:	Kaposiform hemangioendothelioma Tufted angioma Hemangiopericytoma Spindle-cell hemangioendothelioma Glomangiomas Kaposi's sarcoma Angiosarcoma
Vascular malformations	
Simple:	Capillary (C) (port-wine stain, nevus flammeus) Venous (V) Lymphatic (L) (lymphangioma, cystic hygroma) Arterial (A)
Combined:	Arteriovenous fistula (AVF) Arteriovenous malformation (AVM) CLVM (includes most Klippel–Trenaunay cases) CVM (includes many milder Klippel–Trenaunay cases) LVM CAVM CLAVM

called Hamburg classification was developed in 1988 and subsequently endorsed by the ISSVA. In this system, the malformation is described according to the predominant component of the vascular lesion, classified as truncal or extratruncal according to the embryonic stage at which the defect was produced[11,12] (Table 19.2). The Hamburg classification does not include hemangiomas or lymphatic vascular malformations, but is useful for clinical–anatomic diagnosis and treatment planning, and for facilitating communication amongst different specialists.

Waner and Sue[13] introduced two small modifications to the Mulliken classification. They considered the term "arteriovenous malformation" for these lesions to be incorrect, regarding them as capillary malformations, since the small arteriovenous connections are produced in the capillary bed; they described all other characteristic findings (hypertrophy of afferent artery and dilatation of efferent venous system) as secondary effects. They also introduced the term "venular vascular malformation" to designate port-wine stain or nevus flammeus.

Other specialists[14] developed a classification of venous vascular malformations based on their anatomic localization and hemodynamic characteristics, of special value to assess the efficacy of sclerosing treatments. The hemodynamic characteristics of the lesion are defined by performing a phlebography. Thus, venous malformations are divided into four groups:

1. Isolated malformations without peripheral drainage
2. Malformations draining into normal veins
3. Malformations draining into dysplastic veins
4. Malformations draining into venous ectasias.

Types 1 and 2 are easier to treat and show a better response to sclerotherapy.

Finally, the natural history of an arteriovenous malformation was classified by Schobinger[15] into four clinical stages:

1. Quiescence: characterized by a pink-bluish stain and presence of arteriovenous shunt detectable by duplex ultrasonography
2. Expansion: same as stage 1 plus pulsations and evident presence of tortuous tense veins
3. Destruction, same as stage 2 plus presence of dystrophic skin changes, ulceration, bleeding and continuous pain
4. Decompensation: same as stage 3 plus association with heart failure.

The classification of Mulliken and Glowacki[9] will be used in this review, incorporating the aforementioned modifications in the designation of venular and arteriovenous malformations.[13]

Venular malformations

These are divided between midline venular malformations and classic venular malformations, also designated port-wine stain, nevus telangiectaticus or nevus flammeus.

Midline lesions are pink macular stains, sometimes converging, which are present at birth and appear on the midline of the head. They are commonly called "salmon patches," "stork-bites" or "angel-kisses," and occur in

Table 19.2 Classification of vascular malformations (Hamburg 1988)

	Anatomic form	
Type of defect	Truncal	Extratruncal
Preferentially arterial	Aplasia Obstruction Dilatation	 Infiltrating Limited
Preferentially venous	Aplasia Obstruction Dilatation	 Infiltrating Limited
Preferentially A-V shunt	Superficial A-V fistula Deep A-V fistula	Infiltrating Limited
Combined defects	Arterial and venous Hemolymphatic	Infiltrating Limited

A-V, arteriovenous.

40% of white and 30% of black newborns. They are usually transient, disappearing within one year of life in 65% of boys and 54% of girls,[16] especially in cases of anterior location. Unlike port-wine stains, they never progress, and hypertrophy or a cobblestone appearance is extremely rare. When of anterior location, they characteristically extend in a V-shape on the glabella and forehead through areas innervated by supratrochlear and supraorbital nerves.

Classic venular lesions are pink-reddish macular stains that darken over time. Although always congenital, they may not be apparent until several days after birth. They occur in 0.4% of newborns, with no gender preference. In 83% of cases, they appear on the head or neck.[17] Interestingly, a large series showed double the frequency of right than left hemiface involvement.[18]

Pathologically, they are true malformations composed of postcapillary venules of the papillary plexus. In explaining their etiology, the term "sick dermatome" has been used, meaning that the venular malformation is due to a total or partial defect of the sensorial and autonomic vascular innervation at this level, producing growth (hypertrophy) of involved vessels and leading to its typical cobblestone appearance. If the defect is total, the changes are more rapid. Port-wine stains affect one or more facial dermatomes of trigeminal nerve branches. The V2 dermatome is the most frequently implicated (57%), followed by mandibular (V3) and ophthalmic (V1) dermatomes (Figure 19.1).[17] When more than one dermatome is involved, it is V2 with V1 or V3 in 90% of cases. The morphology of the lesion is generally geographic, and there is a better response to laser treatment when the lesion is patchy.[17] At the V2 level, there is usually involvement of mucosa adjacent to, or in continuity with, the skin lesion, for example, labial vermilion, labial mucosa and maxillary and gingival mucosa. Unlike midline lesions, these malformations become darker and thicker with age, acquiring a bluish hue and cobblestone appearance, although this progression is individually highly variable. They can sometimes be associated with small skeletal changes in the form of bone hypertrophy, especially when V2 involvement extends toward gingival and maxillary mucosa. This localized hypertrophy favors separation of the teeth and an increased volume of the affected lip, which is especially conspicuous in adult patients and is the only feature that may require surgical correction. There can be a syndromic association between port-wine stains and phacomatosis pigmentovascularis, eye disorders, Sturge–Weber syndrome, occult spinal dysraphisms or medullar malformations.

Video microscopy of venular malformations shows three models of ectasia at the papillary plexus according to the involvement of vertical or deep horizontal vessels of the plexus or both. The recognition and differentiation of these patterns are important for predicting the response to laser treatment, with the first model responding better than the other two. Venular malformations are classified according to their ectasia grade, from grade I (smallest vessels) to grade IV (largest vessels). Over time, the same lesion can change its grade in this classification.

Lymphatic malformations

Lymphatic malformations have classically been known as lymphangiomas, cystic hygromas, circumscribed lymphangiomas and lymphangiomatosis.[19] Similar to other vascular malformations, lymphatic malformations are

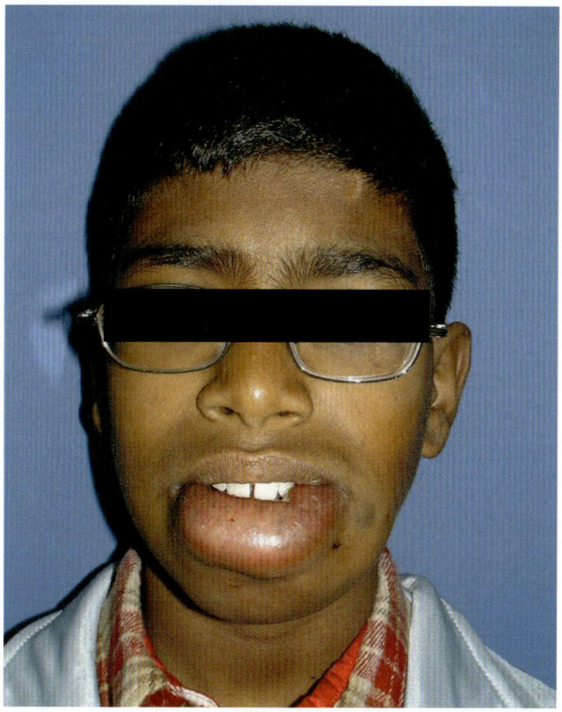

Figure 19.1 Venular malformations can also be treated with sclerosing microfoam, showing an appreciable improvement

always congenital, although only 65–75% are diagnosed at birth, with 80–90% diagnosed by the end of the second year of life.[20] A prenatal diagnosis of large cystic lesions can occasionally be made by ultrasonographic study at the end of the first trimester. The most frequent location is the head and especially the neck (90%),[21] and some authors have ascribed the predominance of this site to the complexity of the cervical lymphatic system.[22] Other typical locations are the axilla, chest, mediastinum, retroperitoneum, buttocks and anogenital region. The clinical appearance varies according to the size, depth and location of the lesion, with the frequent presence of multiple translucid vesicles with viscous content at skin or mucosal level, commonly described as resembling frogspawn. The surrounding skin is normal, often with a bluish hue. These superficial lesions are connected to deeper subcutaneous or submucosal lymphatic cisterns. According to their depth, the malformations are divided between a *microcystic* or *diffuse variant*, also known as *lymphangioma*, characterized by poorly defined borders and massive, generalized edema, and a *localized* or *macrocystic variant* composed of multiloculated cysts. In general, mucosal lesions, which involve the floor of the mouth, buccal mucosa and the tongue, are microcystic and difficult to remove surgically, whereas cervical lesions, the most frequent and also known as cystic hygromas, are macrocystic and easier to excise by surgery, at least in theory. The latter present as painless masses of rubbery consistency, nonpulsatile and generally covered by skin of normal color.

Mild lesions often remain occult for a long time until exacerbated by accidental or surgical injury, intralesional hemorrhage, infection, or hormonal changes.[23] The spread of cervical lesions can compromise the pharynx and, when there is mediastinal involvement, also the trachea. Lesions close to the eye can produce proptosis. The sudden growth of a cervical lymphatic malformation can constitute an emergency by compromising the airway, occasionally associated with respiratory distress. Authors have reported episodes of sepsis in up to 16% of cervical lesions, possibly triggered by oral bacterial flora.[11] Spontaneous hemorrhage is produced in 8% of cases. Skeletal hypertrophy has been described in 83% of patients and distortion in 33%,[25] but these are not explained by an increased blood supply, unlike in other vascular malformations. Specifically, mandibular hypertrophy can cause prognathism and malocclusion. Lymphatic anomalies of the chest, especially of the thoracic duct, can produce pleural symptomatology in the form of chylothorax. In the gastrointestinal tract, they can cause hypoalbuminemia due to protein-losing enteropathy. Large lymphatic malformations on extremities can produce pain, inflammation and gigantism at the expense of skeletal-muscle tissue growth. Pelvic lesions can manifest in urinary obstruction, diarrhea or recurrent infections. Gorham–Stout syndrome, also known as disappearing bone disease, is due to progressive osteolysis induced by a lymphatic malformation in soft tissue and skeleton.[26]

Cases of regression of lymphatic malformations have been reported, theoretically explainable by the appearance with time of a lymphatic–venous shunt,[27] leading some authors to recommend delaying treatment.[11,22,23] On the other hand, it is also likely that many involuted lesions actually correspond to subcutaneous hemangiomas that are following their natural evolution.

Both ultrasonography and magnetic resonance imaging are useful for diagnosis, follow-up and treatment planning in lymphatic malformations.

Venous malformations

Venous malformations are ectatic vessels that are morphologically and histologically similar to veins and all have a low blood flow. In common with other vascular malformations, they are progressive, increasing in size over time and in association with less well-studied factors such as partial surgical resection, traumas and hormonal changes.[11] Venous malformations are classified as superficial or deep and localized, multicentric or diffuse. The skin or mucosa that covers them varies in color according to the depth and ectasia grade of the lesion. The more superficial malformations are purple and the deeper ones are bluer, green or even imperceptible. Besides skin and subcutaneous cell tissue, there is very often muscular, skeletal and visceral involvement. The lesions are soft to the touch, sometimes of nodular appearance, and they empty with compression. In certain positions, the malformation fills with blood, such as in head and neck cases that fill after the Valsava maneuver and others that empty when the affected area is elevated above heart level. Highly ectatic vessels sometimes contain small venous thromboses that can become overinfected and rapidly expand, producing pain and inflammation. Phleboliths, which are used as radiologic markers of this type of malformation, can be present from an early age.

There is frequently involvement of tongue, palate, lip

and buccal mucosa, and infiltration of muscle, salivary glands and even bone structures.

Specifically, mandibular or maxilla involvement is not uncommon, and they are painless masses of slow growth. The most evident sign is dental separation, or the movement or early loss of a tooth with associated intense hemorrhage. Radiologically, involved bone shows a honeycomb appearance.[28] Hypertrophy of soft tissues and perilesional bone is relatively common in large lesions. When the periorbital region or neck is involved, its growth can compromise eyesight or obstruct the airway, respectively. Venous malformations commonly affect the limbs, and their invasion at a deeper level is often greater than evidenced by their external appearance. There is always muscle involvement, and it is not uncommon for joints and bone to be affected. Gonalgia with functional limitation and hemarthrosis is common when the knee is involved, and arthropathy due to hemosiderin can lead to degenerative arthritis. In a series of 176 patients with venous malformations that involved skeletal muscle, the incidence in women was double that in men, with two-thirds of patients being diagnosed at birth and one-third during childhood or adolescence. The most common locations were head, neck and limbs, and pain and inflammation were the main symptoms. Growth anomalies, deformation or pathologic fractures were very uncommon, as were exacerbation or perilesional bleeding induced by hormonal change.[29] In another series of 27 patients with extensive venous malformations of limbs, 100% had muscle involvement and 81% had articular involvement (elbow or knee), with bone changes (thinning, demineralization or lysogenic alterations) found in 63% of the 19 patients in whom this parameter was measured.[30] Another group detected local bone demineralization in 71% of patients[25] and found it to be associated with pathologic fractures.

Venous vascular malformations must be differentiated from glomangiomas and so-called glomovenous lesions. These lesions are true vascular tumors that arise in smooth muscle cells localized in arteriovenous shunts. When multiple, they group as plaques and can spread throughout the limb, acquiring a blue–green color and a cobblestone texture, with a more keratotic appearance than is shown by venous malformations. Characteristically, their size does not modify with changes in position of the affected member, unlike venous malformations.[31]

Coagulation disorders have also been reported in venous malformations and in extensive mixed lymphatic–venous malformations (Klippel–Trenaunay syndrome, see below). These are localized intravascular coagulations, different from the diffuse intravascular coagulation of Kasabach–Merrit syndrome (Figure 19.2). In localized intravascular coagulation, a local consumption of coagulation factors is produced within the malformation or secondary to venous stasis, leading to

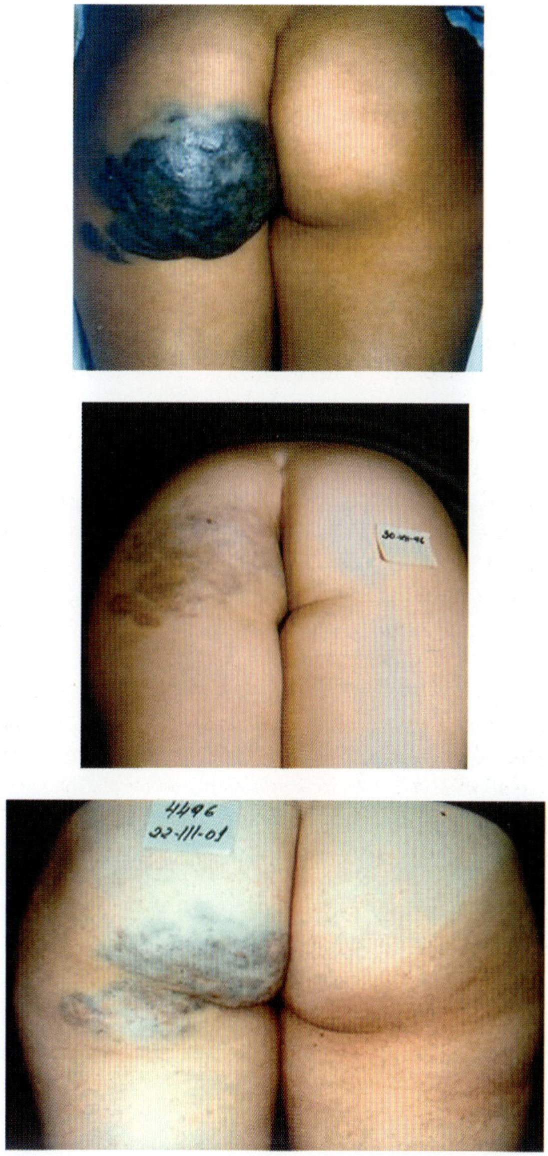

Figure 19.2 This patient with Kasabach–Merrit syndrome had to be admitted to critical care units on three occasions before her successful and stable treatment with sclerosing microfoam

the formation of microthrombi and phleboliths. These patients usually have low fibrinogen (<0.5 g/L) and high D-dimer levels, and measurement of these parameters is useful before undertaking therapeutic procedures. This hypercoagulability state can also be observed in pregnancy, hormonal changes, compression stocking removal, traumas, surgery and sclerotherapy, amongst others. In these situations, which worsen the clinical picture and predispose to a possible thromboembolism, anticoagulation therapy with low-molecular-weight heparin must be initiated. Around half (47%) of these patients also present with deep venous anomalies, including phlebectasia (36%), aplasia or hypoplasia of venous trunks (8%), aneurysm (8%), and incompetence (7%).[3] When these findings are made, a study of the deep venous system of the affected limb is mandatory before any therapeutic procedure is undertaken because of the possible complications.

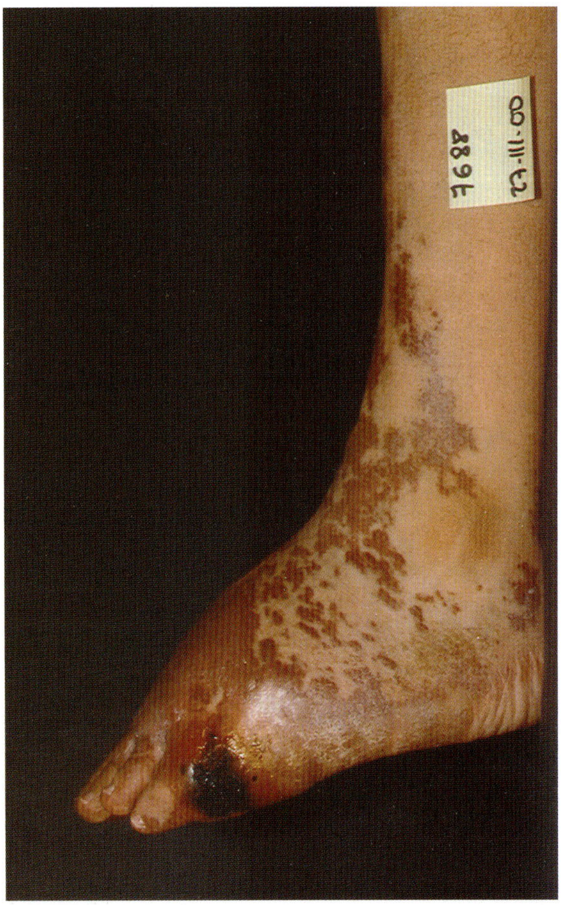

Figure 19.3 Necrosis due to steal syndrome in arteriovenous malformation

The diagnosis and follow-up of malformations can be done with ultrasonography or magnetic resonance imaging according to their size and localization. Phlebography can be useful in malformations of limbs, where the patency of venous drainage must be assessed. Phlebography by direct injection is indicated in treatments with liquid or microfoam sclerosing agents, and ultrasonography is also useful in microfoam therapy to guide the injection of nonvisible areas.

Arteriovenous malformations

Arteriovenous malformations are a group of congenital malformations formed by fistular tracts that communicate arteries with veins. Mulliken and Young[13] restricted the term arteriovenous fistula to the acquired traumatic variant with a single fistula. Histologic analysis of arteriovenous malformations in children and newborns has shown the nidus of the lesion to be composed of capillaries. As the malformation develops, the degree of ectasia increases and the venous dilatation and arterial hypertrophy become visible. The precapillary sphincters are responsible for regulating the blood flow through the nidus. An autonomic innervation defect or some neuroreceptor deficiency at this level may produce arteriovenous malformations. The total or partial nature of the defect will determine the age of presentation and the progression of the malformation. A proximal arteriovenous malformation with high blood flow can increase cardiac output and cause congestive heart failure, whereas a distal malformation is likely to reduce blood flow and produce peripheral ischemia ("steal syndrome") (Figure 19.3).

The most frequent location of arteriovenous malformations is intracranial, followed by head, neck, members, trunk and gut. Despite their congenital nature, the diagnosis of these lesions is generally late, sometimes at the 4th to 5th decade of life.[32,11] They can be confused with hemangiomas and especially with port-wine stains, although they are usually warmer, slightly raised maculae, sometimes palpably beating. Ulceration, intense pain, intermittent bleeding and bone hypertrophy underlying the lesion are also common. Congestive heart failure can be produced in children by large arteriovenous malformations,[33] although the increased output is usually compensated for many years.[34] Unlike venous malformations, these lesions do not completely empty after compression, they refill rapidly and are firmer when palpated. As with other malformations, partial excision, manipulation, trauma or hormonal changes can stimulate their growth.

The natural history of an arteriovenous malformation is documented in the clinical staging described by Schobinger (see above).[35]

The diagnosis and follow-up of arteriovenous malformations can be done with ultrasonography and magnetic resonance imaging, which are improved by the use of duplex ultrasonography and angiographic sequences, respectively. Magnetic resonance imaging is also of great value for surgical treatment planning, to reveal not only the malformation itself, but also its location and relationship with other tissues. However, angiography remains the technique of choice to assess this type of lesion, and the information that it yields is superior to that provided by any other. It is also indispensable for planning and guiding embolization treatment.

Complex or combined malformations

These lesions are almost always associated with an overgrowth of musculoskeletal tissue. We focus on the most important, divided between low- and high-flow malformations.

Low-flow

Klippel–Trenaunay syndrome. This is a well-known eponym for a venous, lymphatic and venular vascular malformation associated with skeletal and soft tissue hypertrophy in one or more extremities.[11,36] Lesions are of sporadic onset and are present since birth. The venular malformation or port-wine stain is usually multiple with a geographic pattern and generally affects the leg (95% of cases), often extending to buttocks and chest. The venous malformation manifests as anomalous lateral veins that become prominent due to their incompetence and to a frequently associated anomaly of the deep venous system. Lymphatic hyperplasia is observed in more than 50% of patients, associated with lymphedema and lymphatic macrocysts. The increased size of the affected limb becomes apparent with age, especially the augmentation of soft tissues and a significant macrodactyly, and specific follow-up and treatment are required. In a small percentage of patients, the affected extremity is shorter or more atrophic than the contralateral. The main complication of Klippel–Trenaunay syndrome is thrombophlebitis, which affects 20–45% of patients[37,38] and causes pulmonary embolism in 4–25% of cases.[39] Pelvic spread of the malformation appears in patients with lower extremity involvement and, although sometimes silent, it can manifest as hematuria, bladder obstruction, diarrhea and over-infection.

Some authors recently classified venular malformations into two groups: geographic and nongeographic. Geographic types are very well-demarcated lesions of irregular shape and a dark, red-purple color, whereas nongeographic lesions have very imprecise borders with normal skin, at least in some areas (not at midline), and are large with a segmental distribution and pink or reddish–pink in colour. For these authors, geographic stains carry a greater risk of association with lymphatic malformations and a higher index of the complications of this syndrome.[40]

The protocol for a patient with Klippel–Trenaunay syndrome includes a multidisciplinary assessment by

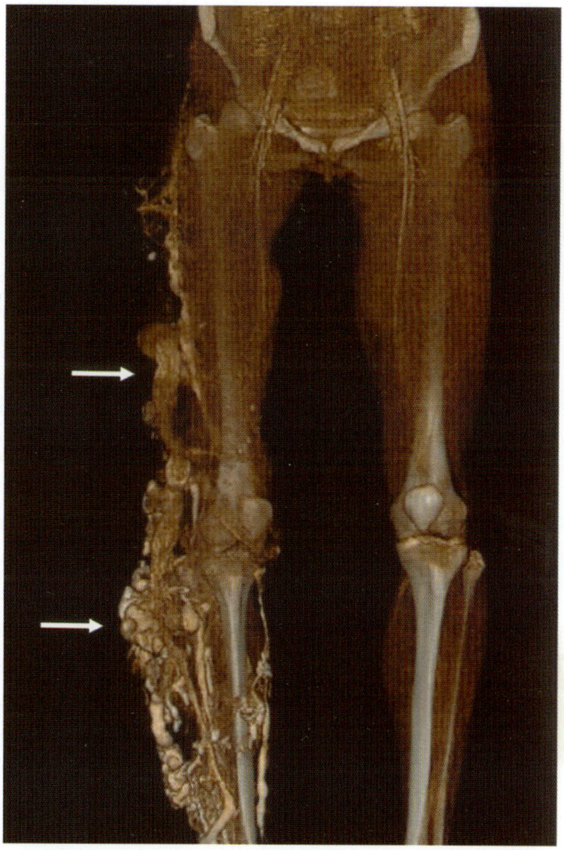

Figure 19.4 Imaging study of patient with Klippel–Trenaunay syndrome, showing absence of deep venous system

specialists in dermatology, traumatology and vascular surgery, with a 6-monthly or annual follow-up, depending on the age of the patient (Figure 19.4). Initially, a complete imaging study is performed, including the deep venous system, establishing its cutaneous and muscular-skeletal limits and possible visceral involvement. Musculoskeletal asymmetry of the affected limb must be prevented and its evolution and treatment programmed. The lateral venous dilatations are treated with microfoam sclerotherapy and, finally, the telangiectatic nevus is treated with pulsed-color or pulsed-light laser.

Proteus syndrome. This syndrome is characterized by the presence of asymmetrical vascular, skeletal and soft tissue lesions of variable size.[41] Possible observations include linear cutaneous verrucous lesions, lipomas and lipomatosis, macrocephalia, asymmetric members with partial gigantism of hand, foot or both, and a characteristic plantar cerebriform overgrowth corresponding histologically to a collagenoma. Asymmetrical body growth and macrodactyly were observed in 98.2% of a series of 55 patients.[42] Vascular lesions occur in 69% of patients, followed in order of frequency by port-wine stain-type venular malformations, micro- and macrocystic lymphatic malformations, and low-flow Klippel–Trenaunay-type combined malformations. High-flow lesions such as those of Parkes–Weber syndrome have never been reported.

Maffucci's syndrome. This syndrome is a congenital and sporadic mesenchymal dysplasia associated with vascular (venous, venular and lymphatic) lesions with exostoses and enchondromas.[43,44] Lesions are more frequently located in the hands and feet and are clinically characterized by bluish subcutaneous soft nodules that often develop phleboliths. The onset of enchondromas causes more or less evident deformities and pathologic fractures. A large percentage of the latter can degenerate into chondrosarcomas. (Figure 19.5)

High-flow

Parkes–Weber syndrome. This is an arteriovenous venular malformation. It appears at birth and most often affects the leg (77%), although less frequently than does Klippel–Trenaunay syndrome. It is characterized by a diffuse, pink–reddish, macular stain with geometric edges that grow symmetrically. It is differentiated from Klippel–Trenaunay syndrome by the high flow of the vascular lesion and the presence of arteriovenous fistulas, whilst anomalous lateral veins are uncommon and lymphatic malformations very rare; there is less musculoskeletal involvement and the location is the arm in 23% of cases. There also tends to be less asymmetry of the affected limb compared with Klippel–Trenaunay syndrome. Instead of thrombophlebitis and risk of pulmonary embolism, the main complication of Parkes–Weber syndrome is the increase in cardiac output, which can produce heart failure and cutaneous ischemia.[11,45]

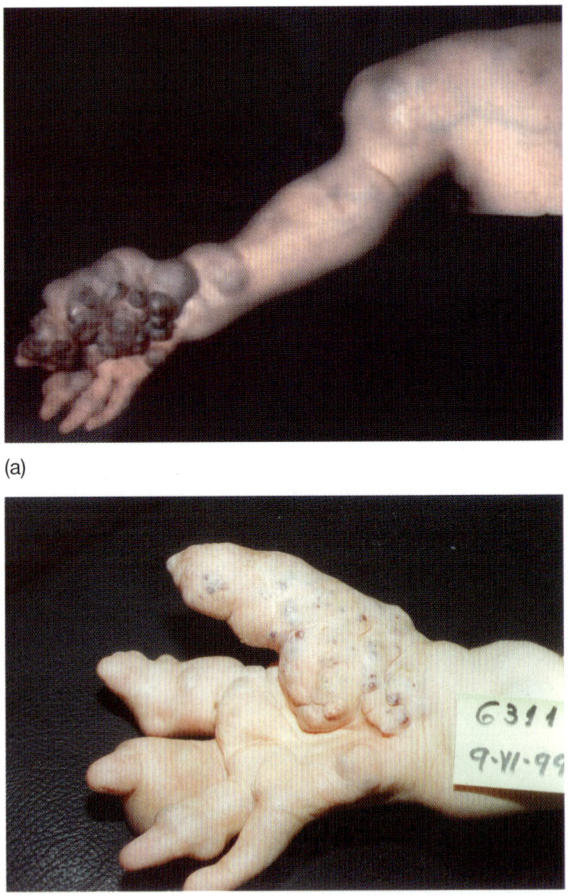

(a)

(b)

Figure 19.5 Maffucci's syndrome: (a) before treatment; (b) after treatment

Treatment

The multidisciplinary approach to vascular malformations was first discussed and introduced at the I Samsung International Symposium for Congenital Vascular Malformations held in Seoul in 1996.[46] It was concluded that vascular malformations should be treated by multidisciplinary units, bringing together all of the specialists involved in their management (Figure 19.6). This new strategy represents a major advance in the treatment of these diseases, since it avoids the excessively partial perspective of a single physician and the extremes of over-conservative or over-aggressive treatments. Thus, congenital vascular malformations are treated by teams able to use all currently available therapeutic tools, including laser, sclerosing, endovascular and surgical treatments. There is also the possibility in the not too distant future of novel medical treatments with antiangiogenic drugs able to limit, control or reduce the development of these lesions. In most cases, it will be necessary to use a combination of treatments, given that the application of a single therapy is usually inadequate.

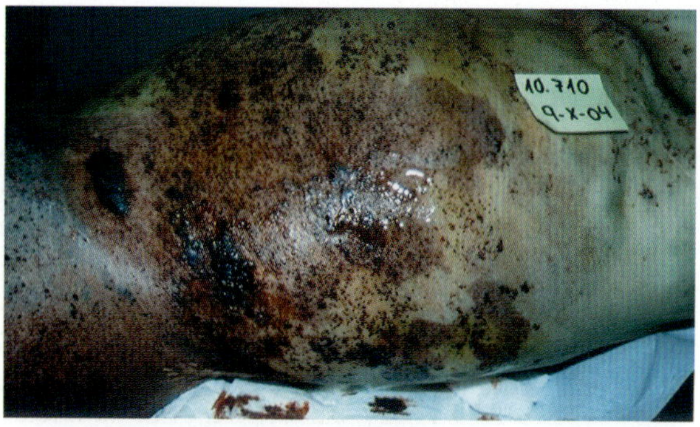

(a)

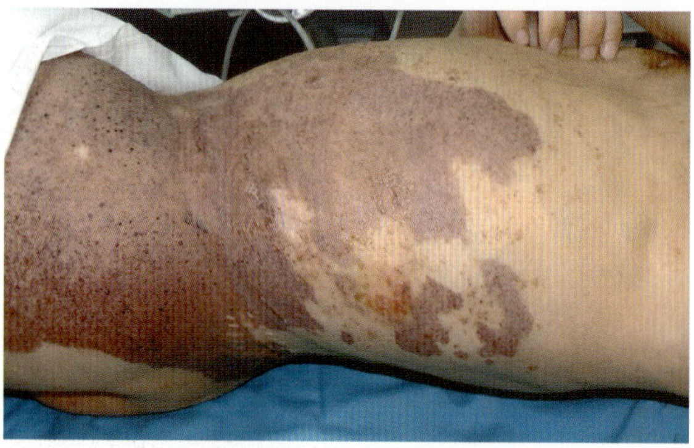

(b)

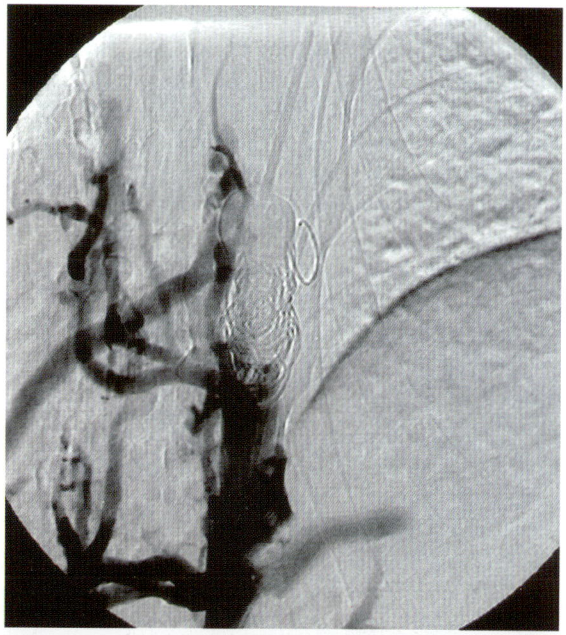

(c)

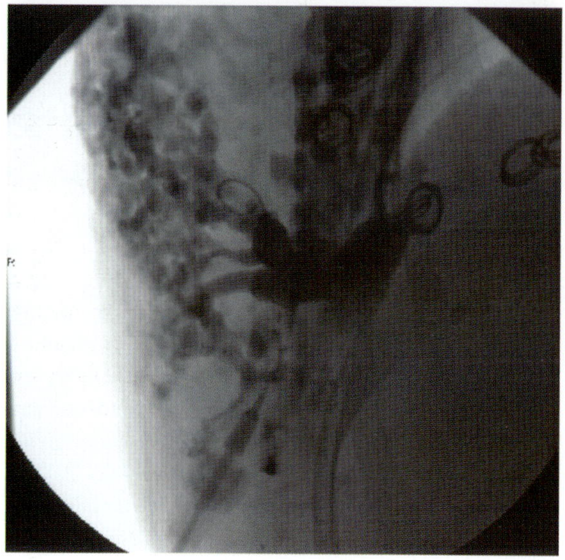

(d)

Figure 19.6 Extensive hemicorporal hemorrhagic malformation subjected to repeated surgery: (a) before microfoam treatment; (b) after several treatment sessions; (c) pre-treatment image showing endovascular occlusion of a large vein with coils in the wall of the thorax before treatment with microfoam; (d) after occlusion of the large vein, the wall vessels were treated with large volumes of microfoam over various sessions (endovascular occlusion)

Surgery

Vascular surgery on its own plays a small role in the management of vascular malformations, and it is usually complemented by plastic and/or orthopedic surgical procedures. Arteriovenous or high-flow malformations are clearly the group of vascular anomalies for which surgery is most indicated and obtains the best outcomes. The objective of treatment is to eradicate the nidus of the malformation, and surgical resection has been considered the only effective option. Exceptionally, isolated embolization can completely resolve the process, although it usually only achieves transient symptomatic improvement or a delay in progression to a higher Schobinger stage. However, embolization should always be considered preoperatively to facilitate the surgery and reduce the bleeding. In fact, a dedicated, patient and experienced interventional radiologist can drastically reduce the rate of surgery in this group of patients.

In lymphatic malformations, especially diffuse ones, it is difficult to find a dissection plane during the excision, since the borders of the lesion are almost impossible to establish. Therefore, the resection should be as wide as possible. Any residual lesion will give rise to short-term recurrence. For this reason, surgery must often be repeated before a satisfactory outcome is obtained.

In mixed malformations, the classic surgical approach of staged ligation can serve as a palliative treatment, although its value is now questioned and it will undoubtedly be replaced by ultrasound-guided polidocanol microfoam sclerotherapy. The outcomes of surgery are poor, and thromboembolic events are 10-fold more frequent than in simple or conventional venous surgery and can leave sequelae of neuropathic pain.[47]

Laser

Use of the laser in the management of vascular malformations is based on the theory of selective photothermolysis, with oxymyoglobin as target chromophore for the light of the laser. Pulsed dye laser is the gold-standard treatment for capillary malformations (port-wine stains), especially in children, because no scars are left. A variable response is obtained, achieving a substantial clearance of the color of the lesion after several sessions. Better outcomes appear to be obtained at earlier ages. One of the drawbacks of early treatment is the frequent need to use general anesthesia (sedation) because of the pain produced by the procedure, which can cause distress and anxiety.

In the case of venous malformations on the skin surface, neodymium–YAG laser can be applied, using one of various cooling systems to minimize the risk of scarring. The neodymium–YAG laser produces a continuous wave of infrared light at 1064 nm that penetrates to a depth of 5–7 mm.[48] The depth of the lesion determines the efficacy of the treatment. Superficial lesions can be considerably cleared after various sessions, although their complete elimination is rarely achieved. In large venous malformations of the mucosa, the presurgical use of laser can remove the superficial component of the malformation and can also create a band of fibrosis that will assist flap mobilization during the subsequent surgery, reducing intraoperative bleeding.[49]

Ablation with carbon dioxide or erbium laser is especially indicated in superficial lymphatic malformations, clinically characterized by the presence of multiple vesicles. Although this is not a curative treatment, it can control the disease and produce an evident improvement in the quality of life of these patients.

Sclerotherapy

Sclerotherapy is the removal of an anomalous venous area by injection of a sclerosing agent, classically a liquid, which produces a chemical irritation of the endothelial cells that coat the interior of the vessel. A thrombus is then produced, and the vein is finally transformed into a fibrous thread that ultimately disappears. This procedure has long been used in the treatment of vascular malformations. We shall provide an outline introduction before focusing on two novel approaches that have appeared in the past few years, namely, sclerotherapy with sclerosing microfoam for the treatment of venous or low-flow vascular malformations, and sclerotherapy with OK-432 for the treatment of lymphatic vascular malformations.

Currently, the greatest therapeutic challenges are posed by venous or low-flow vascular malformations and diffuse lymphatic vascular malformations of large size or extent or those that show infiltration of muscle masses. Because of their invasion of proximal structures, venous malformations usually have a complex morphology and are often associated with anomalies of the deep venous system of the extremities, therefore limiting the possibilities of complete excision by surgery.[50,51] Occasionally, lesions can recur after several surgical interventions, returning patients to their original condition, with a major impact on their state of mind.[52,53] Surgery is indicated in well-circumscribed lesions of moderate size, which have the best possibility of anatomic and functional recovery. Embolization, a useful though delicate procedure for malformations with arteriovenous component, is not effective in extensive pure venous malformations.

The sclerosing agents classically used in the treatment of low-flow venous and lymphatic malformations include 5% sodium morrhuate, sodium tetradecyl sulfate, polidocanol, ethanolamine oleate, ethanol, Ethibloc, hypertonic saline, amidotrizoic acid, bleomycin, dextrose, tetracyclins and OK-432. The selection of agent depends upon the experience and preference of the physician and the morphological appearance and location of the lesion.[54–60]

With respect to the follow-up, it is evidently essential to differentiate between localized and diffuse vascular malformations, since the latter require continuous and prolonged treatment, sometimes for years, at best controlling the lesion but never completely eradicating or curing it.

Vascular malformations associated with arteriovenous lesions are contraindicated for sclerotherapy because an accidental intra-arterial injection can produce extensive necrosis. It must also be taken into account that head and neck veins lack valves and that those in the upper two-thirds of the facial region communicate directly with the cavernous sinus via the superior and inferior ophthalmic veins. Consequently, sclerotherapy is to be avoided at this level.

The general complications of this technique vary according to the agent and dose used. They include allergic reactions (especially with sodium tetradecyl sulfate), brain intoxication (especially with ethanol, which must never exceed a maximum volume of 1.2 mL in patients of about 70 kg),[54] hemoglobinuria with possible renal damage, cutaneous necrosis by extravasation or reflux (10%), and neuropraxia due to extravascular injection near a motor or sensory nerve.

The sclerosis technique must ensure that a precise dose is administered and that the agent is homogeneously distributed on the entire endothelial perimeter of the treated venous segment.[61] It must also ensure that the intravascular concentration of the sclerosant is not reduced by dilution in the blood or that this dilution is minimal but always known. Finally, the sclerosant must remain in contact with the endothelium for the necessary time period. In short, the requirements of sclerotherapy must be met: the intravascular concentration of the sclerosant must be known; there must be a homogeneous distribution within the vessel and control over the duration of contact between agent and endothelia; and, at the same time, sclerotherapy must be selective, that is, limited to the selected venous area. These requirements are not met by conventional liquid sclerosants. Using these, the dosage on the endothelia and therefore the sclerosing action is very difficult to control, and in vessels of a certain volume or flow, the therapeutic effect, besides being unsafe, is generally confined to a short segment.[62]

Conventional sclerotherapy with liquid sclerosants, which is a palliative treatment in most cases of vascular anomalies, offers good outcomes in small malformations.[57] It is indicated before surgery as preoperative support to reduce the size of the lesion or as a postoperative complement.[55] In contrast, conventional sclerotherapy of large malformations is ineffective because of the intrinsic limitations of the injected liquids: their dilution and progressive deactivation in a large blood volume; irregular distribution of the sclerosant on the endothelia of the treated area; difficulties in manipulating and controlling the injected sclerosant; and imperceptibility within the vessels on duplex ultrasonography. Sclerotherapy with ethanol, the most widely used agent in the treatment of these lesions, is highly aggressive and associated with major complications due to lack of control over the injected liquid. Besides its general contraindication in children, reported adverse effects of its use include necrosis of skin and mucosa, deep venous thrombosis in extremities, pulmonary emboli, sensory and motor neurologic lesions, superficial cellulitis, and cardiorespiratory collapse due to bronchial spasm. Moreover, ethanol treatment is not readily repeatable, and this is essential for the sclerotherapy since partial recanalization after the intravascular thrombosis is frequent.[59]

However, the introduction of sclerosants in the specific pharmaceutical form of microfoam has transformed the scenario depicted above, since the microfoam physically displaces the blood contained in the vessels and minimizes dilution, allowing better knowledge of the intravenous concentration. Micronization of the injected sclerosant exponentially increases its surface area with reductions in the bubble diameter, enhancing its therapeutic action and allowing a major reduction in the total dose injected. Moreover, microfoam facilitates a more homogeneous distribution of sclerosant on the endothelial surface and prolongs sclerosant–endothelium contact time. The echogenicity of the microbubbles makes them indirectly visible and the manipulability of the injected microfoam allows it to be steered to areas distant from the injection site. In this way, microfoam allows the intravascular administration of a more precise dose of sclerosant.[63,64]

Aside from its safety, a further benefit of sclerosing microfoam is its manageability. The high internal cohesion of microfoam means that it can be aspirated and re-injected after its initial injection. The color of the aspirated microfoam, visible in the catheter, reveals the degree of dilution or intravascular occupation. It ranges from white when the occupation is exclusive, to pink or red when there is moderate or major dilution. Furthermore, since microfoam can be steered within the vessels, the filling can be intensified or attenuated according to the sensitivity of the venous area under treatment.

Microfoam is made with oxygen and carbon dioxide (CO_2) – physiological gases. A priori, injection of a gas into the blood stream raises alarm about the possibility of a gas embolism. However, CO_2 has been intravenously injected at doses of 50–100 cm^3 as a contrast in radiologic diagnosis since the 1950s.[65,66] Amongst the advantages of microfoam made with CO_2 are its fluidity, allowing the use of fine catheters, the absence of toxicity, even at high doses, and its low cost. For these reasons, there has been renewed interest in the use of CO_2 in angiography of visceral, abdominal and leg trunks.[67] Bendib et al.[68] injected 200 cm^3 of CO_2 into the right heart of 10 000 patients and observed no complications. The intra-arterial administration of CO_2 in angiography started in the 1970s. Fermand et al.[69] injected it, as a contrast medium in aortic arteriography, at a rate of 30 cm^3/s and observed no adverse effects, even after injecting up to 450 cm^3 in a single examination. A report on the use of this gas in more than 700 subdiaphragmatic arteriograms by Kerns et al described no major incidents.[70] Thus, on the one hand, the high solubility of the gas facilitates its metabolism in blood and its pulmonary diffusibility; on the other hand, the micronization increases in exponential fashion the surface area of the gas and facilitates its solubility in bodily fluids. The liquid phase of the foam sclerosant provides an enormous increase in active surface area for making contact with the endothelium in comparison with the small surface area available with the liquid form. In this way, the dosage of sclerosant in microfoam is more precise and its action more predictable compared with the liquid form. The microfoam does not mix immediately with the blood, but displaces it from within the vessel and fills its lumen, so that the sclerosant contacts the endothelia of the veins homogeneously, without dilution and at a known intravascular concentration. Because the vessel can be kept full of microfoam, the sclerosant–endothelium contact time can also be controlled at will.[71,72]

Experience with the treatment of vascular malformations

We treated 50 patients with congenital vascular malformations of venous prominence by sclerotherapy with polidocanol microfoam.[73] Of these patients, 18 were male and 32 female, with an age range of 8–62 years. The patients could be divided into three groups according to the Hamburg classification: the first with infiltrating lesions ($n = 16$), the second with limited lesions ($n = 19$) and the third with Klippel–Trenaunay-type combined vascular malformations ($n = 15$). In some cases, other complementary imaging tests were performed in addition to the ultrasonography study. All patients were treated by ultrasound-guided injection of polidocanol microfoam. At each session, 20–100 mL of microfoam were injected, corresponding to 3–6 mL of 2% polidocanol. The concentration of polidocanol injected ranged from 0.25% to 4%, according to the size of the malformation and the hemodynamic characteristics of the area to be treated. Thus, infiltrating malformations required higher concentrations (2–4%), whereas anomalous lateral veins in patients with Klippel–Trenaunay syndrome were treated with lower ones (0.25–0.5%). The procedure was performed without anesthesia and the number of sessions ranged from 1 to 46 (mean: 12), with only 21 patients requiring more than 10 sessions. The interval between sessions was 2–4 weeks. There was clinical and radiologic improvement in 46 patients (92%), with only 4 patients failing to respond. Amongst the 46 responders, there was total disappearance of the malformation in 18 (39%), a reduction of 50% in 15 (33%) and a reduction of <50% in 13 patients (28%). Out of the 39 patients who reported pain, this disappeared in 25 and was reduced in the remaining 14. Five patients had chronic ulcers, which were all completely closed, and nine had bleeding episodes, which all abated or were reduced. With respect to adverse effects, four patients developed skin pigmentation that spontaneously disappeared. A small necrosis developed in two patients after superficial sclerosis with 0.5% polidocanol microfoam, and another patient had a more extensive cutaneous necrosis after the accidental injection of a distal artery. No case of deep venous system thrombosis, pulmonary embolism or neurologic lesion was documented.[73]

The administration of sodium tetradecyl sulfate or polidocanol preserves the usual benefits of sclerotherapy, that is, its simplicity, speed, economy, outpatient procedure, and repeatability, whilst being relatively innocuous and avoiding major drawbacks. The advantages are even more marked when polidocanol (Aethoxysklerol®, Etoxiesclerol®) is used, because of its excellent local and general tolerance.[60] This drug has been marketed in Europe for more than 20 years for the sclerosis of varicose veins, although it has yet to be approved by the Food and Drug Administration in the United States. These benefits contrast with the aggressive effects of absolute ethanol and/or 5% sodium morrhuate both on the malformation and on neighboring tissues. The injection of these agents is also very painful, and hospitalization, general anesthesia and postsclerosis analgesia are required. Furthermore, sodium morrhuate can produce allergic reactions. These two agents must be administered with great caution.

The best response to microfoam sclerotherapy has been in patients with Klippel–Trenaunay syndrome, with total elimination of pathologic areas in 80% of cases, and only a recurrence of small varicosities (<20% of the original lesion) in ten of the patients (Figure 19.7). The most common surgical treatment in these patients is stripping of the veins and avulsion or excision of the varicosities and vascular malformations, although endovascular laser ablation may also be indicated. With these procedures, it is often impossible to remove all varicosities because of the extent of the involvement, and they will recur in some

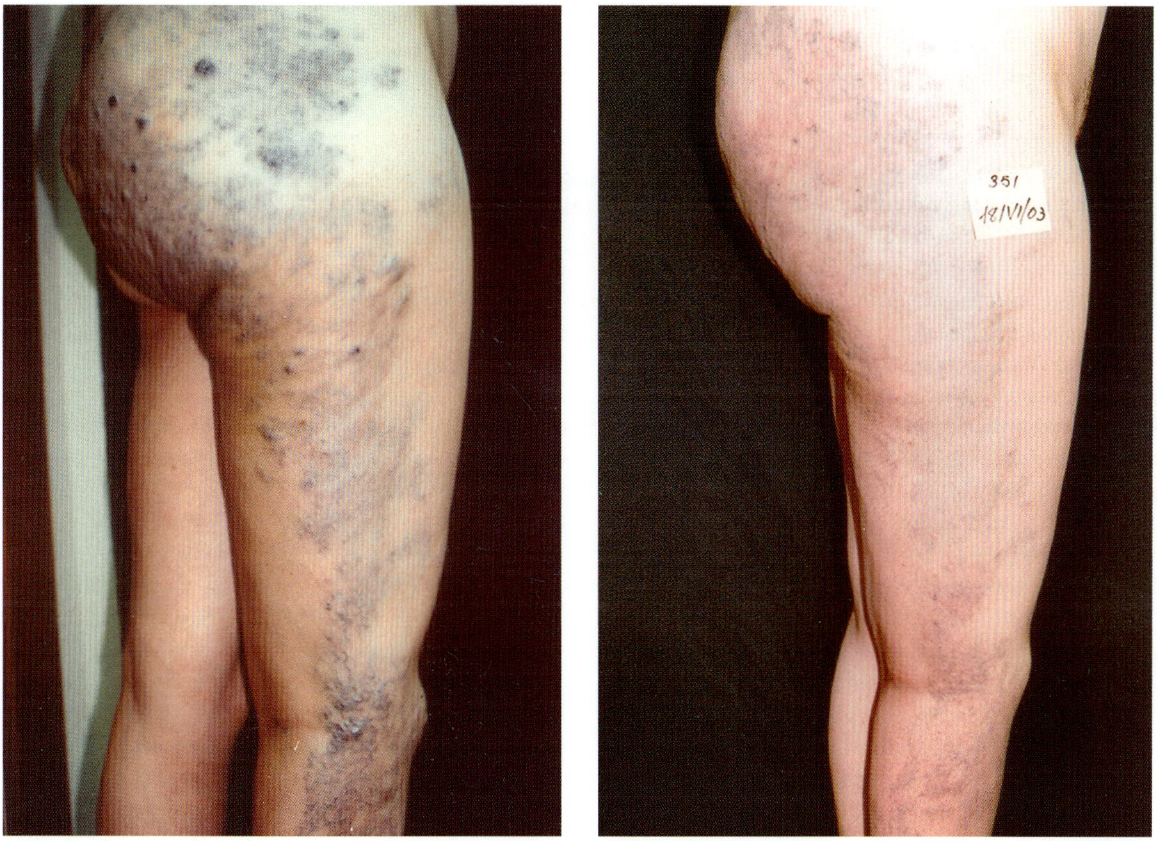

(a) (b)

Figure 19.7 Extensive Klippel–Trenaunay syndrome involving knee: (a) before treatment; (b) good outcome after sclerosing microfoam treatment form in half of the patients. It should be borne in mind that, besides ulcerations and sporadic bleedings, many venous vascular malformations are symptomatic with pain from the malformation itself or as sequelae of the surgical treatment. On the basis of our results in 15 patients with Klippel–Trenaunay syndrome, which have been corroborated in a further 10 patients treated in more recently (data not shown), we believe that sclerotherapy with polidocanol microfoam is the treatment of choice for venous malformations associated with Klippel–Trenaunay syndrome. It is a simple procedure, capable of eliminating or reducing the pain from the very first session. Furthermore, it is easy to repeat should recurrences occur, it is minimally iatrogenic, and it does not involve the risk of neuropathic pain as sequela.

The therapeutic efficacy of polidocanol microfoam depends on its mechanical action in displacing the blood within the vessel. If the blood flow is elevated, dilution of the injected microfoam can result, reducing its effect.

Venous malformations are marked both by the anatomic anomaly of the affected vessels and by their special hemodynamic characteristics, in theory similar but in practice different in each patient, with variability being the norm. This morphologic and functional individuality of lesions requires therapeutic refinements and different techniques to enable administration of the correct dose of sclerosant to each area in each patient. Phlebography must be performed to define the characteristics of a venous vascular malformation. Thus, the lesions can be divided into four groups: (1) isolated malformations without peripheral drainage, (2) malformations that drain into normal veins, (3) malformations that drain into dysplastic veins, and (4) malformations that drain into ectatic veins. Nevertheless, the situation is often not so simple, explaining why Belov placed the term "predominant" before arterial, venous or arteriovenous in his Hamburg classification.[64] In routine practice, duplex ultrasonography can often show some areas in venous malformations with abnormal supplies of pulsatile blood delivered by small arteriovenous communications (Figure 19.8). Therefore, the existence of mixed forms must be accepted – or at least the presence of high-flow areas in malformations that are considered to be low flow. The presence of small arteriovenous fistulas reduces the efficacy of the treatment and the area initially thrombosed after the injection, favoring its early partial recanalization. Attempts can be made to counter this considerable disadvantage by reducing the interval between sclerosis sessions and using a higher concentration of sclerosant. For instance, hand malformations often show a radial artery of increased size and elevated blood flow connected to venous dilatations. In these cases, the high local flow compromises the response to the sclerosant injection, and the technique must be adapted accordingly. For this purpose, we use duplex ultrasonography to identify the most hemodynamically active parts at the start of treatment, compressing the afferent arteries during the injection in order to sclerose these areas of the malformation. Once the lesion is compartmentalized and hemodynamically "disconnected," it can be more easily sclerosed in its entirety by successive sessions. Nevertheless, the stability of the vascular occlusion achieved is more precarious than in pure venous malformations, and recanalization is frequent, so that a more rigorous follow-up is required.

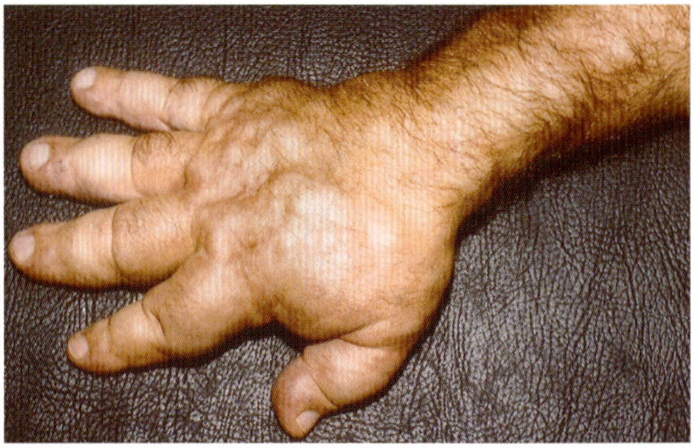

(a)

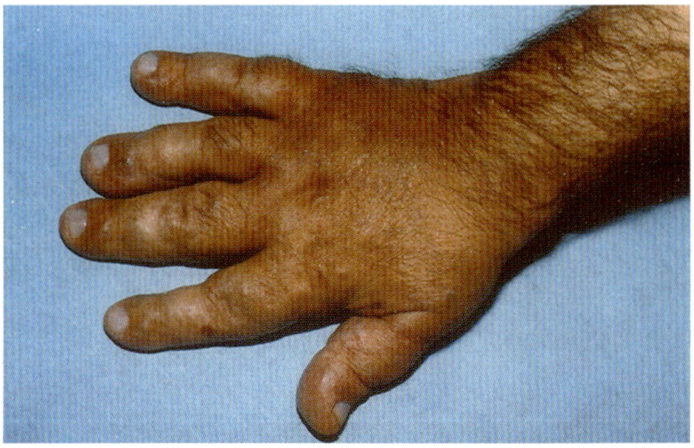

(b)

Figure 19.8 Malformation of the hand: (a) before treatment; (b) after treatment

We can often only helplessly observe the natural evolution of large venous malformations, unable to provide a definitive effective treatment (Figure 19.9). Sclerotherapy with microfoam is a therapeutic option that allows the progression of these lesions to be moderated and their size to be reduced in low-flow cases. We highlight the considerable increase in activity of sclerosing agents in this novel pharmaceutical form, the selectivity of this action on the endothelia, the ability to visualize microfoam on ultrasound and the possibility of predicting the therapeutic effect. Furthermore, it is a well-tolerated technique with no major adverse effects. The simplicity, reproducibility, low cost, safety and strictly outpatient nature of the procedure makes microfoam sclerotherapy the method of choice for the anatomic and functional elimination of a pathologic

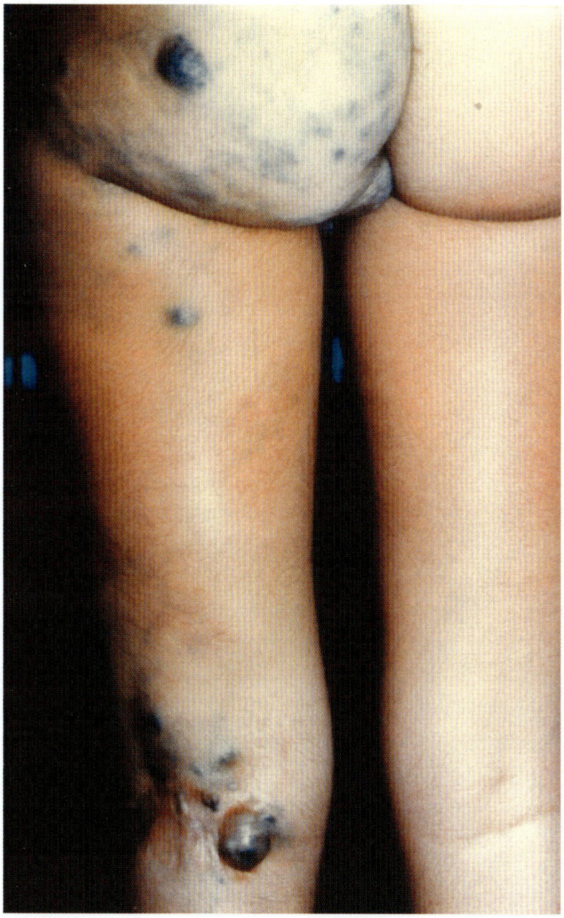

(a)

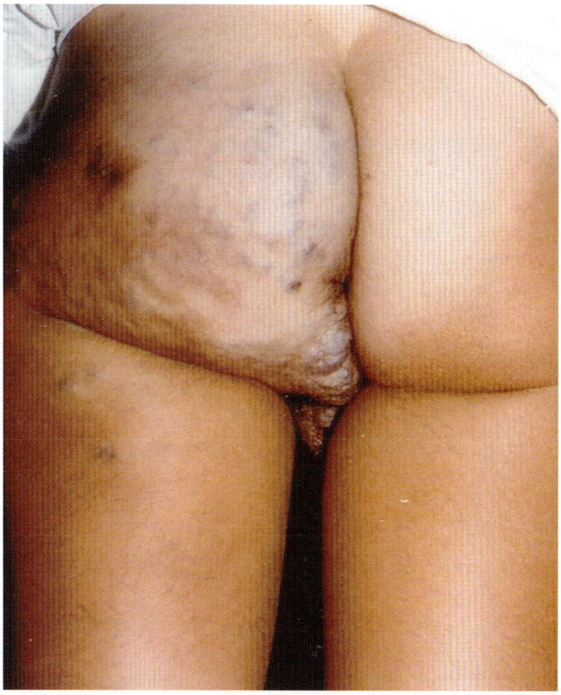

(b)

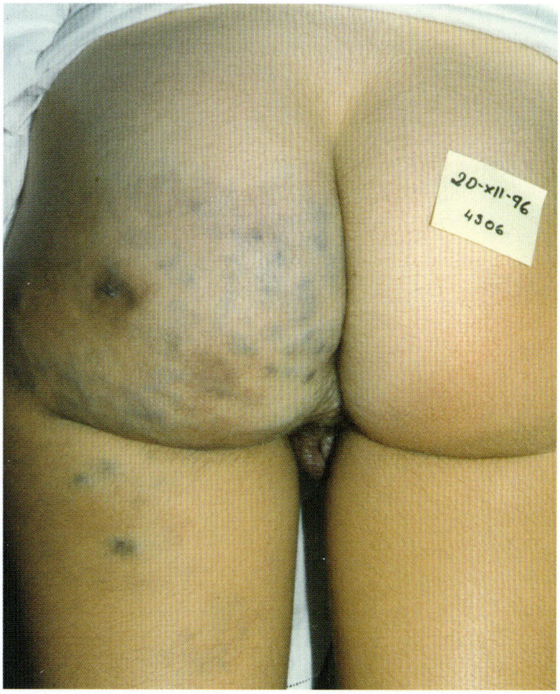

(c)

Figure 19.9 Venous malformation involving the buttock, perineum and genital region and extending to the leg: (a) before treatment – note the popliteal dilatation (post-surgical recurrence); (b) after treatment of gluteal and popliteal dilatation; (c) after 17 sessions of microfoam injections

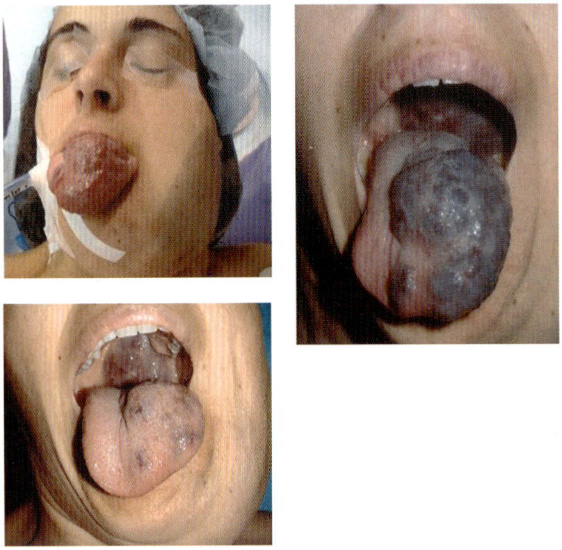

Figure 19.10 Large venous malformation with involvement of tongue, palate and oral mucosa before treatment, and favorable outcome after five sessions of microfoam injection

venous area.[73] As a result of the development of sclerosants in microfoam form, phlebology has entered a new area and can offer hope to some patients with venous or low-flow combined vascular malformations (Figures 19.10 and 19.11).[74]

Sclerotherapy of lymphatic malformations with OK-432

Besides surgery, sclerotherapy with glucose, tetracyclins and OK-432 has been used to treat lymphatic malformations. The mechanism of action of these substances is diffusion to the stroma and production of irritation and inflammation, favoring the retraction and wound contraction of the lesion. Before the injection, the largest possible volume of lymph must be aspirated, emptying the malformation to the greatest possible degree.

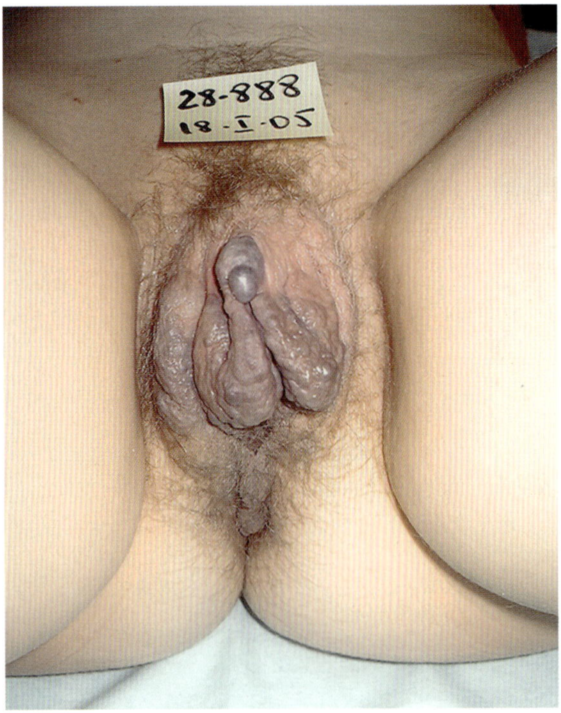

(a)

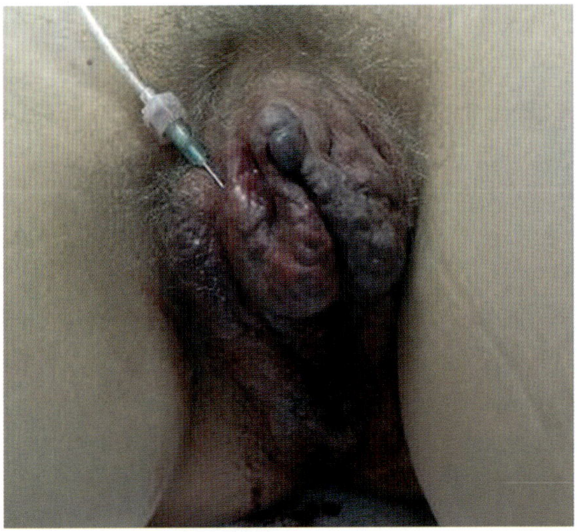

(b)

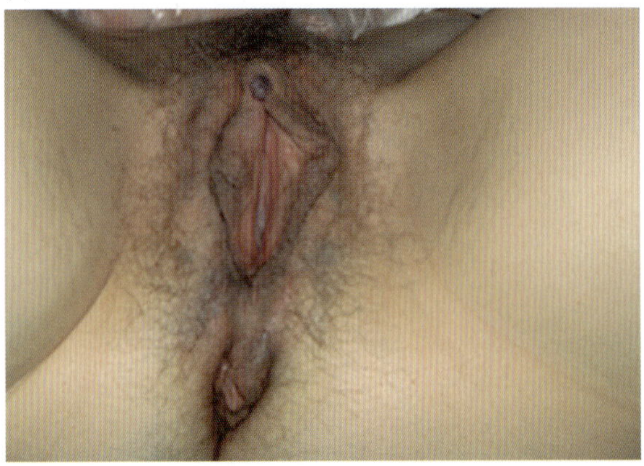

(c)

Figure 19.11 Large vulvar malformation: (a) before treatment; (b) during treatment; (c) after treatment

OK-432 (Picibanil; Chugay Pharmaceutical Co., Tokyo, Japan) is a preparation of dead bacteria obtained by culture of *Streptococcus pyogenes* (group A, type III) of human origin with penicillin G benzathine. The mixture is then lyophilized, resulting in the complete disappearance of streptolysin S. By this means, possible postinjection infection with systemic repercussions is avoided.

Besides its sclerosing action, OK-432 has various immunopharmacologic effects, including increases in the cytotoxicity of natural killer (NK) cells, cytotoxic T lymphocytes (CTL), lymphokine-activated killer (LAK) cells and macrophages, and the stimulation and synthesis of cytokines such as interleukin (IL)-1, IL-2, tumor necrosis factor (TNF), interferon (IFN)-α, IFN-β and IFN-γ. Because of these properties, this substance has been used to modify the biological response in treatments of tumors of the digestive tract, lung, and head and neck, and no major adverse effects have been reported. Its first clinical use was in 1987 to treat nine patients with cystic hygroma, achieving compete regression in eight of them.[75] Subsequent publications by the same group showed excellent outcomes in 93% of cystic lymphangiomas and 47% of cavernous lymphangiomas in series of 23 and 64 patients, respectively.[76,77] Over the years, reports on various patient series by other authors confirmed the efficacy of this procedure,[78,79] and sclerotherapy with OK-432 has been proposed as the treatment of choice for lymphatic malformations, especially those with macrocystic lesions. Although most lesions treated correspond to the cephalic pole because of the natural incidence of this disease, a satisfactory response has been obtained at all sites, including large retroperitoneal lesions[80] and complex locations such as the periorbital region,[81] and there is no age limit for patients. The only exclusion criterion for this therapy is allergy to penicillin.

As part of the OK-432 treatment protocol, the lesion should be measured by an imaging method such as ultrasonography, computed tomography or magnetic resonance. Cystography with contrast can also be indicated to establish the borders of the lesion and its ramifications. OK-432 can be obtained in vials of 0.1 and 0.5 mg. The working solution is prepared by diluting 0.1 mg in 10 mL of physiologic saline, obtaining a concentration of 0.01 mg of OK-432 in 1 mL of saline. After aspirating as much of the content of the cystic lesion as possible, the solution is injected under ultrasound guidance into the lumen of the cyst, using a maximum dose of 0.2 mg (20 mL) per session. If the lymph content cannot be previously extracted, the injection is made at different areas until the lesion is refilled. In the 6 hours after the procedure, the patient suffers a transient fever (38–39ºC) that abates with antipyretic treatment. There can also be a local inflammation 2–5 days after the injection. If there is no response to this treatment, the injection must be repeated at 1 week. If the malformation persists, the next treatment should be applied at 6 weeks. In one case with no initial response to a dose of 0.02 mg, the lesion completely regressed after a new injection with 0.04 mg,[81] indicating that the effect is sometimes dose-dependent. The maximum recommended dose is 0.3 mg of OK-432 per session.[76,82] In general, the lesion regresses, with no scarring or local anatomic changes, and no recurrences have been reported in published series after follow-ups of several years. Regarding its mechanism of action, it has been observed that OK-432 diffuses less readily than other substances used to treat lymphatic malformations, and that the damage remains more confined to the endothelial wall of the lesion. Ogita et al suggested that it has an essential immunomodulatory effect as well as a sclerosing action, and that the leukocytes and cytokines (especially TNF) activated and produced by OK-432 are responsible for increasing the endothelial permeability, thereby accelerating lymphatic drainage and favoring retraction of the cystic cavity.[83]

References

1. Sako Y, Varco R. Arteriovenous fistula: results of management of congenital and acquired forms, blood flow measurements, and observations on proximal arterial degeneration. Surgery 1970; 67: 40–61.
2. Finn MC, Glowacki J, Mulliken JB. Congenital vascular lesions: clinical application of a new classification. J Pediatr Surg 1983; 18: 894–900.
3. Eifert S, Villavicencio JL, Kao TC, Taute BM, Rich NM. Prevalence of deep venous anomalies in congenital vascular malformations of venous predominance. J Vasc Surg 2000; 31: 462–71.
4. Vikkula M, Boon L, Carraway K et al. Vascular dysmorphogenesis caused by an activating mutation in the receptor tyrosine kinase TIE2. Cell 1996; 87: 1181–90.
5. Sato T, Tozswa Y, Deutson U et al. Distinct roles of the receptor tyrosine kinases Tie-1 and Tie-2 in blood vessels formation. Nature 1995; 376: 70–4.
6. Smoller BR, Rosen S. Port-wine stains: a disease of altered neural modulation of blood vessels. Arch Dermatol 1986; 122: 177–9.

7. Rydh M, Malm M, Jernbeck J, Dalsgaard C. Ectatic blood vessels in port-wine stains lack innervation: possible role in pathogenesis. Plast Reconstr Surg 1991; 87; 419–22.
8. Van der Stricht J. Precapillary arterio-venous shunt syndromes: clinical borders between physiology and physiopathology. J Cardiovasc Surg 1972; 13: 503–9.
9. Mulliken JB, Glowacki J. Hemangiomas and vascular malformations in infants and children: a classification based on endothelial characteristics. Plast Reconstr Surg 1982; 69: 412.
10. Mulliken JB. Vascular malformations of the head and neck. In: Mulliken JB, Young AE, eds. Vascular Birthmarks: Hemangiomas and Vascular Malformations. Philadelphia: WB Saunders, 1988: 24–37.

10a. Belov S. Classification of congenital vascular defects. Int Angiol 1990; 9: 141–6.

11. Belov S, Loose DA, Weber J, eds. Vascular Malformations. Reinbek: Einhorn-Presse Verlag, 1989: 25–7.
12. Waner M, Suen JY, eds. Hemangiomas and Vascular Malformations of the Head and Neck: New York: Wiley-Liss, 1999.
13. Puig S, Aref H, Chigot V, Bonin B, Brunelle F. Classification of venous malformations in children and implications for sclerotherapy. Pediatr Radiol 2003; 33: 99–103.
14. Kohout MP, Hansen M, Pribaz JJ, Mulliken JB. Arteriovenous malformation of the head and neck: natural history and management. Plast Reconstr Surg 1988; 102: 643–54.
15. Oster J, Nielson A. Nuchal naevi and interscapular telangiectasis. Acta Paediatr Scand 1970; 59: 416–23.
16. Orten S, Waner M, Flock S, Roberson P, Kincannon J. Port-wine stains: an assessment of 5 years of treatment. Arch Otolaryngol Head Neck Surg 1996; 122: 1174–9.
17. Barsky SH, Rosen S, Geer DE, Noe J. The nature and evolution of port wine stains: a computer assisted study. J Invest Dermatol 1980; 74: 154–7.
18. Levine C. Primary disorders of the lymphatic vessels. A unified concept. J Pediatr Surg 1989; 24: 233–40.
19. Gross RE. Cystic hygroma. In: White M, Dennisson W, eds. The Surgery of Infancy and Childhood. Philadelphia, WB Saunders, 1953: 960–70.
20. Ward GE, Hendrick JW, Chambers RG. Cystic hygroma of the head and neck. Surg Obstet Gynecol 1950; 58: 41–7.
21. Kennedy TL. Cystic hygroma–lymphoma: a rare, still unclear entity. Laryngoscope 1989; 99: 1–10.
22. Broomhead IW. Cystic hygroma of the neck. Br J Plast Surg 1964; 17: 225–44.
23. Nihn TN, Nihn TX. Cystic hygroma in children: report of 126 cases. J Pediatr Surg 1974; 9: 191–5.
24. Boyd JB, Mulliken JB, Kaban LB, et al. Skeletal changes associated with vascular malformations. Plast Reconstr Surg 1984; 76: 789–97.
25. Gorham LW, Stout AP. Massive osteolysis (acute spontaneous absorption of bone, phantom bone, disappearing bone): its relations to hemangiomatosis. J Bone Joint Surg 1955; 37: 986–1004.
26. Sabin FR. The lymphatic system in human embryos, with a consideration of the morphology of the system as a whole. Am J Anat 1909; 9: 43–91.
27. Schmidt GH. Hemangioma in the zygoma. Ann Plast Surg 1982; 3: 330–2.
28. Hein KD, Mulliken JB, Kozakewich HP, Upton J, Burrows PE. Venous malformations of skeletal muscle. Plast Reconstr Surg 2002; 110: 1625–35.
29. Enjolras O, Ciabrini D, Mazoyer E, et al. Extensive pure venous malformations in the upper or lower limb, a review of 27 cases. J Am Acad Dermatol 1997; 36: 219–25.
30. Boon LM, Mulliken JB, Enjolras O, Vikkula M. Glomuvenous malformation (glomangioma) and venous malformation: distinct clinicopathologic and genetic entities. Arch Dermatol 2004; 140: 971–6.
31. Sako Y, Varco R. Arteriovenous fistula: results of management of congenital and acquired forms, blood flow measurements, and observations on proximal arterial degeneration. Surgery 1970; 67: 40–61.
32. Flye MW, Jordan BP, Schwartz MZ. Management of congenital arteriovenous malformations. Surgery 1983; 94: 740–7.
33. Natali J, Jue-Denis P, Kieffer E, et al. Arteriovenous fistulae of the internal iliac vessels. J Cardiovasc Surg 1984; 25: 165–72.
34. Kohout MP, Hansen M, Pribaz JJ, Mulliken JB. Arteriovenous malformation of the head and neck: natural history and management. Plast Reconstr Surg 1988; 102: 643–54.
35. Jacob AG, Driscoll DJ, Shaughnessy WJ, et al. Klippel–Trenaunay syndrome: spectrum and management. Mayo Clin Proc 1998; 73: 28–36.
36. Gloviczki P, Stanson AW, Stickler GB, et al. Klippel–Trenaunay syndrome: the risks and benefits of vascular interventions. Surgery 1991; 110: 469–79.
37. Samuel M, Spitz L. Klippel–Trenaunay syndrome: clinical features, complications and management in children. Br J Surg 1995; 82: 757–61.
38. Baskerville PA, Akroyd JS, Thomas ML, Browse NL. The Klippel–Trenaunay syndrome: clinical, radiological, and hemodynamic features and management. Br J Surg 1985; 72: 232–6.
39. Maari C, Frieden IJ. Klippel–Trenaunay syndrome: The importance of “geographic stains” in identifying lymphatic disease and risk of complications. J Am Acad Dermatol 2004; 51: 391–8.

40. Wiedemann HR, Burgio GR, Aldenhoff P, et al. The Proteus syndrome. Eur J Pediatr 1983; 140: 5–12.
41. Hotamisligil GS. Proteus syndrome and hamartoses with overgrowth. Dysmorphol Clin Genet 1990; 4: 87–102.
42. Cohen MM Jr, Neri G, Wesberg R, eds. Overgrowth Syndromes. New York: Oxford University Press, 2000.
43. Perkins P, Weiss SW. Spindle cell hemangioendothelioma. An analysis of 78 cases with reassessment of its pathogenesis and biologic behavior. Am J Surg Pathol 1996; 20: 1196–204.
44. Cohen MM Jr. Vasculogenesis, angiogenesis, hemangiomas, and vascular malformations. Am J Med Gen 2002; 108: 265–74.
45. Lee BB. What is new in venous disease: new approach to old problem of venous disease: congenital vascular malformation. In: Angelides NS, ed. Advances in Phlebology. Limassol: Hadjigeogiou, 1998: 59–64.
46. Noel AA, Gloviczki P, Cherry KJ Jr, Rooke TW, Stanson AW, Driscoll DJ. Surgical treatment of venous malformations in Klippel–Trenaunay syndrome. J Vasc Surg 2000; 32: 840–7.
47. Werner JA, Lippert BM, Hoffmann P, Rudert H. Nd:YAG laser therapy of voluminous hemangiomas and vascular malformations. Adv Otorhinolaryngol 1995; 49: 75–80.
48. Groot D, Rao J, Johnston P, Nakatsui T. Algorithm for using a long-pulsed Nd:YAG laser in the treatment of deep cutaneous vascular lesions. Dermatol Surg 2003; 29: 35–42.
49. Enjolras O, Mulliken JB. Vascular tumors and vascular malformations (new issues). Adv Dermatol 1998; 13: 375–422.
50. Mulliken JB, Young AE, eds. Vascular Birthmarks: Hemangiomas and Malformations. Philadelphia: WB Saunders, 1988.
51. Jacob AG, Driscoll DJ, Shaughnessy WJ, et al. Klippel–Trenaunay syndrome: spectrum and management. Mayo Clin Proc 1998; 73: 28–36.
52. Baskerville PA, Akroyd JS, Thomas ML, Browse NL. The Klippel–Trenaunay syndrome: clinical, radiological, and hemodynamic features and management. Br J Surg 1985; 72: 232–6.
53. Yakes WF, Luethke JM, Parker SH, et al. Ethanol embolization of vascular malformations. Radiographics 1990; 10: 787–96.
54. De Lorimier AA. Sclerotherapy for venous malformations. J Pediatr Surg 1995; 30: 188–94.
55. Jackson IT, Carreño R, Potparic Z, Hussain K. Hemangiomas, vascular malformations: classification and methods of treatment. Plast Reconstr Surg 1993; 7: 1216–30.
56. Goldman MP, Bennet RG. Treatment of telangiectasia: a review. J Am Acad Dermatol 1987; 17: 167–82.
57. Dubois J, Sebag GH, De Prost Y, et al. The treatment of soft tissue venous malformation in children: percutaneous sclerotherapy with Ethibloc. Radiology 1991; 180: 195–8.
58. Villavicencio JL. Primum non nocere: Is it always true? The use of absolute ethanol in the management of congenital vascular malformations. J Vasc Surg 2001; 33: 904–6.
59. Cadere T. Treatment of varices with ethoxysclerol. Phebologie 1980; 33: 377–8.
60. Belov S. Late results in the treatment of vascular malformations. Int Angiol 1998; 7: 136–43.
61. Weiss RA, Goldman MP. Advances in sclerotherapy. Dermatol Clin 1995; 13: 431–45.
62. Cabrera J, Cabrera J Jr, García-Olmedo MA. Elargissement des limites de la sclerotherapie: Nouveaux produits sclerosants. Phlebologie 1997; 2: 181–8.
63. Cabrera J, Cabrera J Jr, García-Olmedo MA. Treatment of varicose long saphenous veins with sclerosant in microfoam form: long-term outcomes. Phlebology 2000; 15: 19–23.
64. Pascarella L, Bergan JJ, Yamada C, Mekenas L. Venous angiomata: treatment with sclerosant foam. Ann Vasc Surg 2005; 19: 457–64.
65. Meltzer RS, Serruys PW, Hugenholtz PG, Roelandt J. Intravenous carbon dioxide as an echocardiographic contrast agent. J Clin Ultrasound 1981; 9: 127–31.
66. Martinez-Cuesta A, Elduayen B, Vivas I, Delgado C, González-Crespo I, Bilbao JI. CO_2 wedged hepatic venography technical considerations and comparison with direct and indirect portography with iodinated contrast. Abdom Imaging 2000; 25: 576–82.
67. Bendib M, Toumi M, Boudjellab A. CO_2 angiography and enlarged CO_2 angiography in cardiology. Ann Radiol (Paris) 1977; 20: 673–86.
68. Fermand M, Marzelle J, Cormier F, Cormier JM. Aorto-arteriography of the lower limbs using carbon dioxide. Presse Med 1994; 1: 19–22.
69. Kerns SR, Hawkins IF Jr. Carbon dioxide digital subtraction angiography: expanding applications and technical evolution. AJR Am J Roentgenol 1995; 164: 735–41.
70. Bikerman JJ. Foams. New York: Springer-Verlag; 1973.
71. Cabrera J, Cabrera J Jr, inventors; BTG International Limited Assignee. Injectable microfoam containing a sclerosing agent. US Patent 5676962. 16 October 1997.
72. Cabrera J, Cabrera J Jr, García-Olmedo MA, Redondo P. Treatment of venous malformations with sclerosant in microfoam form. Arch Dermatol 2003; 139: 1409–16.

73. Hsu TS, Weiss RA. Foam sclerotherapy: a new era. Arch Dermatol 2003; 139: 1494–6.
74. Ogita S, Tsuto T, Tokiwa K, Takahashi T. Intracystic injection of OK-432: a new sclerosing therapy for cystic hygroma in children. Br J Surg 1987; 74: 690–1.
75. Ogita et al. OK-432 therapy for unresectable lymphangiomas in children. J Pediatr Surg 1991; 26: 263–70.
76. Ogita S, Tsuto T, Nakamura K, et al. OK-432 therapy in 64 patients with lymphangioma. J Pediatr Surg 1994; 29: 784–5.
77. Luzzatto C, Midrio P, Tchaprassian Z, Guglielmi M. Sclerosing treatment of lymphangiomas with OK-432. Arch Dis Child 2000; 82: 316–18.
78. Claesson G, Kuyelenstierna R. OK-432 therapy for lymphatic malformation in 32 patients (28 children). Int J Pediatr Otorhinolaryngol 2002; 65: 1–6.
79. Uchida K, Inoue M, Araki T, Miki C, Kusunoki M. Huge scrotal, flank and retroperitoneal lymphangioma successfully treated by OK-432 sclerotherapy. Urology 2002; 60: 1112xxiv–1112xxvi.
80. Suzuki Y, Obana A, Gohto Y, Miki T, Otuka H, Inoue Y. Management of orbital lymphangioma using intralesional injection of OK-432. Br J Ophthalmol 2000; 84: 614–17.
81. Banieghlbal B, Davies MR. Guidelines for the successful treatment of lymphangioma with OK-432. Eur J Pediatr Surg 2003; 13: 103–7.
82. Ogita S, Tsuto T, Nakamura K, et al. OK-432 therapy for lymphangiomas in children: Why and how does it work? J Pediatr Surg 1996; 31: 477–80.

20 Treatment of venous malformations, Klippel–Trenaunay syndrome and other low-flow lesions with foamed sclerosants

John Bergan and Van Le Cheng

Introduction

Vascular malformations are not rare, but finding an experienced physician to care for them may be difficult. This is because surgical removal may be demanding or impossible, embolization with coils requires an adequate arterial inflow, and closure with ethanol is complex and fraught with complications. Fortunately, a number of specialized multidisciplinary clinics have been formed in the United States and abroad to take care of the small number of under-served patients who harbor vascular anomalies.[1]

Venous malformations are the most common of all vascular anomalies. They comprised 37% of BB Lee's experience at the Sungkyunkwan Vascular Malformation Clinic at the Samsung Hospital in Seoul.[2] Of the 294 cases, 128 were in the extremities (98 in the lower). In the Vascular Anomalies Clinic of the University of California at San Francisco, 62% of patients diagnosed over 10 years of age had venous malformations.

Yakes described 36 such patients in 1994.[3] He called attention to high-flow and low-flow malformations and pointed out that incorrect terms included hemangioma, cavernous hemangioma, venous angioma, phlebectasias, and cavernoma. Yakes used the classification system of Mulliken and Glowacki.[4] In 1982, that system was a step forward away from the chaos of disordered terminology that dominated the 20th century. Mulliken noted that hemangiomas were true endothelial tumors that exhibited a distinct proliferative phase, which was followed by slow involution.

In 1988, a consensus conference was held in Hamburg, Germany under the direction of Stefan Belov of Sofia, Bulgaria. The conference was attended by many of the world's experts on congenital vascular malformations (CVMs), founding members of the International Society for Studies of Vascular Anomalies (ISSVA).[5] Ultimately, this conference proposed an acceptable classification and terminology of CVMs that was properly based on embryologic information that had been accumulating over many years.

The Hamburg classification defined CVMs according to developmental arrest at various stages of embryonic life. This was somewhat modified by consensus at a meeting of these same experts in Denver in 1992. The classification singled out predominantly arterial, venous, arteriovenous shunting and lymphatic lesions in their truncular or extratruncular forms and added the anatomical forms of aplasia or obstruction, dilation, and infiltrating or limited forms. Arterial and venous forms with and without shunts were acknowledged, as were hemolymphatic types.

Extratruncular forms develop from the earliest stages of embryonic life, at the reticular stage. They have embryonic characteristics of developmental potential. This means that, when stimulated by trauma, pregnancy or surgery, they can begin to grow. They are further classified as diffuse and infiltrating, or as limited and localized.

Truncular forms develop from later stages of embryonic life and their hemodynamic impact may be severe. They are further classified as an aplasia type (obstruction, hypoplasia, stenosis, spur or membrane) or a dilation type (localized aneurysm, diffuse ectasia). The Hamburg classification separates vascular malformations from vascular tumors and can decrease confusion regarding these different entities.

Although the Hamburg classification provided a path away from the name-based terminology, some of these eponyms persist even though they remain imprecisely defined. As originally described, the Klippel–Trenaunay syndrome was a triad.[6] This included a cutaneous hemangioma, varicose veins since childhood and limb hypertrophy (Figure 20.1).

Gradually, as various quantities of arteriovenous shunting in these limbs were recognized, the eponym became corrupted into the Klippel–Trenaunay–Weber syndrome. Parkes Weber described "hemangiectatic hypertrophy" and included all hypertrophies of the lower limb.[7] He included limbs not only with varices but also true arteriovenous fistulas. This introduced confusion because congenital arteriovenous fistulas and the Klippel–Trenaunay syndrome are distinctly different entities. Several authorities have described the Klippel–Trenaunay syndrome variously. At the Mayo Clinic, it was described as a limb hemangioma with over-

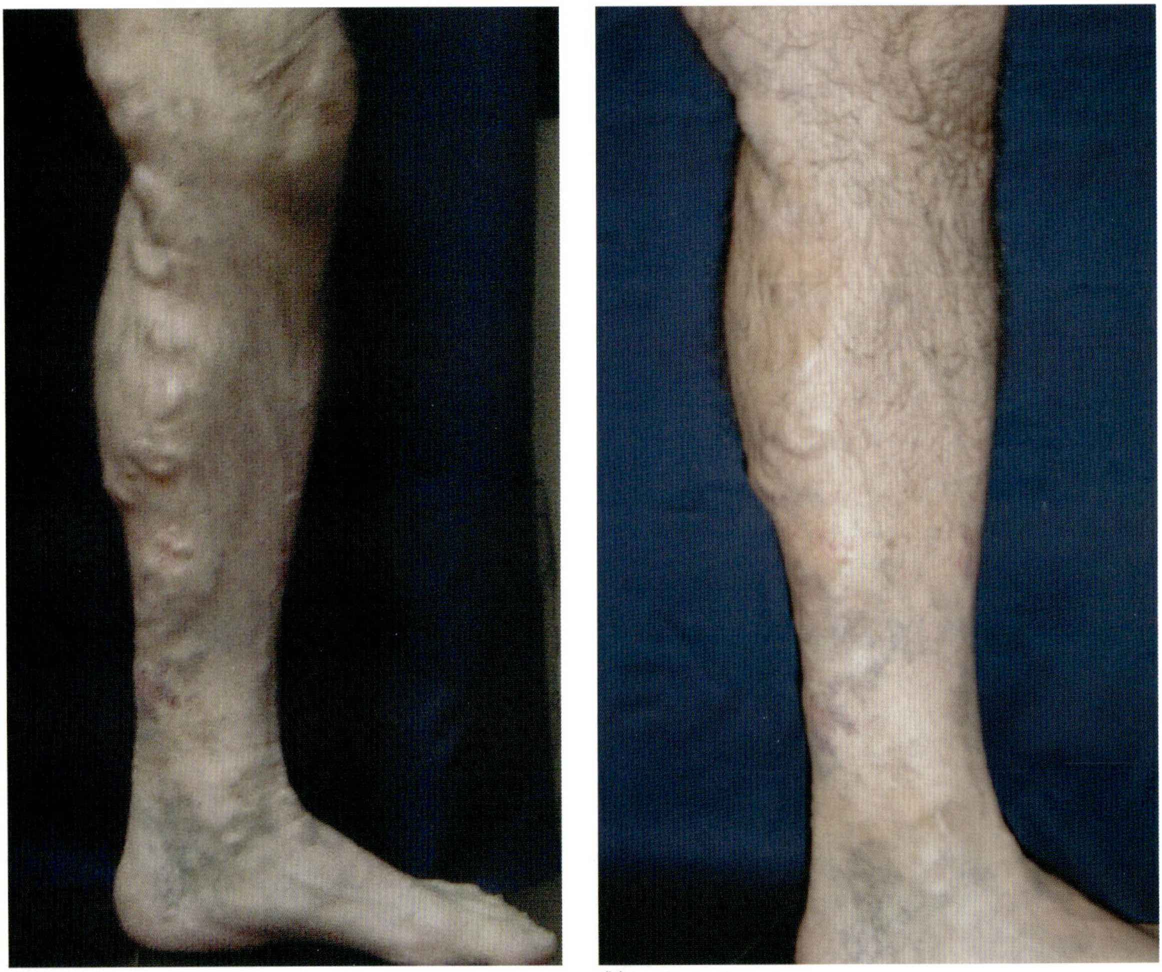

(a) (b)

Figure 20.1 (a, b) Klippel–Trenanauy syndrome in the lower extremity of a 76-year-old physician. Note the presence of a birthmark and enlarging painful varicose veins. He was treated with three injections of sodium tetradecyl sulfate 1.5% equivalent growth of bone and soft tissues in a limb with varicose veins.[8] We favor this definition, thus separating the Klippel–Trenaunay syndrome from high-flow vascular malformations and leaving the syndrome as a venous angiodysplasia.

Probably, the Hamburg classification[9] terminology should be used and the name-based eponyms dropped. But there is a certain historic charm in the use of eponyms, and our interpretation of the Klippel–Trenaunay syndrome is a limb with capillary vascular malformations, soft tissue and/or bony hypertrophy, and varicose veins without gross arteriovenous shunting or lymphatic/soft tissue abnormalities. Some, but not all, of these limbs have abnormal development of deep and superficial veins.

Venous malformations (angiomas) are often present at birth, although they may not be evident until later. They consist of a spongy tangle of veins, and these lesions usually vary in size (Figure 20.2). Treatment of these venous malformations is often requested for cosmetic reasons, but painful ulcerations, nerve compression and functional disability can command care.

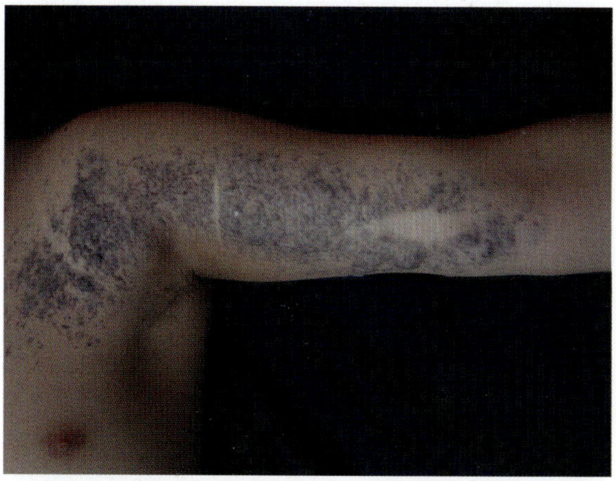

Figure 20.2 This extensive venous angioma did respond well to foam sclerotherapy. Note the scars of ill-advised biopsies, which yielded no useful information

Investigations

Following a focused physical examination, a duplex ultrasound examination can add information about blood flow, volume and velocity of a vascular malformation.[10] If carefully done, it can identify feeding arteries and draining veins. Magnetic resonance imaging has replaced conventional arteriography and phlebography in the initial evaluation of vascular malformations.[11,12] It provides hemodynamic and anatomic information, as well as relationships with surrounding tissues and organs. Lee has found a sensitivity in excess of 97% and a specificity of 91%. It is also useful in assessment of the results of treatment. T1- and T2-weighted images have shown excellent ability to differentiate low-flow shunting from high-flow lesions. Angiography, especially catheter-directed and superselective arteriography, remains useful in pretreatment planning. Magnetic resonance imaging has a distinct limitation in differentiating between lymphatic and vascular malformations.[5]

Personal experience

During a 30-month period, 1321 patients were investigated for venous disorders at the Vein Institute of La Jolla, CA. Fourteen (incidence: 1%) were found to have venous malformations (5 men, 9 women). The age range was 15–76 years (mean: 30.8 ± 18.6). Lesions were classified by the Hamburg system and were primarily venous, extratruncular in 12 patients and combined extratruncular and truncular in 2 patients.[13]

Eight patients, three of them males, had manifestations of lower extremity Klippel–Trenaunay syndrome; six had only venous malformations. Eighteen of the 22 patients were treated.

All patients were studied by Doppler duplex examination. Selected lesions were chosen for helical computed tomographic studies. Magnetic resonance venography was also used to image the lesions, define the deep circulation, note connections with normal circulation, identify vessels for therapeutic access, and determine infiltration of the lesion into adjacent soft tissue.

Foam was produced by the technique of Tessari, using two syringes connected by a three-way stopcock, with the air-to-polidocanol ratio being 4 or 5 to 1. This was used at 1% or 2% concentration, specific for each patient.

The SonoSite 190 Plus duplex Doppler was used for ultrasound guidance whenever deep access was required, and to monitor progress and effects of treatment. A goal was set for each patient before treatment was begun.

The mean number of treatments was 3.6 ± 2.8 (range: 1–10). A primary goal of pain-free healing was set in patients with nonhealing, painful ulcerations or symptomatic varicose veins. This was achieved in all treated patients. Cosmetically, all of the patients were improved, and symptomatic patients were relieved of ulcers and pain.

Sclerosant foam is a satisfactory tool to use in treating venous malformations and the Klippel–Trenaunay syndrome. Use of foam sclerotherapy in this experience has proven the technique to be effective, essentially painfree, and durable in the short term.

Discussion

Absolute ethanol sclerotherapy has been used in the treatment of vascular malformations.[14] Its action is to denature tissue protein, precipitating protoplasm with subsequent obliteration of the vessel lumen. Its use is fraught with complications. The procedures require general anesthesia but are effective. In the Boston Children's Hospital experience, 13% of 40 patients experienced deep ulcerations, 50% had blistering and 28% had hemoglobinuria.[15]

In order to minimize complications, sclerotherapy with liquid sclerosants has been used in the treatment of venous, lymphatic and low-flow vascular malformations. It finds a place in the treatment of small vascular malformations. Over a 20-year period ending in 1995, 157 patients were treated with liquid sclerotherapy in the Dermatology Department of the Humboldt University in Berlin, Germany. The majority of the lesions were hemangiomas and vascular malformations located in the head and neck, and 55% were in children and adolescents. One to three treatments sufficed and the results appeared durable.[16]

Liquid sclerosants, unfortunately, become diluted and inactivated by intralesional blood. Alternatively, the use of sclerosants in microfoam form significantly improves the procedure. The foam displaces blood instead of becoming diluted, and the echogenicity of the bubbles makes them visible on ultrasound surveillance. Foam treatments, in contrast to those using ethanol, can be given on a strictly ambulatory basis.

Yamaki described the use of sclerosant foam in treating a facial vascular malformation of the cheek in a patient with a failed attempt at surgical removal.[17]

Duplex guidance and general anesthesia were used, with the foam being produced by the Tessari technique using 1% polidocanol.

The first report of a large group of patients treated by foam sclerotherapy was that of Cabrera from Granada, Spain.[18] The report included 50 patients, 19 with limited venous malformations, 16 with infiltrating venous malformations and 15 with Klippel–Trenaunay syndrome. Sclerotherapy was by direct injection of 0.25–4% polidocanol microfoam using ultrasound guidance. The therapy was judged to be beneficial in 92% of the patients. Amongst the 46 responders, 18 showed disappearance of treated lesions, 15 had a reduction in malformation size of more than 50% and 13 showed a reduction in malformation size of 50% or less. Of those with severe pain, 25 of 39 patients experienced total relief, and in the other 14, the pain was significantly reduced. No patient reported a major adverse event. There were 4 cases of transient skin pigmentation and 3 cases of skin necrosis.

Cabrera's group has also taken the lead in the evaluation of Klippel–Trenaunay syndrome.[19] Their conclusion was that multidetector computed tomography and three-dimensional magnetic resonance venography are extremely helpful for the global evaluation of patients with Klippel–Trenaunay syndrome. Information regarding soft tissue and bony anatomy, as well as information about superficial and deep venous systems, may be obtained with a single examination (Figure 20.3). In examining 16 patients, persistent embryonic veins were seen in all patients. In one patient, aplasia/atresia of the whole deep venous system was revealed. Half of the

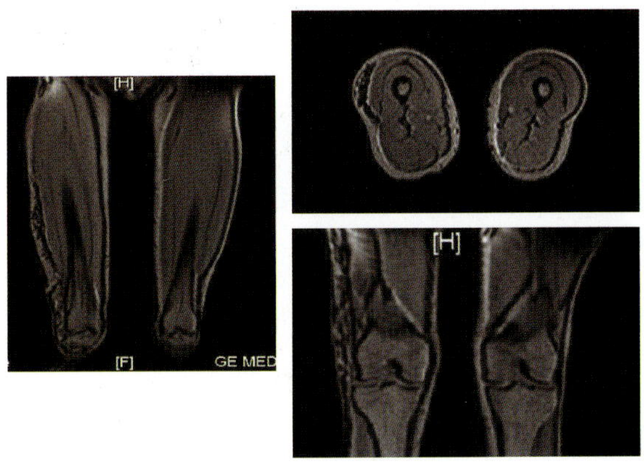

Figure 20.3 Magnetic resonance venogram (MRV) of a patient with an extensive venous angioma on the right lateral thigh. Information regarding soft tissue and bony anatomy, as well as the superficial and deep venous systems, was obtained with a single examination

patients had popliteal venous abnormalities, including aplasia (6 patients) and an aneurysm (1 patient). Other abnormalities in this group of patients included femoral vein hypoplasia in 4 patients, duplication of the femoral vein in 1 patient, and aplasia of the femoral vein in 3 patients.

Conclusions

Foam sclerotherapy holds several advantages over absolute ethanol and liquid sclerosants although, admittedly, it is nowhere near as powerful as ethanol. Neither does it carry the need for general anesthesthia or have the rate of complications of alcohol. The efficacy of a given concentration of sclerosant is greatly increased when used as foam instead of liquid. Also, a small amount of liquid can produce four to five times its volume when made into foam. It is echogenic, a significant benefit that allows foam sclerotherapy of vascular malformations to be moved into an outpatient office.

References

1. Donnelly LF, Adams DM, Bisset GS 3rd. Vascular malformations and hemangiomas: a practical approach in a multidisciplinary clinic. AJR Am J Roentgenol 2000; 174: 597–608.
2. Lee BB. New approaches to the treatment of congenital vascular malformations (CVMs) – a single centre experience. Eur J Vasc Endovasc Surg 2005; 30: 184–97.
3. Yakes WF. Extremity venous malformations: diagnosis and management. Sem Intervent Rad 1994; 2: 332–9.
4. Mulliken JB, Glowacki J. Hemangiomas and vascular malformations in infants and children: a classification based on endothelial characteristics. Plast Reconstr Surg 1982; 69: 412–22.
5. Lee BB, Mattassi R, Loose D, et al. Consensus on controversial issues in contemporary diagnosis and management of congenital vascular malformations: Seoul communication. Int J Angiol 2005; 13: 182–92.
6. Klippel M, Trenaunay P. Du naevus variquex osteohypertrophique. Arch Gen Med (Paris) 1900; 185: 641–72.
7. Parkes Weber F. Haemangiectatic hypertrophy of limbs – congenital phlebarteriectasis and so-called varicose veins. Br J Child Dis 1918; 15: 13–17.
8. Fairbairn II JF, Juergens JL, Spittell JA Jr. Peripheral Vascular Diseases, 4th edn. Philadelphia: WB Saunders; 505 pp.
9. Ernemann U, Hoffmann J, Breuninger H, et al. Interdisciplinary concept for classification and treatment of vascular anomalies in the head and neck. Mund Kiefer Gesichtschir 2002; 6: 402–9.
10. Steven M, Kumaran N, Carachi R, et al. Haemangiomas and vascular malformations of the limb in children. Pediatr Surg Int 2007; 23: 565–9.
11. Lee BB, Choe YH, Ahn JM, et al. The new role of magnetic resonance imaging in the contemporary diagnosis of venous malformation: Can it replace angiography? J Am Coll Surg 2004; 198: 549–58.
12. Laor T, Burrows PE, Hoffer FA. Magnetic resonance venography of congenital vascular malformations of the extremities. Pediatr Radiol 1996; 26: 371–8.
13. Pascarella L, Bergan JJ, Yamada C, Mekenas L. Venous angiomata: treatment with sclerosant foam. Ann Vasc Surg 2005; 19: 457–64.
14. Rimon U, Garniek A, Galili Y, et al. Ethanol sclerotherapy of peripheral venous malformations. Eur J Radiol 2004; 52: 283–7.
15. Berenguer B, Burrows PE, Zurakowski D, Mulliken JB. Sclerotherapy of craniofacial venous malformations: complications and results. Plast Reconstr Surg 1999; 104: 1–11.
16. Winter H, Drager E, Sterry W. Sclerotherapy for treatment of hemangiomas. Dermatol Surg 2000; 26: 105–8.
17. Yamaki T, Nozaki M, Fujiwara O, Yoshida E. Duplex-guided foam sclerotherapy for the treatment of the symptomatic venous malformations of the face. Dermatol Surg 2002; 28: 619–22.
18. Cabrera J, Cabrera J Jr, Garcia-Olmedo MA, Redondo P. Treatment of venous malformations with sclerosant in microfoam form. Arch Dermatol 2003; 139: 1409–16.
19. Bastarrika G, Redondo P, Sierra A, et al. New techniques for the evaluation and therapeutic planning of patients with Klippel–Trenaunay syndrome. J Am Acad Dermatol 2007; 56: 242–9.

Epilogue

Our intention has been to bring together and update our collective experiences with foam sclerotherapy.

We have felt that in doing this we will strongly influence the care of patients with venous insufficiency in the future. No doubt you will have noted that the contributing authors are acknowledged international authorities in the areas that they have addressed, and have demonstrated their skill as experienced teachers of sclerotherapy. It was clear to us – and we trust that it will be clear to you – that these are experienced clinicians whose work is of particular importance to those of us who are students of this art.

We sincerely hope that you, the reader, will have derived as much pleasure and benefit from reading this book as we have had in compiling and editing it.

Index

A

acroangiodermatitis 19–20
adverse events *see* complications and risks; *specific conditions*
air, use as injected air 6
air in carbon dioxide–air mixtures 71, 80, 184, 210
air plethysmography 179
alcohol sclerotherapy 222–3
  transition to foam sclerotherapy 129–40
allergic reactions 149
  contact dermatitis 15–16, 32
allergy testing 21
alpha-galactosidase deficiency 26
angiokeratoma, of Fordyce 25
angiokeratoma circumscriptum 25–6
angiokeratoma corporis diffusum 26
angiomas
  venous malformations 202–4, 221
  see also venous malformations
antiphospholipid syndrome 24
arteriovenous malformations 199–218, 204–6
contraindications for sclerotherapy 209
microvasculature 28
ASVAL (ambulatory selective varices ablation under local anesthesia) 171
ataxia telangiectasia 29
atrophie blanche 16–17, 25

B

Baker's cyst 24, 121–2
'blue leg' 24

C

cannulation, US guided 70–1
carbitol 157
carbon dioxide–air mixtures 71, 210
  and cerebral embolism risk 80
  studies 184
carbon dioxide–oxygen mixtures 90
  eliminating nitrogen 90
CEAP classification 106, 109–10, 141
cerebral embolism risk, carbon dioxide vs air vs mixtures 71, 80
CHIVA cure, role of saphenous veins 163, 166
chronic venous insufficiency (CVI) 13–30
clinical studies 84–5
  comparative trials, sclerotherapy vs laser 148
  randomized controlled trials, polidocanol vs other treatments 105–16
  trials/exercises on safety of foam sclerotherapy 183–91
Cockett's perforating veins 18, 72
complications and risks 97–100, 126–7
  comparison of side effects 147
  German Society of Phlebology guidelines 32–3
  phlebitis 127
  prevention 85–6
rates 151
compounding of sclerosing agents 48–50
compression bandaging 73, 76
congenital venous malformations (CVMs) 129–30, 129–30, 219–20
  see also vascular malformations
consent, patient 70
contact dermatitis 15–16
corona phlebectatica paraplantaris 13–14
coughing, post foam sclerotherapy 75
Cox regression analysis 93, 97, 99
crossectomy
  + stripping + phlebectomy 164
  extended 165
cutaneous lesions 13–30
  contact dermatitis 15–16
  eczematous eruptions 15–16
  lipodermatosclerosis (LDS) 17–18, 120–1
  necrosis 150–1
  venous insufficiency 13–30
  venous malformations 132

D

Darier's sign 29
deep vein reflux 120
deep venous occlusions 97, 100
deep venous thrombosis 24, 33, 86, 151
  distribution and outcome 113–14
  and duplicated segments of femoral vein 184–5
dermatitis, contact dermatitis 15–16
detergent agents 4
discoid eczema 15–16

double syringe system (DSS) 8
  displacing capacity of DSS foams 9
drugs, physician liability 50–1
duplex ultrasound evaluation
  equipment 62
  medium term results 87–101
  right-to-left shunting 185–6
  routine 89, 179
  venous malformations 133
  venous reflux 7, 61–8, 89
duplex ultrasound guided foam sclerotherapy 34–6, 61–8, 79–86, 179–82
  4 phases 81
  rationale 80
  with vs without duplex guidance 79–86
  see also foam sclerotherapy

E

eczematous eruptions 15–16
edema 14–15
efficacy of treatment 75–7, 83, 84–5
  foam sclerotherapy 66, 87–101, 169–70
  German Society of Phlebology guidelines 37–8
  polidocanol 147
  randomized controlled trials 109–12
  statistical analysis of results 93–6
ELLE technique 126
endovenous laser therapy (EVLT) *see* laser therapy
equinus deformity 17
ethanol sclerotherapy 222–3
  transition to foam sclerotherapy 129–39
extravascular injection of sclerosant foams 74

F

Fabry's disease, angiokeratoma corporis diffusum 26
facial telangiectasias 26–7
FDA
  DHSS *warning letter* 50
  drug review steps 46
  legal guidelines for sclerosing agent use 43–52
  summary of history of sclerosants 45
femoral vein, duplicated segments 184–5
Fibro-Vein™ 157
foam sclerotherapy 34–6, 56–8, 61–8, 79–86, 179–82
  4 phases 81
  ablation 82
  assessment of results 66, 87–101
  ELLE technique 126
  vs endovenous laser therapy 2002–2006 88
  first sclerosant foam treatments 58
  foam compared with liquid 97, 177–82
  German Society of Phlebology guidelines 34–7
  hemodynamic variables pre/post treatment 181
  history 3–9
  indications 81–2
  into SFJ or SPJ 126
  large varicose veins 117–28
  legal guidelines for use 50–2
  monitoring 64–6
foam sclerotherapy – *contd*
  needling technique 90–1
    blind needling 91
    closed needle 80–1
  personal review 69–77
  postoperative care and review 125–6
  pretreatment assessment 61–2, 88–9
  protocols: one/two legs 123–4
  randomized controlled trials
    inclusion/exclusion criteria 105
    polidocanol vs other treatments 105–16
    results 109–12
  rationale 80
  relative/absolute contraindications 70
  results 169–70
  safety 80, 117, 183–92
  selection of patients 87–8, 99, 122
  statistical analysis of results 93–6
  with/without duplex ultrasound guidance 79–86
  see also duplex ultrasound guided foam sclerotherapy; foams
foams 56–8
  advantages 145–7
  clinical applications 58
  DSS technique 158–9
  duplex ultrasound monitoring 64–6
  extravascular injection 74
  foam compared with liquid 97, 177–82
  German Society of Phlebology guidelines 34–7
  history 3–9
  mode of use 56–7
  no blood dilution effects 79
  preparation 71, 97–8, 123–4
  production 4–10, 55–9
  properties 58
  randomized controlled trials
    inclusion/exclusion criteria 105
    polidocanol vs other treatments 105–16
  rationale for using 79–8
  stability 8
  substitute for ethanol sclerotherapy 129–39
  volume 73, 89, 107, 122–3
    per puncture 35
    safety issues 122–3
    total 107
  see also foam sclerotherapy; *specific agents*
foramen ovale, patency 85

G

German Society of Phlebology guidelines 31–42
  complications and risks 32–3
  definitions 31
  diagnosis pre sclerotherapy 33
  efficacy 37–8
  indications/contraindications 31–2
  safety 35–6
  sclerosant foam 34–7
  sclerosant solutions 33–4

glycerin, chromated
complications 149
vs polidocanol 146
Gougerot–Blum dermatosis 21, 23
GSVs, testing and mapping 62–4

H
hand, vascular malformations 206, 212
helium 10
hemodynamic theory of venous disease, descending vs ascending 163
hemodynamic variables, pre-/post foam sclerotherapy 181
hemosiderin pigmentary changes 16–17, 33, 76, 127, 150
hereditary benign telangiectasias 28
hereditary hemorrhagic telangiectasias 28
history of foam sclerotherapy 3–9, 55–6, 58
Homan's sign 24
HRT 88

I
informed consent 70
injectable sclerosing agents 3–4
injection site 80–1
injection technique 98–9
extravascular injection of foams 74
intra-arterial injection of foams 150
ischemia, necrosis 204

K
Kaplan–Meier curves 94–6
Kasabach–Merrit syndrome 203
Klippel–Trenaunay syndrome 129, 219, 205–6, 220–1
foam sclerotherapy 210–12

L
laser therapy
vs duplex US guided foam sclerotherapy 2002–2006 88
endovenous (EVLT) 166–7
comparative trials, vs sclerotherapy 148
vs duplex US guided foam sclerotherapy 2002–2006 88
principles 166
results 167
vs sclerotherapy, comparative trials 148
vascular malformations 208
see also endovenous laser therapy (EVLT)
leg telangiectasias 26
lichen aureus 20–1
lipodermatosclerosis (LDS) 17–18, 120–1
livedoid vasculopathy 25
lumps, residual 76
lymphatic malformations 201–2
lymphedema 14–15
lymphoscintigraphy 14–15

M
Mafucci's syndrome 206
Majocchi's disease 21–2
mat telangiectasias 27, 33, 27–8, 33, 127, 150
Medicare, illegally compounded drugs 50–1
migraine-like symptoms 33, 75
mini-invasive surgery, role of saphenous veins 170–1
Mondor's disease 23–4
Monfreux technique 34–5
telangiectasias 58, 145

N
NAS 4 (NIAPROOF 4) 157
necrosis
cutaneous lesions 150–1
steal syndrome 204
needles 90–1
closed needle technique 80–1
neovascularization, recurrence rates of varicose veins 194–6
nitrogen, eliminating, carbon dioxide–oxygen mixtures 90
nodular vasculitis 22–3

O
OK-432 214–15
oral contraceptive pill 88
oral mucosal venous malformations 132–6
Osler–Rendu–Weber disease 28
ostial reflux, and truncal reflux 170
outcomes of treatment 75–7, 83, 84–5
clinical studies 84–5

P
panniculopathies 17
Parkes–Weber syndrome 206
patients
consent 70
selection 87–8, 98–9
Trendelenberg position 188–9
perforating veins
classification 84
Cockett's 18, 72
incompetent 72
injection at a distance 81
re-entries 84
phlebitis, complication of foam sclerotherapy 127
phleboliths 202, 206
phlegmasia cerulea dolens 24
physician liability, illegally compounded drugs 50–1
pigmentary changes (hemosiderin) 16–17, 33, 76, 127, 150
pigmented purpuric dermatoses 20–2
poikiloderma of Civatte 27–8
polidocanol 50, 105–16
compared with sodium tetradecyl sulfate 158–60
complications and risks 148–51
comparison of side effects 147
concentrations/indications 36
degradation in air 9
efficacy 147
first use 3–4
foam vs liquid 97, 177–82
German Society of Phlebology guidelines 34–6
legal guidelines for use 48–50

polidocanol – *contd*
  properties 157–8
    time to settle from foam 159
  vs sodium tetradecyl sulfate 155–62
  stability 8
  vs surgery 105–16
  volumes used 73, 89, 107
post-radiation telangiectasias 26–7
post-thrombotic syndrome 23–4
postoperative complications and risks 97
postoperative management 91
  compression bandaging 73, 76
postoperative reviews 91–6
  assessment of results 66, 87–101
  characteristics of treated patients 92
  medium term results 87–101
  statistical analysis of results 93–6
pregnancy 88
protein S deficiency, livedoid vasculopathy 25
Proteus syndrome 206
pseudo-Kaposi's sarcoma 19
purpuric dermatoses 20–2
  Lowenthal 21–2
  Majocchi's disease 21–2
pyodema gangrenosum 18

R

radiofrequency treatment
  principles 167–9
  results 168–9
  role of saphenous veins 167–9
randomized controlled trials
  discussion 112–15
  polidocanol vs other treatments 105–16
  results 109–12
  study design 106–7
    patient demographic data 109
    patient disposition 108
recurrence rates of varicose veins 75, 117–18, 165, 193–8
  neovascularization patterns 194–6
red cell extravasation, hyperpigmentation 16–17
retrograde sclerotherapy 5
right-to-left shunting
  detection of emboli 187–90
  duplex ultrasound identification 185–6

S

safety of foam sclerotherapy 80, 117, 183–92
  clinical trials/exercises 183–91
saphenous vein incompetence 59
  ablation, traditional/radical surgery 164–6
  ASVAL (ambulatory selective varices ablation under local anesthesia) 171
  ASVAL vs radiofrequency vs traditional surgery 171
  CHIVA cure 163, 166
  endovenous laser therapy (EVLT) 166–7
  hemodynamic mapping 82
  high ligation *x*
  importance in vv treatment? 163–76
saphenous vein incompetence – *contd*
  ligation and stripping 84, 170–1
  mini-invasive surgery 170–1
  preservation/minimal surgery 163, 173
  radiofrequency treatment 167–9
  randomized controlled trials, polidocanol vs other treatments 105–16
  strategy for cannulation 71
  stripping 170–1
    with preservation of SJ 172
    reurrence rate 172
  traditional/radical surgery 164–6
  summary/discussion/conclusions 172–3
saphenous veins 163–76
  accessory SV 64
  GSVs 62–4, 70–1
  SSVs
    search for artery 81
    strategy for cannulation 71
    tributaries 84
Schamburg's disease 21
scintigraphy, whole body blood pool (WBBPS) 135
sclerosant solutions 89
  blood dilution effects 79
  German Society of Phlebology guidelines 33–4
sclerosing agents 209
  compounding 48–50
  injectable 3–4
  injectable agents 3–4
  legal guidelines for use 43–52
sclerotherapy
  compression following 73, 76
  lack of follow-up data on varicose recurrence 170
  principles 169–70
Sclerovein 158
selection of patients for foam sclerotherapy 87–8, 99
'sick dermatome' 201
sodium morrhuate, licensing 44
sodium tetradecyl sulfate
  compared with polidocanol 157, 159–60
  legal guidelines for use 43–52
  properties 156–7
    foam vs liquid 97, 177–82
    time to settle from foam 159
  specifications for impurities (FDA) 47
  volumes used 73, 89, 107
Sotradecol
  standards and validations 47, 156–7
  see also sodium tetradecyl sulfate
spider nevi (ectatic ascending arterioles) 29
spider veins (leg telangiectasias) 26
statistical analysis of results 93–6
  Cox regression analysis 93, 95
  Kaplan–Meier curves 94–6
steal syndrome, necrosis 204
Stemmer's sign 15
Streptococcus pyogenes, OK-432 214–15
superficial thrombophlebitis (STP) 14, 23–4, 121
  great saphenous vein 14

superficial venous reservoir (SVR)
  insufficiency 164
  theory of anterograde evolution of insufficiency 170
  theory of retrograde evolution of insufficiency 164
superficial venous thrombosis 24, 151

T

telangiectasias 26–9, 141–54
  definition and presentation 141
  essential 28
  foam vs sclerosant solutions 58
  hereditary benign 28
  hereditary hemorrhagic 28
  macularis eruptiva perstans 28–9
  matting 27–8, 33, 127, 150
  Monfreux technique 58
  periungual 28
  treatment
    complications, early/late 148–51
    indications/contraindications 144–5
    results 145–8
  unilateral nevoid 28
Tessari-DSS
  advanced version 9–10
  methods 8, 35, 55–6
    3-way tap technique 56
thromboangiitis obliterans 23
thromboembolic events 24, 33
thrombophlebitis
  superficial 14, 23–4
  treatment 74
thrombotic events
  microthrombi 150
  prevention 85–6
tibial perforators, incompetent 18
tongue, venous malformations, treatment 214
Tourbillon technique 7
traditional/radical surgery of saphenous veins 164–6
  frequency of varicose vein recurrence 165
transient visual disorders 149
Trendelenberg position 188–9
Tromboveinᵀᴹ 157
truncal reflux, and ostial reflux 170

U

UGS (ultrasound guided sclerotherapy) *see* duplex ultrasound guided foam sclerotherapy
ulcers 121
  diagnosis 18
ultrasound *see* duplex ultrasound guidance

V

Valsalva maneuver 165
varicose veins
  ablation 82–3
varicose veins – *contd*
  current options 58–9
  etiology and pathogenesis 164
  large
    determining US characteristics 119–20
    foam sclerotherapy 117–28
  recurrence 75, 193–8
  sclerotherapy, guidelines of German Society of Phlebology 32–41
  ultrasound guidance 117–28
varicose veins
Varisolve® (Pol microfoam) 50, 105–16, 188
  see also polidocanol
vascular ectasias 25–9
vascular malformations 129–39, 199–218, 219–24
  alcohol sclerotherapy transition to foam sclerotherapy 129–40
  arteriovenous malformations 204–6
  classifications 199–200, 219–21
  congenital venous malformations (CVMs) 129–30, 219–20
  lymphatic malformations 201–2
  natural history 200
  oral mucosal 132–6
  treatment 207–15
    laser 208
    lymphatic malformations 214–15
    sclerotherapy 208–14
    surgery 208
  venous malformations 202–4
  venular malformations 200–4
vascular tumors 199
vasculitis
  atrophie blanche 16–17, 25
  nodular 22–3
vasovagal syncope 149
veno-arteriolar axonal reflex 24
venous accesses 81
venous eczema 15–16
venous insufficiency
  dermatological manifestations 13–30
  symptoms in large varicose veins 118–19
venous lakes 25
venous malformations 202–4
venous reflux, duplex ultrasound evaluation 7, 61–8, 89
venous ulcers 18
visual disturbances, migraine-like symptoms 33, 75
volume of foam 73, 89, 107, 122–3
  safety issues 122–3
von Willebrand's disease 28
vulvar malformations, treatment 214

W

'white leg' 24
whole body blood pool scintigraphy (WBBPS) 135